T0275918

In early modern England, housewives, clergymen, bloodletters, herb women, and patients told authoritative tales about the body. By the end of the eighteenth century, however, medicine had begun to drown out these voices. This book uses patients' perspectives to argue that changes in the relationship between rich and poor underlay this increase in medicine's authority. In a detailed examination of health, healing, and poor relief in eighteenth-century Bristol, Fissell shows how the experiences of the hospitalized urban poor laid the foundations for modern doctor-patient encounters. Within the hospital, charity patients were denied the power to interpret their own illnesses, as control of the institution shifted from lay patrons to surgeons. Outside the hospital, reforms of popular culture stigmatized ordinary people's ideas about their own bodies. Popular medicine became working-class medicine, associated with superstition and political unrest.

This book is of interest not only to historians of medicine, but also to readers interested in poverty, social welfare, popular culture, and the body.

Cambridge History of Medicine

Patients, Power, and the Poor in Eighteenth-Century Bristol

OTHER BOOKS IN THIS SERIES

Charles Webster, ed. *Health, medicine, and mortality in the sixteenth century*
Ian Maclean *The Renaissance notion of woman*
Michael MacDonald *Mystical Bedlam*
Robert E. Kohler *From medical chemistry to biochemistry*
Walter Pagel *Joan Baptista Van Helmont*
Nancy Tomes *A generous confidence*
Roger Cooter *The cultural meaning of popular science*
Anne Digby *Madness, morality, and medicine*
Guenter B. Risse *Hospital life in Enlightenment Scotland*
Roy Porter, ed. *Patients and practitioners*
Ann G. Carmichael *Plague and the poor in Renaissance Florence*
S. E. D. Shortt *Victorian lunacy*
Hilary Marland *Medicine and society in Wakefield and Huddersfield 1780–1870*
Susan Reverby *Ordered to care*
Russell C. Maulitz *Morbid appearances*
Mathew Ramsey *Professional and popular medicine in France, 1770–1830*
John Keown *Abortion, doctors, and the law*
Donald Denoon *Public health in Papua New Guinea*
Paul Weindling *Health, race, and German politics between national unification and Nazism, 1870–1945*
Ornella Moscucci *The science of woman*
Jack D. Ellis *The physician-legislators of France*
William H. Schneider *Quality and quantity*
John Farley *Bilharzia*

Patients, Power, and the Poor in Eighteenth-Century Bristol

Mary E. Fissell

Wellcome Unit for the History of Medicine
Manchester University

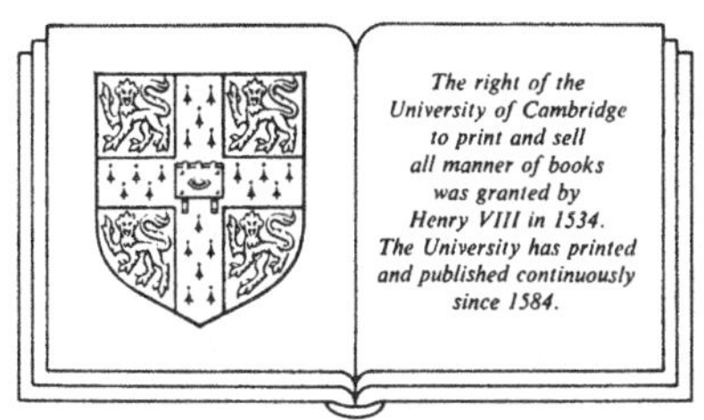

CAMBRIDGE UNIVERSITY PRESS

CAMBRIDGE

NEW YORK PORT CHESTER MELBOURNE SYDNEY

PUBLISHED BY THE PRESS SYNDICATE OF THE UNIVERSITY OF CAMBRIDGE
The Pitt Building, Trumpington Street, Cambridge, United Kingdom

CAMBRIDGE UNIVERSITY PRESS
The Edinburgh Building, Cambridge CB2 2RU, UK
40 West 20th Street, New York NY 10011–4211, USA
477 Williamstown Road, Port Melbourne, VIC 3207, Australia
Ruiz de Alarcón 13, 28014 Madrid, Spain
Dock House, The Waterfront, Cape Town 8001, South Africa

http://www.cambridge.org

First published 1991
First paperback edition 2002

A catalogue record for this book is available from the British Library

Library of Congress Cataloguing in Publication data
Fissell, Mary Elizabeth.
Patients, power, and the poor in eighteenth-century Bristol / Mary
E. Fissell.
p. cm. – (Cambridge history of medicine)
Includes bibliographical references.
ISBN 0 521 40047 3 (hardcover)
1. Medicine – England – Bristol – History – 18th century. 2. Poor – Medical care – England – Bristol – History – 18th century. 3. Poor – England – Bristol – Social life and customs. 4. Bristol (England) – Social life and customs. I. Title. II. Series.
R488.B78F57 1991
610′.92423′9309033–dc20 90-28169 CIP

ISBN 0 521 40047 3 hardback
ISBN 0 521 52693 0 paperback

For my parents
Frederica and William Fissell

Contents

Tables, figures, and maps

TABLES

FIGURES

MAPS

Acknowledgments

Many friends and colleagues have offered suggestions, read chapters, and listened to me try out ideas for this book; it is a pleasure to thank them for their help. My greatest debt is to Charles Rosenberg, who supervised this project as a dissertation and whose masterly editorial skills helped transform it into a book; his belief in the manuscript and his finely tuned ear for language are much appreciated. The many citations to the work of Roy Porter only begin to indicate my intellectual indebtedness to his and Dorothy Porter's work; I am grateful for his encouragement and enthusiasm at all stages of this project. My fellow historians of Bristol, Laura Corballis, Carl Estabrook, and Michael Neve shared their work with me and made the choice of Bristol a felicitous one. Another Bristol historian, Jonathan Barry, read the entire manuscript, as did Bill Luckin and Roy Porter. Their suggestions, however imperfectly incorporated, were of inestimable value. I've also learned a great deal from Tim Hitchcock over the years – more than he probably realizes. Many others read and criticized parts of the book or thesis. Their help was far greater than a mere mention of their names suggests: W. F. Bynum, Sandra Cavallo, Roger Cooter, Susan Lawrence, Lynn Lees, Joan Mottram, Malcolm Nicolson, Margaret Pelling, John Pickstone, Richard Smith, Steve Sturdy, and Adrian Wilson.

I am also grateful to the various agencies whose financial support made this book possible. At Penn, a Pennfield Fellowship and a Mellon Dissertation Fellowship enabled me to do the initial research and write the thesis. The Wellcome Trust's funding of a post in Manchester provided me with time to rewrite and rethink; as my acknowledgments suggest, my Mancunian colleagues are stimulating company. Archivists in the Bristol Record Office, particularly Anne Crawford, made my time there productive and enjoyable. Likewise, I am grateful to helpful librarians and archivists at the Wellcome Institute, the Bristol Central Reference Library, the British Library, the Bodleian Library, the County Record Offices of Gloucestershire, Somerset, and Hampshire; the Royal College of Physicians, the Royal College of Surgeons, the Society of Friends, the Society for the Promotion of Christian Knowledge, and the Bristol University Medical School. Thanks also go to the editors of *Social History of Medicine* for permission to reproduce parts of my argument originally published in their journal.

Finally, two personal votes of thanks. My husband, David Cantor, and my parents helped in innumerable ways known best to themselves. The book is dedicated to my parents, with thanks for their belief in it and in me.

1

Introduction

This study started life as an examination of a local system of health-care provision in early modern England. I was interested in the patient's perspective on medical care, not merely that of the unusual sufferer who left details of his or her encounter with illness, but that of the ordinary person.[1] It seemed to me that patients as well as practitioners structured and shaped medical practice. My focus on the patient provoked questions about how and why individuals made choices among different health-care providers; no simple equation of medical science with "better" health care could be made when a wide variety of different practitioners flourished. Instead, the provision of health care in early modern England resembles some of today's African medical systems, replete with "traditional" healers as well as high technology Western medicine, in which family needs and wishes, religion, and economic factors shape patient choice.[2]

The ordinary, non-elite patient's view is particularly significant for the early modern period because the institutions now central to modern medicine – hospitals and clinics – had their origins, not in provision for the wealthy, but for the poor. Historians of medicine have overlooked the charitable dimension to the origins of institutional health care, and by focusing on practitioners have ignored not only the patients but also the patrons who founded and ran hospitals. By neglecting the meanings of hospitals for those who built and used them, some historians have reduced the significance of hospital utilization to the merely medical, creating a progressivist and noncontextual vision of the institution. Patients' choices of medical care, albeit constrained by poverty, were influenced by their understanding of the hospital's charitable nature as well as the contingencies of ill health.

By examining how patients made choices, how medicine appeared when viewed from the sickbed, an emerging health-care system can be understood not only as a product of altered patterns of charitable provision and attitudes toward poverty, but as the result of a fundamental shift in attitudes toward the body itself. Over the course of the eighteenth century, the very ways people understood and interpreted their bodies altered. What had been a set of shared assumptions, a belief system held by high and low alike in the seventeenth century, became the purview of the poor by the early nineteenth century. But the waning of vernacular medicine was a complex process; to align it with class formation, with modernization, with commercialization, is at once to say all and to say nothing. Certainly as the ties that bound men and women together moved from the vertical chains of hierarchy and patronage to those we construe as the horizontal ones of class, so too did the bonds of a shared understanding of the body crack and break. This gradual process was punctuated by specific moments in which the cultural differences between rich and poor were articulated with special clarity, and those moments owed as much to the expressions of political and religious tension as they did to primitive forms of class conflict.

In other words, the making of modern health care was a part of a more general process of cultural and social change. The respect granted by society's elites to ordinary people's interpretations of their own bodies diminished as a series of reforms of manners in the latter half of the eighteenth century served to isolate and denigrate "popular" medicine. Within this broader shift, the functions of welfare and charity institutions – hospitals, workhouses, dispensaries – became medicalized as ideas about charity were recast. A new style of medical practice was established, increasingly oriented toward modes of diagnosis and therapy alien to vernacular medicine. Medicine was now able to use the charitable institution to emphasize its distance from lay beliefs. But medicine did not create the hospital nor the disparagement of popular culture.

Rather, hospitals and reforms of manners were expressions of the relationship between society's elites and those less fortunate. Historians have usually defined *the poor* in one of two ways. Swayed by the availability of charity and relief records, some have identified the poor as those who were in receipt of funds, from private or municipal coffers;[3] others use the term more vaguely, including most of the laboring classes.[4] But neither usage provides a fully satisfactory analysis. Those based upon records of institutions are seductive; they provide snapshots of individuals, and can illuminate attitudes toward the poor. Such analyses, however, rely upon one group's definition of another, upon benefactors' notions of the "deserving" poor (however constituted) and their recipients' attempts to meet – or subvert – those criteria of worthiness.

This study defines the poor as those who might have been at risk of dependency; rather than basing an analysis on vaguely defined economic criteria, it explores the potentials for poverty, the chances that an individual might become dependent on friends, neighbors, patrons, or institutions. Such an approach derives from demographically inclined historians who have shown that early modern poor relief was very closely linked with life-cycle.[5] For example, recently married couples, with two or three young children, were extremely hard put to pay the bills. The wife's wage earnings were of necessity small, the children too young to earn, the father unlikely to experience a rise in wages sufficient to meet increased expenses. But at other points in the life-cycle, such a family might not be in need of help. Given inferential problems of length of observation in relation to life-cycle, an inclusive definition of poverty is useful.

In addition, the closer one studies the lives of the poor, the more one is struck by the creativity of the economies of makeshift. Distinctions between charity and relief, as well as between receipt of funds and independence, ultimately blur. What to make of an elderly widow who received a loaf of bread a week from a parish-based charity? One loaf a week was obviously not sustaining this woman. Yet such gifts were sought after, and many made do with combinations of charity, relief, use rights, barter, and earnings, details of which will always elude the historian. Rigid definitions of poverty seem inapplicable to the multitude of ways in which the poor managed to keep body and soul together.

Not that the rich are particularly easy to define. In some ways, they are self-identified, the institutions of urban charity and welfare providing a theater for the articulation of social difference.[6] Just as surely as a workhouse distinguished the poor by forcing them to wear badges, so too it denoted middle and upper sorts through their governance of the institution. Both rich and poor defined one another through their interactions, potential and actual, their relationships always those of realization and realignment.[7]

This analysis of welfare and health care is based on a study of Bristol (see Map 1), in the South-West of England.[8] Two rivers –

the Avon and the Frome – flowed through the city, but wealth came from a third: the Severn. Visitors who came by water from the west were treated to the beauty of St. Vincent's Rocks and the deep gorge through which the Avon river linked the Severn to the city. For many, Bristol appeared a city of steeples. For others, it was the small crowded medieval streets and the hills that left an impression. Narrow streets were made narrower by the old-fashioned houses whose upper stories overhung the lower, enclosing noisome streets with open gutters. Daniel Defoe was not the only observer to comment on the odd but necessary custom of transporting goods on sledges within the city; the hills made such measures necessary. The city was only slowly becoming geographically differentiated; it was centered on commercial and residential parishes that housed warehouses, the Exchange, and merchants' houses. Over the course of the eighteenth century, as in many other cities, new socially segregated spaces were created by developers. Thus, Bristol saw Queen's Square, a typical late eighteenth-century large green square surrounded by elegant houses at variance with older cramped dwellings. So too, by the turn of the century the outlying areas of Clifton and the Hotwells were beginning to assume their identities as affluent suburbs.

Bristol's merchants considered themselves second only to those of the metropolis, and until northern cities burgeoned in the latter part of the century, they were probably correct. Almost all of the English trade with the West Indies and with Newfoundland, for example, came through Bristol. The city dominated the African slave trade, although Liverpool overtook Bristol in this regard by the 1770s. However varied and exotic was her long-distance trade, Bristol's economy rested equally on shorter voyages, both to Ireland and inland, the Severn functioning as an important artery to the Midlands in the era before canals.

Bristol's port meant more than just ships and warehouses; local manufacturing was linked to overseas trade. Sugar, for instance, was the most significant manufacture in the city; there were as many as twenty refineries operating in the city at that time. The city served as an entrepôt, distributing wine and sherry from Spain, exchanged for Newfoundland fish in one of the many transatlantic triangular trades. So too, Bristol brass, Bristol glass (some-

Map 1. Bristol

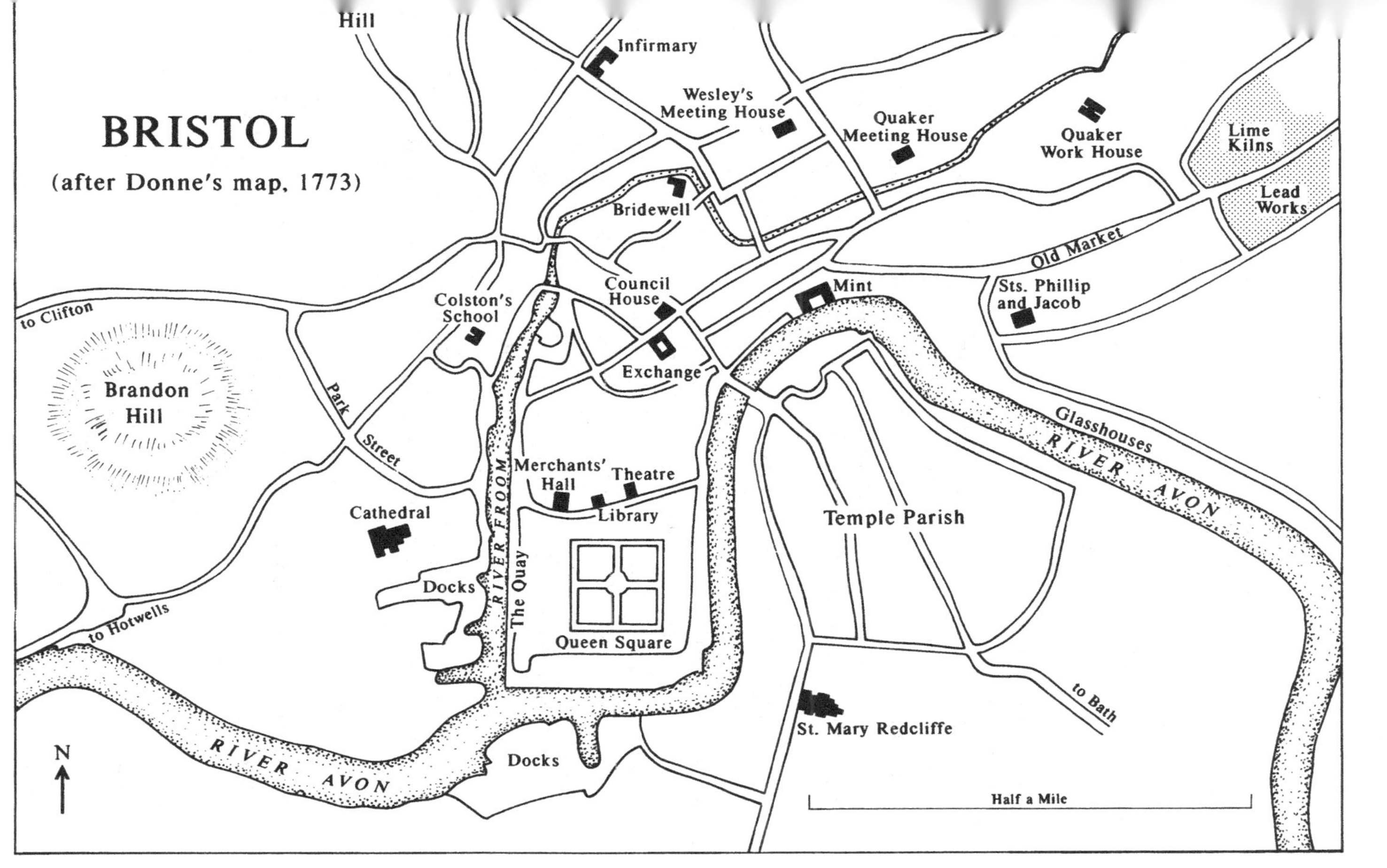
BRISTOL
(after Donne's map, 1773)
Hill
Infirmary
Wesley's Meeting House
Quaker Meeting House
Quaker Work House
Lime Kilns
Lead Works
Bridewell
Old Market
Council House
Mint
Sts. Phillip and Jacob
Colston's School
to Clifton
Exchange
Brandon Hill
Park Street
Glasshouses
RIVER AVON
Merchants' Hall
Theatre
Library
Temple Parish
Cathedral
RIVER FROOM
The Quay
Docks
Queen Square
to Hotwells
to Bath
St. Mary Redcliffe
N
RIVER AVON
Docks
Half a Mile

times containing Bristol water), lead, woollen cloth and numerous other products featured in both distribution and production networks centered on the city's port.

Although contemporaries loved to portray eighteenth-century Bristolians as dull traders thinking only of profit and return – they were reputed to sleep with one eye open so as not to miss an opportunity – the city's residents laid claim to participating in a polite and leisured urban culture. Did not the city have its own spa at the Hotwells? Did not the *bon ton* enjoy a fashionable round of theaters, horse races on Durdham Down, balls, and assemblies? It was from this realm that charity drew one of its inspirations. Like the mayor's installation, the feasts of the City Council, or plays at the Theatre Royal, the annual Infirmary sermon and banquet was a moment of civic show in which the authority and benevolence of the city's ruling elites were on display.

While Bristol had those whose importance and power equaled London's so-called "big bourgeoisie," one of the city's defining characteristics was its extent and range of middling men.[9] Although historians disagree as to the significance of these groups, there was a certain fluidity and openness to the power structures in Bristol, which meant that the "small" bourgeoisie had important civic roles to play. At the most basic level, Bristol had a wide-open electorate; as many as 80 percent of the city's male heads of households voted in the parliamentary elections of 1696. Although middling sorts were unlikely to become one of the city's forty-three councillors or a member of the Society of Merchant Venturers, they participated in parish vestries, city companies, and after 1696, the Corporation of the Poor. On occasion, Bristol's elites deferred to the city's middling men, courting their allegiances in an attempt to present a united and prosperous face to the city.

But the city was far from united. The other key to Bristol's charitable munificence lay in the bitter sectarian divisions that characterized much of the city's civic life. Both church and party divided the city, but the fracture lines created by religion probably ran deepest. Bristolians' penchant for religious deviance is sometimes traced back to the Lollards, and by the latter half of the seventeenth century, the city was renowned for its variety and extent of religious difference. Baptists, Independents, Presbyterians, and Congregationalists all had their followers. The city's population included the highest percentage of Quakers anywhere in England,

and harsh fines and imprisonments had characterized the Friends' experiences of the 1670s and 1680s. Even after the 1689 Toleration Act, memories were far too grim to permit any deep or long-lasting unity in the city. Indeed, the Society of Merchant Venturers, the center of the trading community, did not admit its first Quaker until 1720.

In a place so marked by difference, charity could scarcely be neutral; institutions were quickly characterized by factional interest, even if founded in a spirit of unity. For example, the city's workhouse, founded in 1696 by amalgamating all seventeen city parishes into a single corporation for poor relief, was soon perceived as the tool of Whig and dissenting interests, although alliances subsequently shifted. Such an equation was not difficult to make, because the ideological roots of the project lay in Interregnum approaches to poor relief and in the Low Church interest in the reform of manners.

But Bristol's unusual workhouse owed something to the city's expansion as well as to the politics of religious difference. For as in London (which tried to imitate Bristol's Corporation of the Poor), the rich and poor were becoming geographically distinct. Prior to the foundation of the workhouse, the rich and tiny inner-city parishes had already been turning over some of their funds for poor relief to the larger and much poorer parishes, because the industrial populations of St. James, SS. Philip and Jacob, and Temple parishes were growing faster than their relief mechanisms, based upon Elizabethan statute, could respond.

Although Bristol's foundation of a hospital in 1737 was less exceptional than her Corporation of the Poor, it too was quickly subsumed within urban rivalries. Historians of British hospitals have focused on their role in polite culture, with various provincial cities emulating one another's new foundations. But analyses of Continental institutions suggest that hospitals also served as sites for the negotiation and mediation of power by local elites.[10] Bristol's Infirmary represented a place where individuals could maintain networks of patronage, the recommendation from a hospital supporter required by a prospective patient a form of social exchange in a face-to-face society.[11] The hospital provided an arena for the mediation of social power, both directly through individual patronage, and symbolically through civic ritual and display.

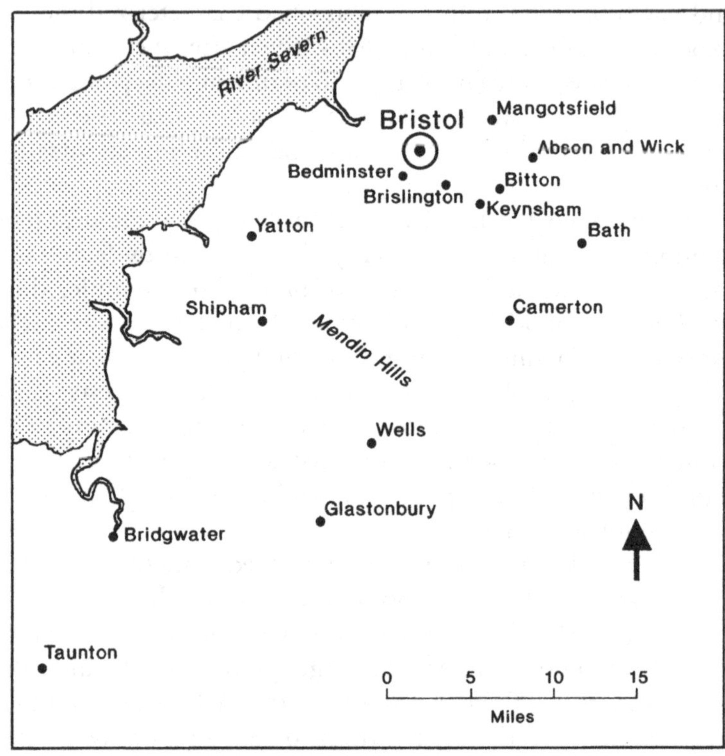

Map 2. Bristol's environs

But there is another side to these charitable institutions. For it was not just their founders who made them; clients used institutional health care in ways unforseen by their benefactors.[12] This study focuses on two parishes, one rural and one urban, in order to delineate the factors shaping institutional populations. Abson and Wick, the rural parish, was seven miles from Bristol, just to the north of an imaginary line drawn between Bristol and Bath (see Map 2). It was made up of four hamlets and had a mixed industrial and agrarian economy. It was tiny compared to its urban counterpart, SS. Philip and Jacob. Like Abson, Philip and Jacob housed many industrial workers. But if a poor person fell ill in the city, he or she had a wider range of options than did a rural denizen. As in the country, there was the Poor Law, but in the city, this might mean incarceration in the workhouse, which had a medical staff, rather than so-called out-relief, payments for medical attendance, rent, food, heating, and other necessities. The urban worker might also try to get a recommendation for a lengthy stay in the infirmary, or the equivalent of out-relief in the outpatient department of the hospital or a dispensary.

In the city parish, an individual was also more likely than in the country to be without family or friends for support. Patterns of local desperation, of family economies gone wrong, of immigrant isolation, led people to make use of new institutional resources. So too, connections with urban elites provided the means by which individuals sought help, so that institutional utilization was mediated by the circumstances of neighborhood, of workplace, of church or meetinghouse.

Just as charity has most often been discussed from the perspective of its benefactors, so too has medicine been understood as the creation of its practitioners. Recent years have seen the study of eighteenth-century British medicine reinvigorated as a focus of scholarly attention. Often, however, this new intellectual vitality has been granted through attempts to integrate British medicine into a Continental, especially Parisian, model.[13] But British infirmaries never aspired to be the Hôtel-Dieu, and the search for the Paris model of medicine – accomplished through the bodies of thousands upon thousands of destitute patients as well as a revolution – seems to have led some historians to a narrow perspective on British medicine.

Instead, the vitality and strength of local traditions of medical practice were far more significant to experiences of illness and infirmary growth than any developments across the Channel.[14] In Bristol, barber-surgeons' and apothecaries' companies provided a structure for urban practice that integrated their members into the city's civic rituals and functions. The leaders of these companies commanded high apprentice fees and trained the sons of merchants and gentlemen. Only as patterns of apprenticeship changed did the infirmary come to adopt an educational function similar to that of Parisian hospitals. A local focus on medicine as it was practiced, rather than on the national and supranational construction of the identity and bureaucratic structures of a profession, presents an alternate view of early modern medical practice to those based upon Continental models.

However, the patient's view reveals that even these formally trained practitioners represent only a fraction of the city's health-care providers. Many understood how to maintain health and treat illness; medical knowledge was a part of everyday discourse. There were wig-makers, blood-letters, inoculators, itinerant venereal disease doctors, druggists, and "cunning women," purveying health care which competed with domestic medicine provided by patients themselves. As Roy Porter and Irvine Loudon have shown, health care was an economic free-for-all, an open market, an exemplification of the consumer revolution.[15] But such openness was not solely predicated on a cash economy; in a world in which most people were capable of practicing the rudiments of domestic medicine, the utilization of protoprofessionals needs to be explained on a deeper level than mere emulation of others' consumption.

In a local study such as this, some of the dimensions of the relationship between healer and healed can be traced out in detail. For instance, some of Nicholas Jewson's schematic views of an eighteenth-century medicine dominated by the desires of the patient rather than the practitioner can be supported with examples from Bristol.[16] But over the course of the century, the relationship between healer and healed shifted as the cultural role of lay medicine altered.

In the late seventeenth century, vernacular medical knowledge was extensive and tenacious. For lay practice, interpretations of the causes and precipitants to illness were as significant as therapeutics. These interpretive frameworks owed much to religion, be it Anglican orthodoxy or dissent. One of the keys to these belief systems was the importance placed on signs inscribed on the body's surface. Such concepts were congruent with cultural norms about signs and wonders, from the appearance of monsters to the healing virtues of plants; the outside reflected the inside, and interpretation was open to all.

Later in the century, the shared basis of these beliefs was attacked by those who would impose a rationalistic and class-specific order upon belief and behavior.[17] But the persistence of a supernatural component to these vernacular healing practices calls into question the seventeenth-century replacement of magical beliefs by a more rational, secular outlook.[18] Nor was this process gradual and imperceptible; it was punctuated and stimulated by specific issues and debates. Thus, in the 1740s and 1750s, concerns about Jacobitism and dissent were voiced in terms of the opposition between "polite" and "vulgar" beliefs and behaviors. In the 1780s and 1790s, a new wave of reformers attacked cultural expressions associated with an emergent working class. In both periods, modes of interpretation of the body that emphasized signs visible to all came under particular attack as they were easily associated with forms of deviant "enthusiastic" popular religion.

Medical men were not prominent in any of these reevaluations of the body. And yet such processes served to augment medical authority by denying poor patients' abilities to interpret illness in ways sanctioned by dominant cultural norms. Within the hospital, parallel processes denied patients a voice as medical men closed ranks and defined themselves as the products of a dissection-oriented anatomical training. No longer were patients' own narratives of illness and interpretations of external signs the key to diagnosis; no longer were the moral meanings of illness central to medical as well as vernacular practice. Instead, truth lay deep inside the body, accessible only to the trained observer, sometimes apparent only at the postmortem dissection so loathed by patients.

Medical men were able to take control of the process of illness interpretation within the hospital because the authority of the infirmary's benefactors devolved upon them in an unexpected way. As hospital governors slowly abandoned their direct day-to-day control of the institution, surgeons inherited the apparatus of management. But medical men did not create the hospital; they medicalized it.

Such an analysis serves, of course, as comment on and critique of Michel Foucault's *The Birth of the Clinic.* Other historians have tried to map Foucault's discussion of French Enlightenment medicine onto Britain, without great success.[19] But Foucault's analysis is suggestive on a deeper level. His perception of the ways in which power can be inscribed on the body, however schematic, is a model for understanding some of the means by which English medical men came to dominate their patients. But this domination comes at the end of our story; control over the hospitalized body had already been derived from the infirmary's origins in the workhouse. Perhaps it is Foucault's *Discipline and Punish,* which illuminates how early modern institutions contained and concealed deviance, to which historians of English medicine must turn. Like bridewells, workhouses, and prisons, hospitals were designed to reform their inmates and engage them in the world of productive labor – in this case, by mending their bodies, making them fit for work. Medical men's power over their patient's bodies depended upon incarceration; only slowly was such power mediated through medical knowledge as the hospital became central to medical thought and practice.[20]

This is a book about Bristol, but it is also intended to have more general relevance. Thus, for example, Chapters 2, 3 and 9 discuss aspects of English medicine, often relying on examples from the South-West, but making a larger argument. Although Bristol's wealth and size may make it atypical of English provincial cities and towns in this period, the city experienced much in common with its smaller counterparts. The pattern of infirmary development was similar to that in other old cities, and there were connections to other hospitals through figures such as Alured Clarke and Sir James Stonhouse (associated with the Winchester and Northampton infirmaries). Given the paucity of historical work on English provincial medicine and welfare in this period, it is also instructive to compare Bristol with Continental and American cities. Certain themes link Montpellier and Philadelphia and Turin with Bristol, suggesting commonalities to ancien régime experiences of medicine and urban welfare.

One of the most apparent features of charity and poor relief in eighteenth-century Bristol was its commitment to moral reform. So too in other cities; the poor were to be brought to godliness as well as protected from starvation. Thus, for example, in Montpellier (home of the leading French provincial medical school), poor-relief institutions, including the Hôtel-Dieu, emphasized their roles in transforming the shiftless into the saved. As a member of the board of Montpellier's Hôpital Général declared, *"cette maison a toujours été regardée comme un azille pour les moeurs aussi bien qu'une ressource contre la misère."*[21]

As in many other cities, the key to Montpellerian reformation lay in work and in community. Colin Jones has illustrated how the regular life of the community in poor-relief institutions was intended to reform inmates, however perennially subverted by them. Similarly, Philadelphia's responses to poverty emphasized work and community. Thus, for example, the so-called Bettering House was founded in 1766, a combination almshouse and workhouse whose name indicated its reforming function. Like its European counterparts, it housed a range of individuals, the invalid, the beggar, even the petty criminal. Although England was rapidly losing faith in the ability of the workhouse to cope with poverty, Philadelphians looked back to English models, to the ideal communities of John Bellers, in their attempts to improve the poor.[22] Not surprisingly, their experience echoed Bristol's: managers of the workhouse found that inmates could not earn sufficient through their labor to offset running costs. But work was more than just wage earning; its functions in inculcating discipline and godliness were equally significant. Inmates were kept picking oakum or spinning wool for reasons far beyond finance.

If institutions provided reformation as well as relief to their inmates, so, too, they performed a range of functions within the city. As Sandra Cavallo has shown for Turin, hospitals and workhouses served as centers for the negotiation and exercise of patronage.[23] Such power was manifested in public display. Thus, for instance, in Catholic countries the remnants of baroque piety promoted funerals ornamented by large numbers of paupers in attendance, while in Protestant England charitable institutions stage-managed public processions to anniversary sermons and the like. The public role accorded philanthropy mirrored the private power which it conferred upon donors who could use their control of institutional admissions to support their own clients. The recommendation system was in wide use on both sides of the Atlantic and the oft-distinguished "worthy" poor were validated through their connections with local patrons.

In cities with more than one institution, this system could mean a certain level of differentiation. Thus, for example, in Philadelphia, a three-tier system separated the most worthy (who could make use of the Dispensary founded in 1786) from those who utilized the Hospital. Both were preserved from the elderly and infirm in the Bettering House who were in turn distinguished from the beggars and vagrants in that same institution. However, as Colin Jones has pointed out in his analysis of Montpellier, segregation and differentiation did not occur along modern medical lines, but in accordance with social dictates.[24] So too, in Bristol, even within the city workhouse there are hints that the respectable elderly enjoyed medical out-relief while those less fortunate in acquiring local patronage only received medical care as inmates.

Thus the ancien régime institution, often old, almost always multifunctional, looks back to a tradition of moral reform and local patronage and piety. From such a perspective, it is easy to see why any sort of medicalization proceeded slowly and incompletely. In Montpellier, for example, the nursing sisters allied themselves with poor-relief administrators in opposition to the introduction of certain features of clinical medicine. In Philadelphia, in Montpellier, in Bristol, the stories of grave robbing and its counterpart, patient resistance to dissection, are virtually interchangeable. But such opposition was countered as patients lost power, often in local and specific ways. Thus, for example, it was only with the French Revolution and the dismissal of the nursing sisters that the Montpellier medical men were able to use patients as clinical objects. In Bristol, changes in apprenticeship structured the advent of clinical medicine. But in each case, despite a certain retrospective flavor of inevitability, charity and welfare components of the institution resisted the objectification of the inmate by clinical medicine, and often change was accomplished through nonmedical agency.

The local focus of this study presents a history in which doctors assume less significance than in many other accounts. By starting with the patient, we arrive at an alternate version of the development of medical institutions and professional authority. By situating the early infirmary in the context of charity, the relationships between rich and poor mediated by that institution become apparent. So do the ways in which those social divisions came to be expressed through that powerful and emotive medium, the body itself. This process almost inadvertently granted the medical professions an increased authority, one which derived in part from the hospital setting, a transmutation of the benefactor/client relation into that of practitioner/patient. Medical men, however, did not make this opportunity; they were the unexpected beneficiaries of changes within charity and those cultural shifts that made vernacular medicine a mode of expression suitable only for the plebians.

Such an argument also suggests a reevaluation of the interactions between rich and poor. Once again, the patient's view provides an alternate understanding of charity and welfare institutions, suggesting that the poor negotiated some small powers to themselves. Although few could struggle against the bonds of deference, many could utilize institutions for ends never intended by their benefactors.

Finally, a cultural analysis of health and illness that starts from the patient's view creates an alternate understanding of the ways in which the body itself is subject to policing. Infirmary surgeons granted the inmates of hospitals peculiarly opaque bodies, which only the powerful could read, and robbed the patient of his or her understanding of illness. But they were the inheritors of a more substantial tradition. Whereas reformers of manners at the end of the seventeenth century saw discipline of the body as a means to discipline the soul, later devaluation of lay beliefs inscribed power relations on the body in a more insidious fashion, denying the poor ownership of themselves.

2

Everyone their own physician

In the early modern period, much of English health care was provided by nonprofessionals, by mothers and housewives, by cunning women of local repute, by clergymen carrying out charitable works. Such lay practice was not merely a congeries of specific remedies, a set of hand-me-downs, remnants from antique and medieval learning preserved by the common people long after their betters had discarded them. Rather, vernacular medicine was a coherent system capable of multiple meanings and interpretations, but organized around a few basic principles that extended fairly widely throughout late seventeenth- and eighteenth-century English society.[1] Indeed, many of the tenets of vernacular health care were familiar elements of the medicine practiced by surgeons and apothecaries as well as that provided by lay people.

An analysis of three different types of sources reveals strong similarities in medical and lay ideas and practices. First are diaries, letters, and manuscript remedy books that detail what people actually did for their own health – vernacular medicine in action. Although references to health in these are not abundant, they are significant because they are the only extant indicators of actual healing practices. A much broader range of evidence is provided by popular printed works, both medical and nonmedical. During the latter half of the seventeenth century popular health books, explicitly intended for a lay audience, enjoyed a publishing boom.[2] Of course, it is difficult to know how these texts related to vernacular practice. However, such books were sold in large numbers, and presumably read. The medical ideas contained within them are clearly related both to the evidence we have of actual practice, and to those ideas about health and illness contained in popular nonmedical works, such as chapbooks, proverbs, ballads, and the like. In other words, certain ideas about the body had a very wide currency in the popular literature, medical and nonmedical, of the day. Many of these ideas also underlay the medicine practiced by surgeons and apothecaries, those medical men trained through apprenticeship, rather than at a university, as were physicians. Printed manuals and reference works for these practitioners, as well as manuscript notebooks kept by them, indicate that they shared many of the precepts of vernacular medicine.

Lay medical knowledge was thus not the province of the uneducated or even the nonprofessional; large numbers of early modern people held in common many ideas about the body. Such medical knowledge was intimately related to styles of practice; patient-practitioner encounters were predicated upon the fact that patients knew a good deal about medicine. Negotiation over diagnosis and prognosis, as well as therapy, militated against professional autonomy and reproduced a very open medical economy.

Two principles formed the basis of vernacular and professional health care: sympathy and equilibrium. Both had long histories. That of equilibrium was related to a humoral medicine, which emphasized the body's balance of the four humors. In lay medicine this concept centered on the antitheses of hot/cold and wet/dry. The second basic principle of vernacular medicine, the idea of sympathy, also had a long history; particularly significant was its Renaissance manifestation in the concept of man as microcosm of the larger universe.[3] These two fundamentals, however, provided only a minimal structure for the elaboration of systems of medical thought or specific remedies appropriate to local resources. Flexibility rather than dogmatism was medicine's hallmark.

One of the most frequently mentioned principles of early modern health care was the maintenance of bodily equilibrium regarding temperature and moisture. These concepts resonated with physicians' age-old humoral theories. They also had much in common with many other systems of folk medicine.[4] It was thought that sharp contrasts between hot and cold or between being wet and dry had deleterious effects on health. For instance, James Lackington, an artisan, got very ill taking a coach: "I was so very cold, that when I came to the inn where the passengers dined, I went directly to the fire, which struck the cold inward, so that I had but a very narrow escape from death."[5] Similarly, John Bennett, a Bristol house carpenter, recounted how, "being at a house at work in Clifton, it was very hot, and I drank some cold water, then I was laid up for a week with a bad Stummick."[6]

Testimonials, an extremely popular advertising strategy in this period, provide further evidence of such hot/cold reasoning. The veracity of some of these "puffs" is open to question; but whether "genuine" lived experience or no, these tales followed the conventions of vernacular medical belief. For instance, Charity Bull, from the Somerset town of Chewton Mendip, went to a spa in Glastonbury during its brief vogue in the early 1750s. She had had smallpox when a young woman, and disliking the redness it left in her face, she dipped her head in cold water a few times every day for a whole summer: "The consequence was, that she got a severe pain in her Head and Jaws, lost most of her Teeth, became short-breathed, and grew Deaf of her Right Ear." She then suffered the consequences of vanity and cold water for fifteen years before finding relief at the spa.[7]

Hot/cold, wet/dry reasoning was not used solely by lay people. A Bristol printer's apprentice, Charles Manby Smith, described the illness of his fellow worker:

> he had caught a chill through incautiously bathing while hot and the doctor had warned him that the consequences might be serious, if not fatal, unless he used great caution. As he used none, the admonition became a veracious prophecy; the cold settled upon his lungs, and he soon fell into a rapid decline.[8]

Here, both doctor and patient agreed, linking illness to a contrast of hot and cold, coupled with carelessness on the part of the sufferer.

Similarly, manuals for surgeons, which often included the rudiments of physic as well as surgery, utilized hot/cold explanations. Richard Wiseman, author of one such seventeenth-century manual, explained that "A man of about thirty six years old, after a hard Journey on horse-back, sitting on a cold bench, was seized with a pain in his right Hip."[9] So too, the Bristol surgeon's apprentice Alexander Morgan described a patient in his 1720s notebook: "The third Day after the Wether happened to be very warm he changed his Thick Waistcot for a Linning one & being careless sat a quarter day in a Room that was wett the same evening he found himself not well & a little Feverish & thirsty . . . "[10] A 1685 digest of the practical aspects of the works of Dr. Thomas Willis, the rational physician, taught that those with tender constitutions must be "careful to avoid all injury from outward Cold."[11] In other words, the extremes of hot and cold, wet and dry, provided a framework for understanding the body; both professional and lay people made use of this simple prescription and explanation for health maintenance.

Just as this hot/cold wet/dry schema could explain the causes of illness, so too it might point to cure. In the words of Nicholas Culpeper, author of a number of early modern popular health texts, "All Medicines . . . perform their office, by heat or cold, moistening or drying."[12] Thomas Willis, for instance, induced sweating in a patient who was hot, in part to rid the body of noxious humours but also to rid it of heat.[13] In sum, as in many other systems of medicine, hot/cold wet/dry reasoning both elucidated the cause and pointed to the cure of illness.

Sympathy was the other pillar of early modern medicine. Obviously, the idea that men mirrored aspects of the natural world was of great antiquity; it remained a powerful explanatory strategy well into the eighteenth century.[14] As Nicholas Culpeper explained, "Sympathy and antipathy are the two Hinges upon which the whole Model of Physick turns; and that Physician which minds them not, is like a Door off from the Hooks, more like to do a Man Mischief, than to secure him."[15] For physician, surgeon and patient alike, sympathetic reasoning underlay disease explanation and treatment.

Sympathy enabled people to cure their illnesses by transferring them to other objects. In the South-West, for example, those near Exeter who had the ague would visit the nearest crossroads and secretively bury an egg in the ground, and be cured. The underlying principle seems to have been the transfer of the disease to the egg, although the magical component of crossroads burial (where, after all, suicides were buried so that they would not rise again) cannot be overlooked.[16] Similarly, sufferers in eighteenth-century Devon gave a dog a salted cake of bran in order to transfer a malady to the animal.[17] Although the patients might not have known it (or the writer may have sanitized the story) this practice was clearly derivative of one recorded in Nicholas Culpeper's popular health text, *Last Legacy*. Here, the principle of the transfer of illness, in this case, the quartan ague, was made explicit. A cake was to be made of the sick person's urine, mixed with flour, and fed to a dog, which then contracted the illness. Culpeper emphasized that it should be a female dog for a woman who was sick and a male dog for a man.[18]

John Cannon, who grew up in rural Somerset in the 1680s and 1690s, recorded in his memoirs how his brother was sympathetically cured of a rupture. He was passed through a slit cut in a young ash tree three times on three Monday mornings before dawn. The ash was then bound up, and as it grew back together, so did Cannon's brother. Some years later their father decided to move the tree, and it was transplanted, after which it died in a dry summer. As Cannon explained, "and some time after, my brother grew Bad again, which confirmed ye Opinion some held concerning ye aforesaid Value in an ash."[19] Although his comments, written in the 1740s, are tinged with hints of skepticism, it seems there were few doubters in 1688, when Cannon's brother was healed.

Such sympathetic transfer of illness was not confined to vernacular practice. For example, Richard Wiseman, in his manual for surgeons, discussed the very common procedure of rubbing warts with a piece of beef, and then burying the beef, another example of the transfer of an ailment to a quasianimate object.[20] In the digest of Thomas Willis's works, sympathetic explanation is melded with Willis's own acid/alkali theories. He wrote, "The other cure of Jaundice at a distance, is said to be done by I know not what sympathy or secret manner of working." The procedure was to take the patient's urine and mix it up with ashes in order to make three equal balls. These were placed in front of the fire, and when they dried out, the disease went and the patient was cured. Willis explained that when the lixivial salt in the ashes was mixed with the urine, it set the volatile salt in the urine free:

> and at the same time that this is done in the icterical Urine, it happens by sympathy that the volatile salt also in the Blood of the Patient gets free from the Dominion of the fixed salt and Sulphur, and consequently the Icterical Dyscrasy of the Blood vanishes.

Although Willis provided other direct cures for jaundice, he claimed that this one had worked when all others had failed.[21] Sympathetic explanations were thus very flexible, capable of almost endless accommodation to other theoretical approaches. Such flexibility may have contributed to their popularity with patient and doctor alike.

In the case of jaundice and many other ailments, color was a very significant mode of sympathetic treatment. For instance, Thomas Willis used yellow remedies to heal jaundice. Of the nine specifics he cited, eight include yellow ingredients, such as saffron, celandine (which has yellow flowers), turmeric, "the outward yellow coats of oranges and lemons," and the like. Willis characteristically explained that these were specifics for jaundice because they promoted the separation of choler from blood and augmented the excretion of bilious elements in sweat and urine.[22] Nevertheless, the yellowness of these remedies would have been very apparent to patients whatever explanatory framework Willis offered.

Moving to a text intended for lay readers, Nicholas Culpeper recommended a decoction of earthworms, celandine, and ivy berries for jaundice, but added that if "you add a little saffron tyed up in a rag, 'twill be the better."[23] John Wesley, whose *Primitive Physick* was a best-selling lay health text in mid-eighteenth-century, also had a penchant for yellow remedies for jaundice, although he did not make explicit claims for their efficacy based on color. For instance, he suggested wearing celandine leaves under the feet. Decoction of dandelion was another yellow recommendation.[24] Again, these writers did not always make sympathetic claims for their yellow remedies; rather the flexibility of such explanations enabled them to be used in conjunction with a number of different frameworks.

Sympathy could work either by likes (as in yellow remedies for jaundice) or by opposites. Thus, for example, Nicholas Culpeper explained some of his remedies for bleeding: "Toads, Spiders and Frogs, or their Spawn . . . do it by antiphony, because blood flyes from its enemy; and therefore if a dried Toad be but held, in the hand of one that bleedeth, the blood presently ceaseth, and retireth back to the Centre."[25] Thomas Beddoes, a Bristol physician in the late eighteenth century, noted down an example of the "like" sympathetic remedy:

> Yet the powder occasionally found within the cavity of flints is still used as a remedy for calculous complaints in our chalk counties; I met with an instance of this kind within these few days. It was probably conceived, in both cases, that one kind of grit would draw or drive the other out of the body.[26]

This vernacular remedy was of long standing. Culpeper, for instance, had recommended dried and powdered eggshells for stone, on the same principle of using stonelike substances to expel stones.[27] In Bristol, sufferers were using preparations of ground-up oyster shells, another stonelike substance.[28]

Sympathetic styles of explanation were related to astrological medicine and the concept of man as microcosm.[29] As "Aristotle," the pseudonymous author of a best-selling health manual, explained, "Man is said to be a Microcosm (or little World) and in him the Almighty has imprinted his own Image . . . "[30] With "Aristotle," many other authors of vernacular health texts relied upon astrological explanations and cures, as did some manuals intended for surgeons and apothecaries.

Nicholas Culpeper, for example, often delineated which herbs were governed by which planets in his vernacular health texts. If a headache were due to the actions of Venus, for example, fleabane (a herb of Mars) would be an appropriate cure. "Aristotle," in common with other vernacular books, reprinted a woodcut of Zodiac Man, which illustrated parts of the body governed by different planets.

One of the chief vehicles for vernacular astrological explanations of illness were almanacs. A 1710 one claimed that

The Heaven's a Book,
The stars are Letters Fair,
God is the writer
Men the Readers are.[31]

But the *Vox Stellarum,* the most popular almanac of the eighteenth century, took a somewhat more moderate view, "Men may be inclin'd, but not compell'd to do good or evil by the influence of the stars."[32] By 1740 the same almanac was quite sarcastic about using astrology for prognostication, saying "The fifth House tells ye whether Whores be sound or not; when it is good to eat Tripes, bloat herrings, fry'd Frogs, rotten Eggs, and Monkey's Tails butter'd."[33] Despite this indication of astrology's fall from grace, elements of astrological healing remained embedded in almanacs. For example, this same 1740 edition of the *Vox Stellarum* indicated which diseases were prevalent in particular months, a kind of vestigial form of astrological medicine. A South-West almanac, made in Wiltshire for 1692, was more straightforward and less witty. It included discussions of the weather, parts of the body likely to be at risk at various times, the chief roads in the area, and a table for gauging the contents of barrels, hogsheads, and butts.[34] In contexts such as this, astrology was just one means of understanding the world; the table to figure out the contents of barrels

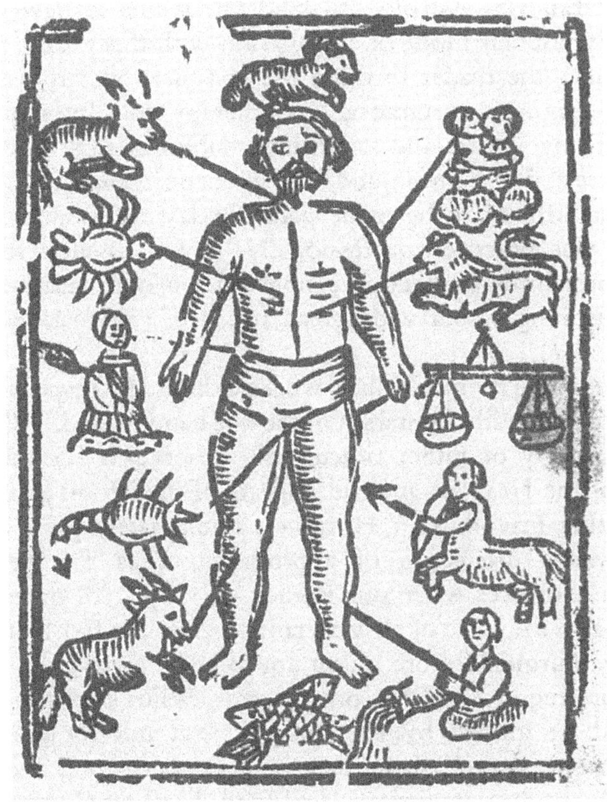

Figure 2.1. Zodiac Man (Wellcome Library, London)

was given rhetorical weight equal to the picture of Zodiac Man (Fig. 2.1). Almanacs, whether humorous or plain, relied upon astrological conventions and ideas and presumed that their users were familiar with such concepts.

Astrological explanations also featured in books meant for mixed audiences of lay and professional healers. These could range from William Salmon's *Synopsis Medicinae,* which provided both astrological and humoral explanations for all ailments, to the work of Thomas Willis, which made only occasional reference to astrology. Salmon, as befitted a colleague of Nicholas Culpeper, emphasized the demystification of professional practices. Like Culpeper, he published in English and reflected a revolutionary antiprofessional monopoly stance common to several authors of manuals written in English. Astrological medicine seems to have been a particularly popular mode of explanation with this group.[35] Thus Salmon takes the reader through the complex operations of astrological diagnosis, prognosis, and therapy step by step, with appropriate star charts and logarithmic tables as aids to learning and practice.[36] For Salmon and Culpeper, no technique was too obscure or difficult to be made plain for lay readers. Although astrology was practiced professionally, it was an ideal form of analysis for Salmon to make accessible to lay people because astrological reasoning was a widespread mode of explanation in lay culture.

The digest of Thomas Willis's works exhibited a more ambivalent relationship with the stars. On the one hand, it said, "Whereas some religiously or rather ridiculously observe in Bleeding the Position of the Heavens and the Aspects of the Moon and Stars, it's altogether Frivolous."[37] However, immediately prior to this passage was a discussion of appropriate times for bleeding, "About the Solstices when our Bodies are very cold, or hot, the Blood, as also the Juice of all Vegetables being in a fixt State, and apt for any Turgid Motion, ought not to be let forth unless some urgent cause requires it."[38] In other words, Willis said that bleeding should be guided by the solstices, but not by the stars. Although he was emphasizing that the depths of winter and summer were inappropriate times to let blood, he phrased this idea in terms of man's relation to the sun. He then quickly denied that bloodletting should be guided by the stars. In other words, even a medical writer generally unsympathetic to astrological explanation expressed himself in ways that could be made consonant with a microcosm-macrocosm frame of reference.

The relationships of astrology, vernacular health care, and lay beliefs are complex. It seems that astrological thought remained a significant aspect of vernacular healing well into the eighteenth century.[39] Writers for a medical audience tended to abandon explicit astrology before lay texts did so, but often their interpretations of illness were not wholly alien to astrological interpretation by a reader so inclined.

Sympathy and astrology shaded imperceptibly into beliefs now considered supernatural.[40] Examples of "supernatural" beliefs are tantalizing; they tend to illustrate the potential range of ideas rather than conveying the norm.[41] At best, we can only show that magical beliefs were held by rather ordinary working men and women, and, like other medical ideas discussed here, were flexible and highly adaptable to local circumstance.

For example, Thomas Perks of Mangotsfield, outside Bristol, supposedly conversed with spirits in the early 1700s. He was a blacksmith, who studied astrology extensively, and he invited the local clergyman Arthur Bedford to come and see his spirits. He drew a chalk circle at a crossroads, chanted words from the Bible, and produced several tiny women, eighteen inches high. As time went on, however, his control over the spirit world slipped, and he was troubled by "dismal Shapes, like Serpents, Lions, Bears etc., and hissing at him, or attempting to throw spears, or Balls of Fire at him."[42] Perks consulted a Bristol apothecary, Mr. Jacobs (whose existence is verified by apprenticeship records), but to no avail: "These Methods cost him his Life in this World." Perhaps this was a complete fabrication by the author, invented to warn the unwary of dabbling in the spirit realm, although Bedford's other writings make this improbable. But even if it were fiction, it is suggestive that such warnings were thought necessary.

Other evidence suggests that magic was, if not commonplace, far from unusual. John Cannon, whose brother had been healed by the sympathetic ash tree, had a good friend who engaged in magical practices, on one occasion impressing Cannon by making the sky grow dark at his bidding.[43] This friend, one John Read, spent his spare time in heavy drinking and heavy reading. When he left Somerset he buried a copy of Cornelius Agrippa's *Occult Philosophy* for Cannon to collect. But Cannon claims to have "utterly despised anything sounding of Magick or Occult Science" and did not recover the book, despite being an avid reader.[44]

Although the extent of popular magical practice will probably never be ascertained, several local manuscript remedy books contain cures that might be deemed magical. To take just one, a mid-eighteenth-century book included charms for a burn, to stop bleeding, for the ague, for the prick of a thorn, and to catch thieves. For example, for a burn or scald, one was to say "Mary mild as burned her child and on a Spark of Fire out Fier in Frost in the Name of the Father Son and holy gost Amen Amen Amen."[45] Again, it is impossible to know if the writer tried or believed in such things, but they were recorded, and in this text, given equal status with more mundane recipes and cures. In 1751 a woman in

Bristol wore a doctor's prescription around her neck rather than having it filled, believing that it was just as efficacious as a charm.[46] Of course such a newspaper report might be apocryphal, intended as a joke, but even in jest, it hints that such practices were well-known.

A final example of magical beliefs comes from the letter book of the Champion family, Bristol Quakers influential in local charity. In a 1761 letter to her brother, Miss Champion recounted:

> It happened to a poor Man at work in a field just by, which I will tell as it has just been related me. How that on a certain day as he was just going to work with his fellow labourers, it happened that he found a white wand and when they went home they burnt this white wand, and so a little while after the old woman that own'd it came to discover the matter, that this man dreadful to relate fell sick, so that they could find no relief till a Neighbour more knowing that the rest found out the Cause and nature of his Distemper and told him he was bewitch'd.[47]

The story had a happy ending, at least for the laborer. The old woman was brought before two magistrates, and they spared her life on the condition that she transform herself into a hare every morning for their sport. This last whimsical touch suggests that no one took this tale too seriously, but Miss Champion wrote, "I really believe the Country People would think one an atheist to disbelieve it. It is amazing to think how superstitious they are." John Latimer, in his annals of Bristol, recounts that in 1730 in the Somerset town of Frome a poor elderly woman suspected of witchcraft was drowned by a mob at the suggestion of the local cunning man, using the ancient custom of swimming a suspected witch.[48] Almost as startling as the death of the "witch" is the evident power of the local cunning man.

It was not just assumptions about illness causation that doctors and lay healers shared; both employed the same remedies. Physicians may have been discussing the body according to corpuscular theory, or later might adhere to Cullen's nosology emphasizing the role of the nervous system, or might pledge themselves to any number of other systems of thought. But, as in the example of Thomas Willis's yellow remedies for jaundice, the therapies they provided were easily assimilated to those proffered by lay healers and popular health texts.[49]

The Bristol physician Arthur Broughton took careful notes in his London and Edinburgh materia medica courses, which list what remedies elite medicine could offer in the middle of the eighteenth century. These notes provide a counterpoint to domestic medical texts, particularly Nicholas Culpeper's *English Physician Enlarged* and John Wesley's 1747 *Primitive Physick,* as well as a number of local manuscript remedy books, and handbooks for surgeons. Although therapeutics in these varied sources are by no means identical, there is considerable overlap.

For example, almost all sources agree about the uses of the plantain in healing, although they argue their cases in characteristically different ways. For Culpeper, this was a herb of Venus. Consequently, it cured heat by antipathy, and venereal problems through sympathy – Venus, of course, governed the genitals. Because of its antipathy to heat, plantain was especially good for stopping fluxes, or any other kind of sudden bleeding from wounds, or even spitting up blood from consumption. As Culpeper summed up, it was a "singularly good wound herb to heal fresh or old Wounds or Sores, either inward or outward."[50] John Wesley, too, recommended plantain (either its seeds, or its leaves boiled up, or its juice) for a flux, although he typically declined to give any reasons for its effects.[51]

On the practitioners' side, surgeon's guidebooks also recommended plantain to stop sudden effusions of blood. William Salmon, for instance, cited it as a good wound herb, and said that the seed stopped fluxes and spitting up blood.[52] Five of the eight juleps that Thomas Willis's manual recommended to stop the spitting of blood in phthisis contained plantain water.[53] So too, both of Arthur Broughton's instructors cited plantain for bleeding. His London teacher (there are no clues as to whom it was) taught that plantain was an astringent; hence it was good for hemorrhages.[54] In Edinburgh, Broughton learned materia medica from Francis Home at the University. Home spoke up for the humble plantain as well, claiming that it was an inspissant (meaning that it thickened bodily fluids) and hence was good for phthisis, fluxes, ophthalmia, and ulcers.[55] In other words, all of these rather varied authorities shared a certain core of beliefs about the therapeutic properties of this plant. It healed sudden bleeding, be that due to ulcers, or spitting up of blood in consumption, or in a flux (a sudden discharge of blood). The rationales for its efficacy were different, but therapy was the same.

Looking at an illness rather than a specific plant also reveals many links between popular and professional healers. For example, remedies for gravel (small kidney or bladder stones) are similar in "lay" and "medical" sources. Unfortunately, both of Broughton's teachers listed very few specific remedies for gravel; some of their recommendations must be inferred. Culpeper, on the other hand, listed twenty-seven different cures, and several more for the stone, a similar problem.[56] Basically, all authors agreed on two sorts of cures: diuretics and preparations of umbelliferous plants. Culpeper and both of Broughton's teachers, for instance, cited butcher's broom, a diuretic, as useful. Culpeper, Wesley, and Francis Home (Broughton's Edinburgh teacher) all thought that a wildflower, pellitory of the wall, considered a diuretic, could be used for gravel. So too did a letter writer to the *Gentleman's Magazine* in 1731, who recommended a tea of marshmallow leaves, saxifrage, herb mercury, and pellitory of the wall.[57] William Salmon and Thomas Willis recommended pellitory of the wall as well, each for characteristic reasons – because it was diuretic and emollient (Salmon) and because of its acid salt (Willis).[58]

Almost all authorities, lay or medical, claimed that kidney stones might be remedied by a preparation of an umbellifer, a group of plants with tiny flowers, similar to the American weed called Queen Anne's lace or the British cow parsley. In London, Broughton's teacher included wild carrot seed in his list of diuretics, all of which were more or less appropriate to gravel. Wild carrot is a common umbellifer; it looks similar to the wild parsleys. So too, Willis mentioned wild carrot seed and stone parsley as diuretic remedies suitable for the stone.[59] William Salmon also included wild carrot, the suggestively named stone parsley, and carrot in his list of remedies.[60]

Moving into the realm of popular texts, John Wesley, in his *Primitive Physick,* suggested wild parsley seeds for gravel. A century earlier, Nicholas Culpeper had recommended parsley-piert for gravel. This plant, although not an umbellifer, has parsleylike leaves, which makes it similar in appearance, albeit in miniature, to wild carrot, and other of the umbellifers used for stone. Its other name, parsley breakstone, points to its use in healing. Cow parsnip, or hogweed, a very common large umbellifer also linked to healing the stone, was sufficiently well-known in Somerset to have two dialect names: "lumper-scrump" and "old rot."[61]

There is evidence that this umbellifer remedy complex was actually used in and around Somerset. In the 1780s and 1790s, William

Falconer, M.D., F.R.S., practiced in Bath, where he developed his cure for gravel, called the Aqua Mephitica, a sort of carbonated water. He published a book describing his remedy which includes case histories that discuss what his patients did prior to seeking his help. These individuals downed prodigious quantities of patent remedies, used mechanical aids to restore the patency of the urethra, and took opiates for the pain when all else failed. Of the sixteen whose own therapeutic efforts he chronicled, five included decoctions of wild carrot seed, an umbellifer.[62] Finally, a barely literate Gloucestershire farmer, whose manuscript remedy book dealt mostly with animal disorders, included a recipe for "Collick and Gravel" that contained wild parsley roots.[63] In other words, this remedy complex, which centered on a group of commonly available weeds, seems to have extended from rural farmer right through elite London medicine.

These similarities are suggestive rather than definitive. They imply, first of all, that physicians, surgeons, and lay people shared, in some vague way, certain ideas about what plants could be used medicinally, and for what purposes. For instance, virtually every local plant mentioned by either of Broughton's instructors could be found in Culpeper. This overlap also suggests that, whatever their differences, elite physicians and lay healers might have been purveying – and employing – the same remedies, albeit with varying explanations, and at a range of prices.

These commonalities among practitioners and between practitioners and their patients mitigated against the creation of professional autonomy and power within a doctor-patient encounter. Similarly, the ways in which knowledge reproduced the social relations of medicine is particularly apparent in the early-modern emphasis upon reading the body's surface for indications of disease. Margaret Pelling has discussed the relationship of Tudor surgical practice to a cultural focus upon the outside surface of the body. She said, "medical practitioners and the laity alike placed great stress on disfiguring conditions, especially those affecting the face."[64] She went on to suggest that because Elizabethan and Jacobean clothing was designed to conceal much of the body, it highlighted deformity, disease, or bad smells in those parts of the body which remained visible. Medicine, of course, profited from this emphasis on the outside of the body. The barber-surgeon served as a custodian of the body, whose functions included wig-making, teeth-cleaning, and syringing ears, as well as treatment of the disfiguring pox, venereal disease.[65] Concern with the surface of the body continued to be a significant theme in vernacular and professional ideas about health. In the eighteenth century, popular health texts and practices reiterated that a person's external self, his or her body surface, revealed important inner truths, just as plants revealed their healing virtues in their outer forms and colors.

Perhaps the clearest example of this concern with outward appearance is in popular texts' explanations of, and fascinations with, monster births.[66] Often, the only pictures in a cheap popular health text are three or four rudimentary woodcuts of monsters. The woodcuts change from edition to edition, but their message remains the same. It is an attempt to understand the relationship between outward appearance and inner qualities. "Aristotle" emphasized that meaning was to be drawn from such instances:

Of monstrous Births some Instances I'll Shew
Which, tho' they frightful seem unto our View
Yet they by their mishapen Forms may preach.[67]

Such interests were a part of the larger culture; they were by no means exclusively or even mostly medical. Thus, for example, an eighteenth-century chapbook recounted the tale of Sarah Smith from Darken, in Essex. She had been brought to bed of a monster, and subsequently died. Her funeral sermon was included lest any reader miss the point, describing Smith as "a very wicked Liver, and disobedient to her Parents, and one that was mightily given to Wishing, Cursing, and Swearing."[68] Her sad tale was certified by the local churchwardens, as were miracle cures and vagrants' passes.

These curiosities were important for what they revealed of their Maker. An early eighteenth-century broadside makes this point in its advertisement for a combined show of a horned woman and an amazing clock that sang like birds: "Is to be seen a Miracle in Nature, being a Woman that has a Horn growing on the back part of her Head . . . Also the greatest piece of Art ever the World produc'd, being a spring Musical Clock; or a curious Piece of Machinery . . . "[69] The problem of monsters was neither obscure nor irrelevant in a hierarchical society whose ultimate governor and architect was divine. Hence the association between a clock, made by man, and a freak, made by God; both were examples of

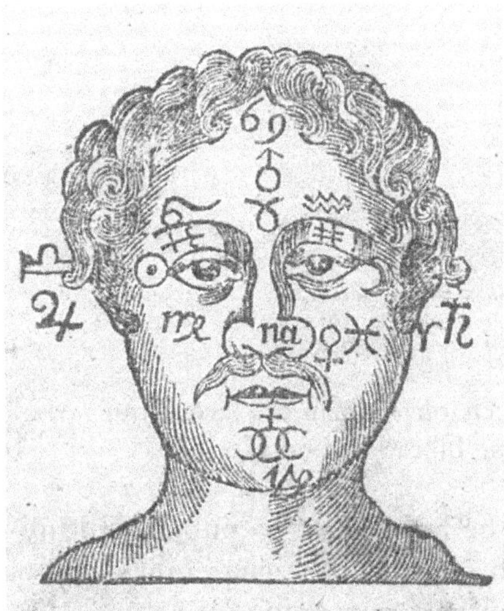

Figure 2.2. Zodiac Face, a form of astrological physiognomy (Wellcome Library, London)

unusual artifice. As in the case of Sarah Smith, many early explanations of monsters moved from the craftsman to the sinner as the key.[70] In other words, the divine artificer only permitted the imperfect in the context of sin and personal responsibility, where it might serve as lesson and punishment. In any case, the lesson could be read from the outside of the body.

In more mundane examples, both chapbooks and popular health texts in the late seventeenth and early eighteenth centuries emphasized how an individual's character and attributes were reflected in his or her personal appearance (Fig. 2.2). The ubiquitous Zodiac Man indicated not only what planets ruled parts of the body in regard to illness, but also what various body parts revealed about character. Thus, for example, "Aristotle" discussed hair:

Thus does wise nature make our very Hair
Shew all the Passions that within us are,
If to the Bottle we are most inclin'd
Or if we fancy most the Female Kind
If unto Virtue's Paths our Minds are bend
Or if to vicious Ways our Footsteps tend,
A skilful Artist can unfold the same,
And from our Hair a certain Judgement frame;
But since our Periwiggs are come into Fashion
No Room's left for such an Observation.[71]

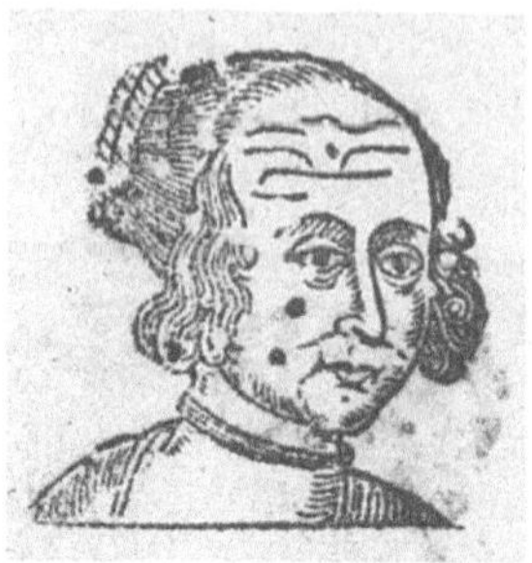

Figure 2.3. Reading character from the face, from "Aristotle's" *Masterpiece* (Wellcome Library, London)

Virtually all the parts of the body open to public scrutiny could provide the observer with clues to character, unless the barber-surgeon or wig-maker had been improving on nature.

Medical works, too, emphasized the knowledge that was apparent at the body's surface. William Salmon advised his readers, "The Countenance like itself in Health is a good sign; but contrariwise evil: as if the Nose is sharp, the Eyes hollow, the Temples fallen, the Ears cold and drawn in . . . it foreshews Death to be near."[72] The able medical practitioner could thus make his disclaimers and prepare the patient for his or her demise.

Again, such preoccupations with appearance, especially facial signs, were by no means peculiar to medicine (Fig. 2.3.). A chapbook entitled *The Egyptian Fortune Tellers Last Legacy* provided a zodiac map of the face, in order to divine the significance of moles. This book, like others of its kind, also supplied advice about dream interpretation. It was related to the genre of courtship books, which included recipes for love powders, directions for making enchanted rings, and the like.[73]

Physical characteristics hinted to the reader of popular literature about character. In a black-letter ballad from the seventeenth century, facial details indicated truths about character. This song tells the tale of Mrs. Jane Reynolds, a West Country woman who betrothed herself to a sailor, and married someone else when he did not return home. In the text, she is described physically only by the rather nondescript words "fair maid." But two woodcuts illustrate this song; one of a ship, the other a portrait of Jane Reynolds. A careful observer would know that Reynolds was not to be trusted; she is shown with two facial warts and some odd wrinkles in her forehead.[74] And she did come to a bad end, taken away on a ghost ship by the spirit of her former lover. Marks on the face (which, of course, were emphasized by the extent of clothing) seem to have been afforded especial significance. A West Country edition of popular sayings, for instance, said "Five things that will hardly be hidden: Poverty in pride; wantonness in lust; a wart in the face; wildfire in the dark, and a painted whore in a shop."[75] The other items, such as painted whores and wantonness, emphasize the negative connotations of facial marks. This sort of physiognomy was commonplace. John Cannon, for example, wrote of one woman, "she being truly a meer strumpet, being black graind small share of beauty of a middle stature, light and wanton."[76] For many such as Cannon, moral worth was easily equated with physical appearance.

Popular medical works, of course, also provided remedies for such outward blemishes. To take just one text, Nicholas Culpeper's *English Physician Enlarged* listed cures for such disfigurements as hair loss, bloodshot eyes, webs and pins in the eyes, smallpox scars, freckles, redness in the face, superfluous hairs, and many others.

For medical practitioners, one of the most significant aspects of this attention to the body surface was the power that it gave to the patient. Just as Sarah Smith's tale was attested by her churchwardens, so too were advertisements of cures in the newspapers. Quite specific instructions were given about finding the person who had been cured, so that one could verify the treatment oneself. The cured person was analogically related to monsters or freaks; one whose inner state could easily be revealed by outer inspection. Although such testimonials are obviously rhetorical devices to add verisimilitude, this usage also implied that any ordinary person could judge medical matters on an equal footing with a doctor. If illness' meaning were to be read from the body's surface, anyone could be the reader.

These meanings of illness were often cast in historical terms. One of the most striking features of early modern accounts of illness is their very long time span. The most trivial of events might trigger a deathly illness. For example, the Bristolian William Dyer recorded in his diary the pathetic story of a man who accidentally swallowed a cherry pit which lodged in his throat. It stayed there for several years, increasingly obstructing the passage until the man died of starvation.[77] A woman from Ashton Keins, in nearby Wiltshire, explained to Dr. Rice Charlton in Bath how she'd gotten caught in a sudden shower ten years earlier, on Michaelmas. This provoked scorbutic ulcers, which she had treated with purges for five years before they went away.[78] These lengthy tales highlight the importance of chronic, long-term illness; dramatic epidemic killers like fevers were balanced by quotidian misery. The time span of these accounts also emphasizes the importance of understanding illness' roots; people searched far back into their memories to find the events which underlay sickness, gave it meaning, and afforded some measure of control.

This deeply historical perception of disease had several functions. First, recounting how they fell ill enabled patients to understand their bouts of sickness, to make sense of the seemingly random incidence of disease. For example, this is what Samuel Sholl, a poor silk weaver, recounted in his autobiography:

> my bedfellow scratched my right leg with his toenail; being young and unacquainted with anything of the kind, I did not attend to it; it festered and became so bad that I was obliged to apply to different surgeons, but all in vain, indeed, I was apprehensive it must be cut off; however, as I knew something of medicine, I set about trying some means myself, and I have every reason to be thankful that it answered the end. I cured it, to my unspeakable joy, in about four months, after its being bad between eight and nine years.[79]

For Sholl, this was a tale of resourcefulness. He wanted to emphasize that he was young and knew nothing, or the initial scratch would have been better seen to. But with more advanced years and wisdom, Sholl was able to understand his illness, and even to cure himself.

Resourcefulness was not the only theme to such narratives of illness.[80] Again and again, patients searched far back in time to understand what had befallen them, a quest often cast in religious terms. After all, one of the forms of narrative familiar to many an early modern was the spiritual autobiography.[81] Such an examination of one's daily life for signs of God's providence or displeasure, events which seemed trivial but which revealed a divine plan to the awakened – such a framework was easily adaptable to untangling the meanings of illness. This style of analysis was most consonant with enthusiastic religion, including Quakers, and with inheritors of the Puritan tradition of self-examination.[82]

Samuel Sholl, for example, reiterated his theme of youthful innocence in his discussions of a visit to a surgeon. He had bad ulcers inside his mouth. He started his narrative with a snowball fight that had happened when he was a boy, sixteen years earlier. Having been hit in the face with a snowball, he reasoned, was the underlying or initiating cause of his ulcers.[83] This tale of unintended consequences and youthful ignorance can be read on many levels. Motifs of innocence and redemption, error and salvation, provided a framework in which Sholl could understand what had befallen him. Note also that the surgeon, who ultimately helped to heal Sholl's ulcers, takes a very minor part in the story. He is but an instrument, a technician, rather than a decisive actor. The interpretative burden of sickness is Sholl's, and once he has understood cause and effect, the cure – and the curer – is of lesser significance.

Such a portrait of early modern relations between patient and practitioner should not be read as an idealization, as a plea for talking rather than treating. To articulate illness causation is not to cure. But nor should we overlook the ways in which medical and social power could be disaggregated in situations where patients maintained interpretive autonomy. As we shall see, when medical and social authority were united in the hospital, poor patients were doubly dispossessed.

In sum, the content of medicine embodied a world of practice in which physicians, surgeons, and apothecaries lacked professional autonomy and power. Not only did vernacular medicine rely upon the same theoretical constructs as that practiced by full-time medical men; the same kinds of remedies were favored by a wide range of lay and quasiprofessional healers. Medical knowledge, be it vernacular or learned, inscribed the significance of illness on the surface of the body, accessible to all. Like many other aspects of the natural world, the meaning of illness was apparent – to see was to know. This openness was related to two aspects of people's experiences of illness. First, as discussed, there were few privileged opinions about health. Most ideas about the body were common to many if not most early modern English men and women. Full-time medical practitioners lacked the power, or perhaps the inclination, to make illness' meaning unseen, to maintain a privileged interpretation of the body based upon its inaccessibility.[84]

Such openness was also related to the interpretive framework of inadvertence and God's providence that many early moderns relied upon to explain illness. Had Samuel Sholl been wiser, he would not have suffered for years from mouth ulcers but would have treated the wound made by the snowball in his youth. But in time the redemption offered all sinners and sufferers was his. For the patient, this sacramental understanding of illness placed primary importance on the untangling of meaning and the integration of the causes of illness into the narrative, usually spiritually-oriented, of one's life. In other words, stories of sickness began much earlier, went on much longer, and depended much less upon professional healers – indeed upon healing at all – than those we are used to constructing.

3

The marketplace of medicine

Someone who fell ill in eighteenth-century England found a profusion of health-care providers eager for his or her custom. Apothecaries, surgeons, bonesetters, druggists, midwives, and a wealth of other practitioners plied their trades in city and country. Rather than seeking help outside the home, however, many early modern Englishmen and women turned to self-medication, to remedies concocted at home or perhaps purchased in a shop. Few people seem to have hesitated to play a therapeutic role; medical knowledge, or at least recipes for cures, were a part of everyday conversation, and lay health manuals enjoyed large sales. In a world in which illness' meanings could be interpreted by all, it is not surprising that illness could also be cured by all.

For example, an early nineteenth-century compiler of recipes for coughs and colds cited forty different sources for his or her set of remedies.[1] The list included medical authors such as Andrew Pitcairn or John Fothergill, lay authorities such as Jonas Hanway or the *Gentleman's Magazine* as well as local doctors. But it also included eighteen women, many of whom were evidently known personally to the writer. No particular textual authority was granted to one group or another. Friends and relations rubbed shoulders with renowned medical figures. It seems that the sharing of remedies was a common practice, a form of social intercourse not unknown to later generations. Thomas Beddoes, the iconoclastic Bristol physician, often inveighed against self-medication, which he considered the worst sort of quackery. In an advice book for the middle classes, he used sarcasm to combat domestic medicine:

> many of these people . . . have strong upon them, the passion for snapping up verbal and written recipes for every current *name* of disease. I

have seen some of their pocketbooks as full crammed as the cloth hall at Leeds, during our dispute with the Northern Powers. Some treasure up these stores for family use. Others are public-minded, and know no greater pleasure than in drawing from their magazine for the benefit of every acquaintance within reach of a call or note.[2]

Beddoes had strong and rather idiosyncratic views on medical care and quackery, but his belief that ordinary people practiced a good deal of medicine is borne out by other sources.[3]

An examination of the healing practices of William Dyer, a Bristol clerk who left a detailed diary, shows how giving and receiving medical advice was a part of everyday social life.[4] Dyer was probably more diligent and interested in medicine than many – he had very briefly been apprenticed to an apothecary, and was a great reader – but he was not considered exceptional. For example, Dyer had been sending a powder for spitting up blood to a Mr. Clarke in London. Mr. Clarke had:

inscribed his case in one of the magazines, and thereupon Bro. John sent him 1/2 doz doses in a Frank. I likewise have since supplied him. He desired to make an acknowledgement but as that was not expected nor accepted; I recommended John Payne's volume of sermons, & his new translation of Thos a Kempis; which Mr Clarke accordingly applied for & purchased, as Mr Payne informed me.[5]

The chain of connections in this tale of healing was complex; Mr. Clarke had evidently published details of his ailment in a magazine, whereupon John Dyer sent him some of his own secret remedy. Before John died of consumption, he revealed the secret to his brother, who continued to send Clarke the remedy. When Clarke wished to pay for the cures in some way, Dyer suggested that he buy a worthwhile book written by an acquaintance.

Like most of his contemporaries, Dyer saw no real distinction between proprietary remedies and those made at home. For example, he prescribed Dr. James's Powders (one of the century's most popular fever remedies) for a friend and for his father, boiled up a decoction of bark for his mother, and "after Dinner prepared pills of Balm Gilead for Bro John" – all within three weeks.[6] In September 1762, Dyer became deeply involved in preparing remedies from hemlock. He had read a book on hemlock, and discussed it with his friend Mr. Peglar, who was suffering from a leg ulcer.[7]

Peglar asked Dyer to write to London for him, to obtain two ounces of the hemlock extract. Three days later, Dyer "set about preparing extract of Hemlock for Miss Roe, she having sent me some of the plant."[8] Hemlock seems to have been of some use to Peglar, but Miss Roe was visited by Dyer at least three times a week during the next month. In October Dyer went to Bedminster (a suburb of Bristol) "in quest of hemlock," and then went to see his friend Capt. Cheyne "to inspect some Green hemlock which he has procured."[9] For Dyer, his social and medical lives were completely melded, "visited Sukey Cox and drank tea there with AD [his wife] & advised a vomit of 25 gra Ipecacuanha steep'd 10 minutes in a Cup of Tea."[10] Unfortunately there is no record of what Sukey Cox or Dyer's wife thought about this tea-time conversation, but it was typical of Dyer.

It seems that Dyer was far from singular in his access to and interest in knowledge about health. As Roy Porter has shown, lay medical knowledge was extensive and commonplace, particularly among the literate.[11] A Taunton shoemaker, for example, had in his home the Bible, Watt's Hymns and Psalms, Foot's tract on Baptism (he was an Anabaptist), Culpeper's *Herbal, The History of Gentle Craft,* and "an old imperfect volume of Receipts in Physic, Surgery etc and the Ready Reckoner."[12] In other words, in a home with very few books, one or two might be domestic medical texts, although the extent of systematic lay knowledge is almost impossible to estimate.

Of course, the meanings and uses of these texts are open to historical question. John Cannon, for example, growing up in rural Somerset in the last decades of the seventeenth century, found *Aristotle's Masterpiece* and Nicholas Culpeper's book on midwifery a spur to adolescent lusts. He bought a copy of the *Masterpiece* for a shilling, "which I got to pry into ye Secrets of Nature Especially of ye Female Sex".[13] "Aristotle's" depiction of female anatomy led Cannon to investigate for himself by spying on a maidservant. Curiosity unabated, he then obtained a copy of Culpeper's midwifery text, "which only served for a further inlett into Youth's forbidden Secrets of Nature" – but his mother found him reading it, and confiscated the book.[14] It is impossible to fathom if Cannon's access to popular texts was typical of his generation, although he was a more eager reader than some of his contemporaries.

Certainly authors of popular health texts assumed rudimentary medical and botanic knowledge on the part of the reader, and sometimes a great deal more. For example, in Nicholas Culpeper's seventeenth-century *The English Physician Enlarged,* the author provided detailed descriptions of local plants and their therapeutic uses. Sometimes Culpeper told where it was to be found, such as for Wall Rue, "it groweth in many places of this Land, at Dartford, and the Bridges at Ashford in Kent, on Frammingham-Castle in Suffolk, on the Church-Walls at Mayfield in Sussex, in Sommersetshire, and divers other places."[15] However, for 102 different plants, he did not give any description, saying that they were so well known as to preclude the need for any details of their appearance. This list suggests that Culpeper considered most of his readers to have some measure of botanical knowledge. Some of the plants he mentioned were common foodstuffs, such as wheat and rye, others were garden flowers, such as roses and marigolds, or trees like cherry and oak. But he also cited plants with strictly medical uses, such as wormwood, savin, and knotgrass. This list suggests, first, that its readers had a fairly good knowledge of local plants. Given Culpeper's avowed purpose to demystify professional medicine, this assumption of lay knowledge is all the more striking. Second, the inclusion of food items highlights the similarities between cooking and making remedies; both employed similar processes and ingredients. Cookery books from this period, both printed and manuscript, included recipes for preserves and other delicacies, veterinary remedies, hints on household management, and remedies for common human ailments. In both content and form, domestic management and domestic medicine went hand in hand.

However, over the course of the century, such medical remedy books came to include an increasing number of ingredients that could only be obtained commercially. Culpeper represents a particular political approach to domestic health; he wrote to emphasize the availability of remedies in native plants. Other remedy books relied upon both local and exotic, imported remedies. The popularity of Culpeper's work suggests that people did in fact make use of local resources in preparing remedies, as Dyer did in seeking out hemlock. But by Dyer's time, a century later, many manuscript and published remedy books came to rely on purchased ingredients. For example, this cure for a sore elbow, from a Gloucestershire farmer's notebook of the late eighteenth century illustrates a more commercial style of remedy:

furst let blud
2 peniyworth oyle of spicke
2 of the oyl of turpodine
2 of linsed oyle
Mix it up in a bottle and Steack it together and rub a little on morning and evening then use it neat drunck.[16]

None of these ingredients would have been made at home; they all must have been purchased. Indeed, the measure of a "pennyworth" became increasingly common at the end of the century, a sure indicator of the commercial origin of the remedies' components.[17]

Among the more memorable extensions of this process of commercialization was the marketing of artificial peas for issues, a common therapeutic measure in which a cut was made and kept open by the insertion of a small round object, such as a dried pea. In an advertisement, carefully turned artificial orange "peas" were offered at four shillings a hundred, along with plasters to cover the issue.[18]

The passion for pills seems to have extended fairly far down the social scale. Itinerant occasional practitioners may not have taken advantage of new marketing techniques by creating unique named medications, or engaged in expensive advertising, but they were selling their own remedies nonetheless.[19] In his popular antidrink story, *The History of Isaac Jenkins,* Thomas Beddoes describes an epidemic of spotted fever in a small village. Isaac Jenkins's wife wanted to send for the doctor, but "he lived at a distance; and she could not pay him for his medicine, much less his journey." However, a quack doctor had provided some nameless white powder.[20] The family couldn't scrape together the money to use the quack again, although his preparations were cheap. Anything Beddoes says about "quackery" is suspect; this type of practice was one of his lifelong bugbears. But most of this little tract seems to have been drawn from Beddoes's actual experiences in fighting an epidemic, so perhaps his observations can be trusted. If so, even the rural poor had access to commercial remedies, and could participate in the medicine boom of the latter half of the century.

Stereotypically, we imagine country people such as Jenkins making country remedies, brewing up herbs, preserving old traditions, while their city counterparts make use of druggists, chemists, and the apparatus of commercial medicine. As late as the 1840s, in *Mary Barton,* Mrs. Gaskell shows us the newly urbanized workers walking out to the countryside, gathering herbs for remedies. In popular health texts, learned authors emphasize the tenacity of rural healing practices. But this rural/urban, traditional/commercial paradigm breaks down upon closer examination of rural healing practice. First, as discussed in Chapter 2, there were strong unities underlying vernacular and professional health care. The urban/rural divide seems less strong when various remedy complexes were common to city and country alike. Second, remedies in the country as well as the city became increasingly commercialized in the latter half of the century.

To take a rural example, Hugh Smythson's *The Compleat Family Physician,* published in 1781, integrates commercial with traditional domestic remedies. He recommended his book to "the many humane and benevolent characters among the *country gentlemen* and *resident clergy,*" especially in the remoter provinces. For jaundice he suggests time-honored remedies – eating lots of eggs, wrapping the feet with celandine, decoctions of the inner bark of the barberry – all "yellow" remedies that could have been found in health texts a century earlier.[21] But he also gives descriptions and recipes for Daffy's Elixir, Dr. James's Powder, Maredant's Drops, Ormskirk Medicine, and many others. Similarly, in a manuscript remedy book from Bristol, there is a recipe for Staughton's Drops, a popular medicine, and elaborate directions for the use of Ching's Worm Lozenges.[22] As noted above, William Dyer often busied himself making commercial remedies at home, such as the Cordial Balm of Gilead.

Even Nicholas Culpeper's list of plants "familiar to all" does not suggest a rural bias toward herbal remedies or knowledge. One did not need to go out to the countryside and grub around under hedgerows to collect these familiar herbs because many were cultivated as garden plants, not wild ones.[23] In other words, the presumption that country folk continued to use herbal remedies because they were easily obtainable is dubious. Many of Culpeper's cures were as likely to be found in an urban garden, or even a market garden, as they were in the countryside.

Culpeper's "Known to All" Plants

Alexander
Alder tree
Angelica
Garden Arrach
Anemone
Ash tree
Balm
Barberry
Barley
Bay tree
Beans
Beech tree
Blackberry
Borage/bugloss
Broom/broomrape
Burdock
Cabbages
Colewort
Chamomel
Carduus benedictus
Carrots
Cherry tree
Chestnut tree
Chickweed
Chives
Columbines
Costmary
Cowslips
Cucumbers
Daisies
Ducksmeat
Dragons [a plant]
Earthnuts
Elder tree
Elm tree
Ferns
Fennel
Fig tree
Flower-de-luce
Furze
Garlic
Clove gillyflower
Gooseberry
Hearts-ease
Hazelnuts
Hawthorn
Hemp
Hyssop
Hops
Houseleek/sengreen
Holly
Ivy
Juniper
Knotgrass
Lavender
Lettuce
White lillies
Mallows
Marjoram
Marigolds
Mulberry
Nettles
Oak
Oats
Onions
Parsley
Pear tree
Pennyroyal
Plantane
Plums
Garden purslane
Primroses
Roses
Rosemary
Rue
Rushes
Rye
Saffron
Sage
Winter and Summer Savorys
Savin
Service tree
Smallage
Sow thistle
Southernwood
Strawberries
Tamarisk tree
Tansy
Wild tansy
Thistle
Black thorn
Time [thyme]
Wild time
Meadow trefoil
Vine
Violets
Wallnuts
Wheat
Willow
Woodbind
Common wormwood

Indeed, even in the countryside, by the late eighteenth century, herbs were sometimes purchased rather than picked. For instance, when William Holland, the Somerset parson and diarist, wanted some chamomile flowers to treat his biliousness, he bought them from an apothecary in a nearby village, rather than picking the flowers in the wild or cultivating the herb. He had a garden, and a gardener of sorts, but by 1800 it was not uncommon to purchase what had formerly been homegrown remedies like chamomile and rhubarb.[24]

The commercialization of domestic medicine had paradoxical effects on the relationship between professional healers and their patients. On the one hand, it further blurred the distinctions between "professional" and "lay" healing by making "professional" remedies like Dr. Ford's pills available without the professional Dr. Ford's consultation. In this sense, commercial remedies merely expanded the options for patients, who had never hesitated to mix lay and professional healing.

For example, John Addington, a surgeon who published an essay on gonorrhea, treated a thirty-five year-old man, a "healthy mechanic" for two months. He had not been improving while on Addington's gentle cure, and brought the doctor a recipe from a friend, demanding that it be tried. Addington was forced to agree, and the laborer proceeded to take three grains of corrosive sublimate of mercury in rectified spirits of wine daily.[25]

As domestic health care became increasingly commercialized, patent medicines and home remedies were used side by side. For instance, patients of Dr. William Falconer, in Bath, took a motley array of cures for the stone. One, for example, had tried castor oil, fomentations, emollients, and warm baths. He then went on to opiates for the pain, and next tried Chittick's Recipe for the stone, and finally Perry's Solvent. Another first tried Adam's Solvent and then used infusions of marshmallow and other home-made softening and lubricating remedies. The stone was a painful and long-term condition; many of these people had conscientiously tried a dozen or more remedies.

So, on the one hand, commercial remedies represented an expansion of the domestic healing repertoire. Such cures easily fitted into a system in which patients had a good deal of choice in health-care matters. However, the expansion of choice was not without its paradoxical effects. Ultimately, the boom in commercial remedies may have limited choice by the poorer members of society.

By the latter half of the century, Bristolians had a wealth of choice in patent medicines advertised in local newspapers. In the 1770s there were at least half a dozen druggists in the city, who did not practice as apothecaries but ran drugstores. A few years later, Brown's Medicinal and Stationery Warehouse had opened, selling medicines wholesale and retail. Prior to the development of druggists, an important source of remedies had been book- and newspaper-sellers. Not only could one purchase drugs from the newspaper office, but it was advertised that remedies were also to be had of "the men who carry the news" – distributors of the papers. Three things can be noted about remedies sold by newsmen: they were plentiful, expensive, and specific to a particular range of illness.[26]

In 1786, William Pine, a leading printer in Bristol, published a list of the medicines he sold. This list represents only one supplier (albeit a major one) of patent remedies in Bristol (see Table 3.1). Other newspaper publishers advertised other remedies. It is clear from advertisements that Bristol was well-integrated into a national market by the middle of the eighteenth century; almost none of Pine's list were local specialties. Most of these remedies were for a few non-life-threatening ailments – coughs, colds, toothache, cuts, and bruises – or for fevers or venereal disease. These remedies served to complement other types of practice; surgeons and apothecaries were treating slightly different ranges of ailments.[27] Venereal disease represents an exception to this; it was treated by surgeons, apothecaries, and (to judge by the advertisements) a range of patent medicines.[28] Such remedies offered the advantage of secrecy; one advertisement in Bristol claimed, "Persons afflicted may cure themselves with the utmost privacy and even without the Knowledge of a Bed Fellow."[29]

A significant aspect of these medicines is their very high cost. Most of these remedies were out of reach for the average laborer, who might bring home five or six shillings a week.[30] Many of these medicines represent just such a week's wage. And most came in very small sizes – one that advertised a box of forty pills for 1s.2d. was clearly atypical – making them even more costly. Irvine Loudon has pointed out the extraordinarily high levels of spending on drugs in this period, and advertisements certainly bear this out, although as Roy Porter adds, even half a dozen pills in a box may have looked like a bargain when compared with the day-by-day dispensing of single doses by apothecaries.[31] But the poor could not have sustained such high levels of spending, at least in absolute terms.

Table 3.1. *Medicines sold by William Pine, 1786*

Name	Cost (s/d)	Cure	Name	Cost (s/d)	Cure
Adam's solvent	6/9	stone, gravel	Leyden Pills	6/6	anti-venerial,
Orient. Veg. Cordial	5/2	cholic, bowel	Dr Armstrong's Pills	2/9	scorbutic
Stoughton's Bitters	1/2	"	Jesuit's Drops	2/10	"
Dalby's Carminative	1/10	"	Friar's Drops	3/8	"
Dr James' Powders	2/9	fevers	Leake's Pills	2/1	"
Dr Norris' Drops	2/9	"	Velno's Veg. Syrup	11/6	"
Bateman's Drops	1/2	colds, coughs	Steer's Opodeldoc	2/	cuts, bruises
Squire's Elixir	1/8	"	British Oil	1/2	"
Greenough's Lozenges	1/10	"	Jackson's Tincture	1/2	"
Dawson's Lozenges	1/2	"	Friar's Balsam	1/2	"
Hill's Honey Balsam	3/2	"	Patent Ointment	1/10	itch
Essence of Coltsfoot	3/9	"	Volatile Essence	1/6	"
Crawcour's Dentrifice	2/10	teeth	Wheatley's Ointment	1/10	"
Asiatic Tooth Powder	2/2	"	Spilsbury's Drops	5/	scurvy, gout
British " "	1/2	"	Snell's Ointment	6/	"
Toothache Tincture	1/2	toothache	Hill's Ormskirk Med.	5/6	mad dog bite
Hamilton's "	2/10	"	Wace's Asthmatic Drops	3/8	asthma
Maredant's Drops	5/5		Vandour's Nerv. Pills	2/10	nerves

Table 3.1. (*cont.*)

Name	Cost (s/d)	Cure	Name	Cost (s/d)	Cure
Hypo Drops	4/2		Hooper's Female Pills	1/2	female maladies
Inglish's Scots Drops	1/4		Arabian Oil	2/2	sprains, rickets
Wilson's Pills	1/2		Godfrey's Cordial	8d	painkiller
Analeptic Pills	4/6		Cephalic snuff	10	headache
Turlington's Balsam	2/1		Thompson's Ague Tinc're	1/4	ague
Daffy's Elixir	1/8		〃 Antiscorbutic Pills	1/10	scurvy
Dr Becket's Restorative	11/		Corn plaster	1/2	corns
Sticking Plaster	6d	bandage	Franklin's Cornsalve	1/6	〃
Smyth's Restorative	11/6	?VD?			

In conclusion, home health care was thriving in eighteenth-century Bristol and Somerset. The ideology of "every man his own physician" so often used in titles of domestic health books seems to have been a reality if translated into "every man – or maybe every woman – his own apothecary." However, over the course of the century, domestic remedies became increasingly commercialized, and the boundary between domestic medicine and patent remedies, between commercial and noncommercial medicine, became more difficult to divine.

But home remedies represented just a part of the medical market in eighteenth-century England. Throughout the century, an extensive array of medical men and women offered their services to the injured, unwell, and worried. They ranged along a spectrum from those whose careers as healers were full-time and long-term to those who were occasional practitioners, whose careers are ill-represented in historical records. It has sometimes been assumed that there were relatively fewer sorts of practitioners in the early modern period than in the medicalized late twentieth century, and that they were relatively thin on the ground. However, an examination of the diversity of practitioners, both full-time and occasional, suggests that this period was characterized by an abundance of diverse healers. In particular, Margaret Pelling's work on London and Norwich has revealed large numbers of practitioners of many types in both cities, and Bristol resembles both cities in this as in many other regards.[32] In fact, although the numbers can only be approximate, it seems that the number of healers per capita may have actually fallen over the course of the eighteenth century.[33] Bristol enjoyed a robust ratio of as many as one healer to every 106 people at the beginning of the eighteenth century. By 1800, this ratio had declined to a still-generous 1 to 312, although this decline may reflect incomplete sources rather than such a precipitous drop. These figures suggest that demand for health care was high, and practitioners did not hesitate to meet this demand. Moreover, the number of practitioners was multiplied in effect by the use of apprentices, who have not been included in these calculations.

Apprenticeship was far more than entry to a healing career; it was an institution that continued to structure all medical and surgical practice.[34] For most of the century, although full-time practitioners labeled themselves as barber-surgeons or apothecaries, the common structure of apprenticeship was more significant than distinctions between them. It fostered a style of practice based upon frequent, even twice-daily, visits to a patient's home, and the administration of complex and often-changed remedies, over periods of weeks or months. The apprentice made up the medicines or surgical dressings, kept the shop tidy, visited patients when his master was out or disinclined, and provided the manpower for a highly labor-intensive form of medical practice.

In Bristol, as in other ancient cities, apprenticeships were governed by the remnants of a medieval guild structure. Apprentices were registered with the city upon indenture, and were bound to their masters for seven years. They were subsequently able to join the appropriate city company, such as that of barber-surgeons, and become freemen of the city, entitled to practice their trade and, unusually, vote for the city's two members of Parliament. In theory, those who were not members of the appropriate city company could not practice their trade within the city, although by mid-eighteenth century, the entire apprenticeship system was disintegrating, and prosecutions for such practices became fewer and fewer.[35]

The status of one's master seems to have been more significant than his occupational title, at least as far as future practice was concerned. Masters tended to take a succession of boys from similar social backgrounds, and thus well-off apothecaries resembled well-off surgeons more closely than they did struggling apothecaries. For example, William Cook, a barber-surgeon, took only two apprentices, but both were sons of gentlemen. Benjamin Fox, an apothecary, took four: three sons of gentlemen, and one son of a serge-maker (presumably a manufacturer). Samuel Pye, a barber-surgeon, took twenty apprentices. At the start of his career, they came from families headed by merchants, curriers, and other surgeons. By the end of his career, he was training the sons of gentlemen who paid £200 for the privilege.[36]

A similar pattern of upward mobility is illustrated by James Ford, a surgeon at the Infirmary, who had also followed the traditional apprenticeship training. After serving his time, he went to Paris and pursued further training at the Hôtel Dieu and the Charité. In 1743 he became an Infirmary surgeon, and took his first apprentice, John Castelman. Castelman's family had chosen wisely. Ford went on to treat Lord Bute at the Hotwells Spa in Bristol in 1756, and thus made his name. Bute was so pleased with

Ford's performance that he promised Ford he'd make his fortune if Ford would move to London. Ford acquiesced, and Bute was as good as his word; the surgeon acquired an extremely successful practice and became Accoucheur to the Queen.

But back in 1743, when Ford apprenticed Castelman, he was struggling to make ends meet. In his pocket notebook, he gleefully calculated that taking on John Castelman had enabled him to clear £198.18s.6d after expenses – a doubling of his income.[37] Not only did an apprentice represent a tidy sum in cash, he also served for seven years, starting with humble tasks like sweeping the surgery, but quickly moving up to patient care. Of course, not all practitioners were so well-off or attracted the sons of merchants and gentlemen. John Crocker, for instance, also a barber-surgeon, took thirteen apprentices, whose fathers' occupations included mariner, clerk, house carpenter, gardener, silk dyer, cordwainer, brassman, baker, wig-maker, and laborer. The highest recorded premium that he received was £20. In other words, within the structure of apprenticeship, there was a great deal of individual variation in family background, level of education, and ultimately, type of practice. Given such variation, the different medical occupations might not be most usefully thought of as nascent professions; rather, they were a jumble of different types of practitioners who, for reasons of civic administration, fell into the same category.

Thus, it is difficult to fit Bristol health care practitioners into Geoffrey Holmes' model of the professions. Holmes argues that medicine, in step with law and the clergy, began to assume the status and identity of professions in the early eighteenth century.[38] Irvine Loudon has expanded on Holmes, claiming that eighteenth-century medicine (physic, surgery, and pharmacy) was a lucrative, well-regarded, although quite fluid, profession.[39] In some senses, Bristol fits Loudon's case well, if he would avoid the term "profession." It implies an internal cohesion, a united front, a set of shared values, that the diverse array of Bristol practitioners do not seem to possess, at least prior to the nineteenth century. It seems improbable that men such as James Parsley, who dressed wigs, shaved, let blood, and drew teeth, saw themselves allied with an elite Infirmary physician. It seems even less likely that gentlemanly physicians considered themselves akin to Parsley.

Loudon adopts a version of Holmes' model in part because he wishes to emphasize the interactions among practitioners, rather than between practitioners and their patients. He takes issue with the work of Nicholas Jewson, who suggested that much of eighteenth-century medicine was based upon an aristocratic patron-client relationship between patient and doctor.[40] Although it is certainly true that most eighteenth-century patients were neither aristocrats nor patrons, this is not the central point of Jewson's argument. Read more broadly, Jewson is suggesting that patients in a free-market medical economy could, in some measure, control their practitioner-clients. If they did not like their treatment, they could go elsewhere. Thus patients, by choosing among practitioners, exerted their influence upon the social and cognitive structures of medicine. As discussed in Chapter 2, the system of beliefs about the body current in early modern England articulated and embodied a world of healing in which the patient maintained a substantial measure of interpretive control.

However arbitrary were occupational categories, Bristol was undoubtedly a city of surgeons. Throughout the century, they always outnumbered apothecaries, often by two or even three to one. (See Fig. 3.1 for the distribution of types of medical practitioners in Bristol.) In the year 1700, for example, there were about thirty-five apothecaries and almost ninety barber-surgeons practicing within the city. Such an imbalance may not have been typical; perhaps Bristol's role as a port, with attendant numbers of ships' surgeons, contributed to this emphasis upon surgery.[41] In Somerset, numbers of apothecaries and surgeons were more closely matched: we know of seventeen apothecaries and fourteen surgeons who practiced in rural areas of the county at the beginning of the century. (see Fig. 3.2 for Somerset practitioners.) Over the course of the century, the most important change in the practice of surgery in the city was the replacement of apprentice-trained barber-surgeons with hospital-trained surgeons, a development discussed in detail in Chapter 7. In both city and country, medical men increasingly practiced as surgeon-apothecaries, while the apothecary met with competition from the druggist.

In day-to-day practice, barber-surgeons provided their clients with a wide range of services. As their name suggests, they shaved and cut hair. Henry Haines, for example, advertised in 1754 that he "shaves each person for two pence, cuts hair for three halfpence, and bleeds for sixpence. All customers who are bled he treats with two quarts of good ale, and those whom he shaves or cuts their

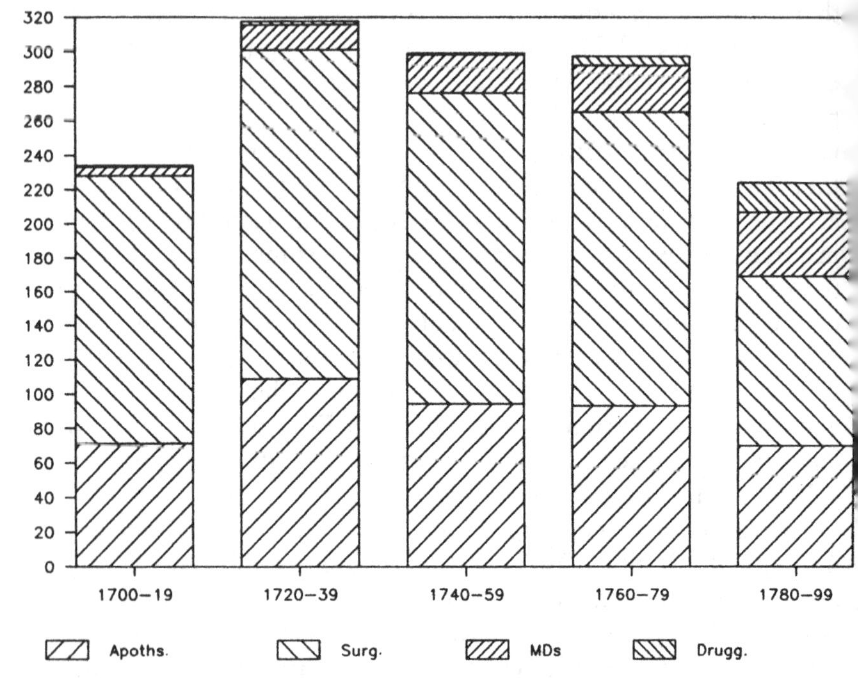

Figure 3.1. Medical practitioners in Bristol

hair with a pint each."[42] Haines was at the cheaper end of the market; bleeding could cost several shillings. However, not all who shaved were competing for the custom of the working man. Thomas Hellier, a prestigious barber-surgeon who treated the city's merchant community, head of the Barber-Surgeons Company, billed a client for three years worth of shaving at thirty shillings a year.[43] Bloodletting was a major part of surgical practice; James Ford bled 190 people in 1754, at fees ranging from half a crown to two guineas, making for a yearly income from bloodletting of perhaps £100. This figure should be compared with Ford's operations for the stone (one of the most common types of surgical operations in this period), which amounted to fifteen people over a period of seventeen years, yielding £221.[44] Such operative surgery formed only a very small proportion of a surgeon's practice. Surgeons functioned almost as a sort of body servant, shaving, bleeding, drawing teeth, treating disfiguring skin condi-

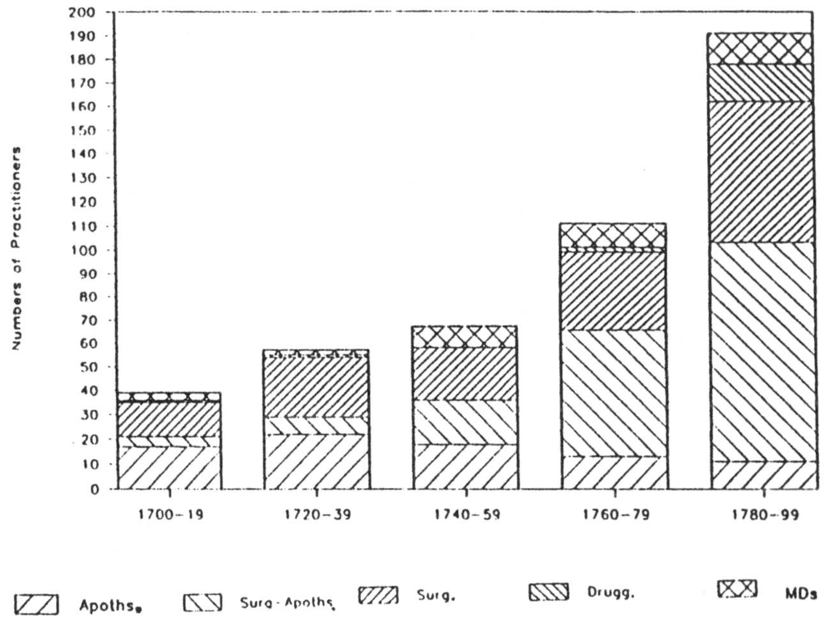

Figure 3.2. Medical practitioners in Somerset

tions, as well as providing care for wounds, ulcers, fractures, and the like. (See Fig. 3.3 for Samuel Pye's trade card.)

A detailed casebook kept by a barber-surgeon's apprentice in Bristol illustrates the daily routine of a surgical practice in the first half of the century.[45] Alexander Morgan, the son of a mariner, was apprenticed to Jeremy Deverell in 1716. At that point, Deverell had three other apprentices, including Thomas Hellier mentioned above, and ran a very busy practice. Morgan seems to have spent his days going from house to house, usually changing dressings on wounds, ulcers, or inflammations, bringing a purge ordered by Deverell, or seeing an emergency.

The dressings used by Deverell and Morgan were complicated mixtures, although the basic procedures for dealing with wounds and ulcers were fairly standard. A typical case was that of a young man who had been fighting and had had a chunk of flesh ripped out of his forehead. Morgan cleansed the wound, and dressed it with oil of turpentine and a pledget of basilicon unguent, one of

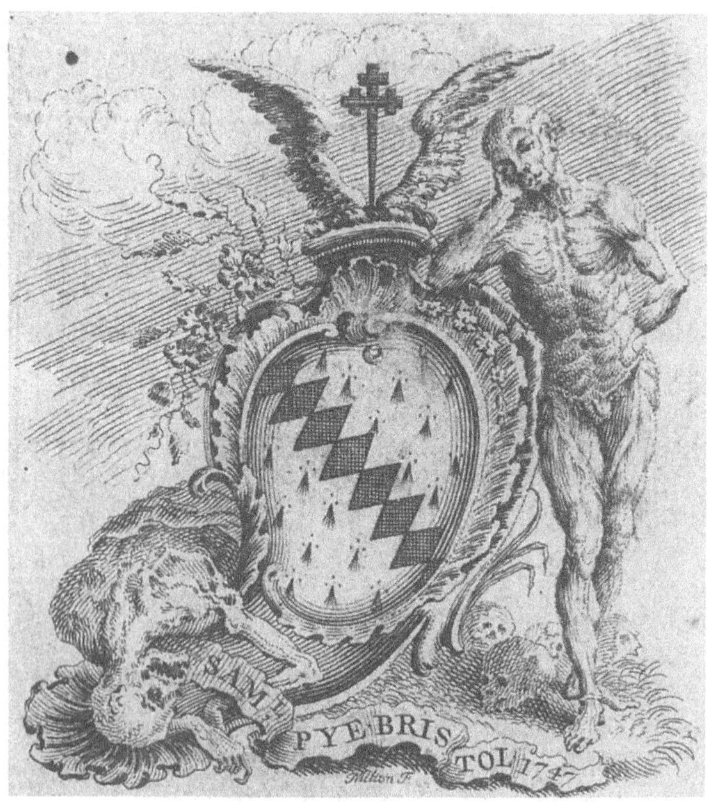

Figure 3.3. Shop culture – the Bristol barber-surgeon Samuel Pye's trade card (Bristol Record Office)

the most common treatments for wounds or sores. The man also had a swelling on his forehead, which Morgan rubbed with spirits of vinegar, and then dressed with a soap plaster. After bandaging up the patient's head, Morgan let twelve ounces of blood. The next day, the wound was treated with a common digestive, and re-dressed. On the third and fourth days, two new dressings were used, and then the wound was re-dressed every day for the next eight days. Finally, the proud flesh in the wound was treated, the wound cicatrized, and the man considered cured.[46] Nine different preparations were used, almost all made in Deverell's shop, and the patient visited daily. Other cases required such daily attendance for weeks, even months.

Unfortunately, no comparable casebook to Morgan's exists for a Bristol apothecary for this period. Historians of provincial medical practice have used the Bristol surgeon Richard Smith's memoirs, in particular his twelve-page essay, in their analyses of apothecaries.[47] Smith claims that apothecaries enjoyed a "golden age of physic" in the mid- to late-eighteenth century, but were then eclipsed by dispensing druggists.[48] In some respects, Smith's tale is borne out by other records, but not in all; like any other author, Smith was defending his own interests, which need to be understood in order to evaluate his assessment of Bristol medical practice.

First, Smith was a snob. As a part of the first generation of hospital-trained surgeons, he proclaimed their superiority to barber-surgeons, or, more often just left barber-surgeons out of the story altogether. For instance, in his essay on apothecaries, he said that there were thirty-five apothecaries and twenty surgeons in Bristol in 1793. In fact there were about fifty surgeons in the city, as well as a dozen barber-surgeons still in practice. But Smith clearly overlooked the men he did not consider appropriate practitioners. One of the most often quoted passages from Smith's memoirs is his comment on the last barber-surgeon:

> the last remnant of Barber-Surgery dropped with Old Parsley, who lived next door to the Guildhall in Broad Street so lately as the year 1807 – This man dressed more wigs, drew more teeth, and spilled more blood than any man in Bristol – at his window, and by the side of his door hung immense double strings of teeth, drawn by one terrible jerk, having never used a gum lancet in his life – thousands of people yet alive can testify by this, for he regularly brought his patients to the door, either for the sake of a good light or for notoriety.[49]

Although exceptional by 1807, this man was a typical practitioner of the mid- to late-eighteenth century. James Parsley, the son of a blacksmith, was apprenticed to Isaac Bretherton, a well-respected barber-surgeon, in 1741, and went on to take his own apprentices as late as 1786. Compared with some of his contemporaries, who fled the city for debt, or abused their apprentices, he seems to have had an uneventful and even prosperous career.

But Richard Smith saw himself as a rather different kind of surgeon. In particular, he despised apprenticeship training, saying, "That, as a body, the Physicians had the advantage, both as Gen-

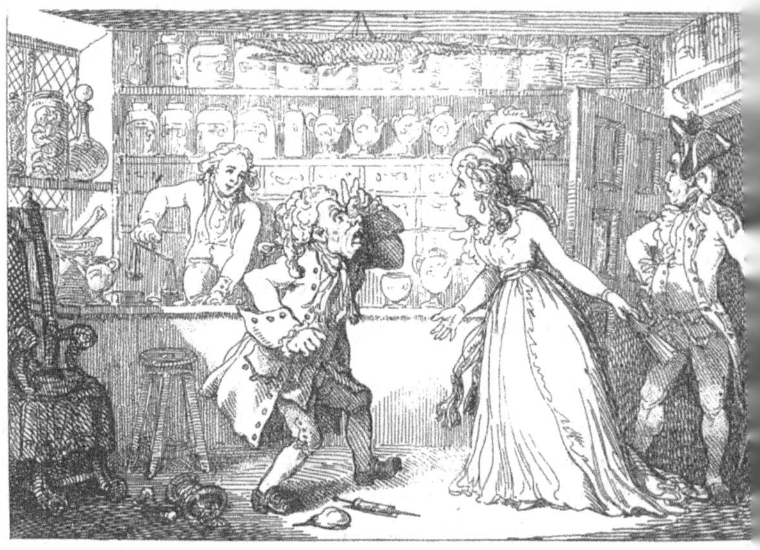

Figure 3.4. Shop culture – Rowlandson's representation of an apothecary's shop (Wellcome Library, London)

tlemen and in point of intellect there could be no doubt, since with two or three exceptions the great majority of Apothecaries were not men of education very many had absolutely been shopmen and mortar boys." In fact, Smith's own father had been a "shop man"; or had minded the shop when an apprentice. Smith's disparagement of such training should not be taken at face value; it was a part of Smith's self-identification with gentlemanly physicians rather than trading apothecaries. (See Fig. 3.4 for illustration of an apothecary's shop.)

For all of Smith's criticism of apothecaries, there is also envy; he claimed that they had made a great deal of money. But this claim, like his disparagement of shop training, needs to be read carefully. All evidence from Bristol, and Britain more generally, points to the consumption of heroic quantities of medicines in the eighteenth century.[50] However, both surgeons and apothecaries dispensed, as did Smith himself; all benefited from their patients' predilections for pills. Smith cites only one spectacular example of apothecary wealth – William Broderip. Broderip, it seems, did make money hand over fist; he bought a fancy country estate (nicknamed Gallypots Hall by the locals) and an elegant carriage, although he later lost his money.[51] But few other apothecaries could match this success, and there were also surgeons such as James Ford, eventually made Accoucheur to the Queen, who became wealthy gentlemen.[52] Thus, Smith's portrait of the golden age of physic, in which the apothecary was king, was colored by a combination of nostalgia for possibly fictive times gone past, and the yearnings of a marginal man for better status.

The less meteoric careers of other apothecaries remain largely unknown.[53] The diary of William Holland, a clergyman in a Somerset parish near Bridgewater, provides a brief portrait of an apothecary who did not enjoy William Broderip's wealth. Lewis was a shop-based apothecary, of whom Holland wrote, "One might clap him and all his medical goods in one's pocket and carry them all off without much inconvenience or fatigue."[54] Despite being located in a rather small village, Lewis had competition from one Forbes, whom the diarist refers to as a surgeon. Neither medical man got much respect from Holland, although he did continue to patronize them both. Forbes, he wrote, "is the very Deuce of a man for Visits Physicks and Charges."[55] It is clear that both Forbes and Lewis practiced as surgeon-apothecaries, despite the way Holland refers to them. Lewis dressed leg ulcers and the like and Forbes prescribed. A typical apothecary was perhaps more like Lewis than like Broderip.

Although Richard Smith may have exaggerated the ease with which apothecaries made their living, nevertheless, in Bristol, apothecaries stayed a remarkably constant group throughout the century: there were almost always between thirty and forty practicing at any given time. In rural areas, almost all apothecaries practiced as surgeon-apothecaries by the latter half of the century, and perhaps earlier. As early as 1733, Samuel England, apprenticed to a surgeon near Taunton, in Somerset, learned the rudiments of physic as well. He explained, "there are but few apothecaries now a Days living in the Country who confine themselves to ye Practice of Pharmacy; and since they frequently live remote from Physicians upon which ye generality of people can't have their Advise by reason of ye Expense . . ."[56] England went on to explain that his master was far from any physician, and hence practiced medicine as well as surgery. In the city, apothecaries tended to take far fewer apprentices than did their surgical counterparts, and also continued using apprenticeship training after surgery had come to be taught within the hospital.

Although he overstates the case of the apothecary, Richard Smith's assertions about the rise of the druggist are borne out by evidence from Bristol and Somerset.[57] By the 1780s and 1790s, almost a dozen druggists had opened shops in the city and were selling remedies. As Irvine Loudon has suggested, these practitioners were a sort of commercialized, sedentary form of apothecary.[58] Where apothecaries increasingly united physic and surgery, visiting patients to dress wounds as well as to prescribe, the druggist took the shop side of pharmacy and transformed it from the context of guild-style practice to the newer retail store.[59] In the city, this process was gradual, and marked by many a hybrid establishment. John Till-Adams, for example, was a respected apothecary and man-midwife, who was associated with the city's Dispensary. He took an M.D. in 1779, and continued to undertake what was in essence a general practice. His wife had always dispensed his prescriptions, and by the 1780s, she ran her own druggist's shop. Other druggists entered the market as retailers from the start; Cornish and Howe, for example, sold paints as well as medicaments.

Even in rural areas, druggists became increasingly common. By the end of the century, there were at least fifteen druggists practicing in rural Somerset; that is, in rural parts of the shire, excluding Taunton and Bath. Obviously, most were in the larger towns: two in Bridgewater, two in Frome, one each in Yeovil, Chard, Crewkerne, and Shepton Mallet. But the relatively small-sized town of Wellington supported two druggists in 1791, and a third by 1798. Even tiny Widcombe had its own druggist. The "rise of the druggist" therefore looks both forward and backward. It reflects the increased commercialism of the medical marketplace of the second half of the eighteenth century, but the druggist's roots in the apothecary's shop point to the market orientation of apprenticeship-based practice.

The third major group of health-care practitioners were the midwives. Unfortunately, because they were both female (and thus often excluded from formal apprenticeship) and occasional practitioners, few records of their activities remain. The careers of two Somerset midwives, almost a century apart, serve as indicators of the extremes between which most midwifery was practiced.

Roger Langdon, born into a very poor Somerset family in the early 1820s, wrote an autobiography late in life that provides a portrait of his village's midwife, Nanny Holland.[60] Holland was a terrifying figure to the young Langdon, "Nanny was a sort of oracle in the village, besides being a kind of quack doctor, and what with her superior cunning and evil temper, always excited more or less with gin, she held most of the poor women under her thumb."[61] Not only did her strong personality hold the women in sway; she also possessed the only oven in the village, and therefore anyone wishing to bake bread had to stay on good terms with her.

Nanny Holland was, in anachronistic terms, the primary care practitioner in this village. "Nanny had been known more than once to set a broken leg, or arm, when the doctor was too busy, or, which was often the case, too drunk to attend."[62] She had also enjoyed the reputation of being a very skilled midwife in her younger days. But by 1829, when Langdon was a boy, she was an imperious figure few dared antagonize.

For instance, Holland managed smallpox prevention. It was this village's practice to put a healthy child in bed with one sick with smallpox. The healthy child would then contract the illness, his or her mother better able to manage if it were planned rather than epidemic. When Roger Langdon was eight, he was taken to a nearby family, and put in bed with a boy dying of smallpox. Langdon did not catch the disease, and "Nanny soon began to see about 'knockleheading' the children, and when she turned to me first, and I saw her coming towards me, with her surgical knife, my hair stood on end from fright."[63] Holland cut a tiny flap of skin, put some matter on the wound, replaced the flap, and told Langdon, "Now youngster, if you scratch that off, I'll kill thee."[64] Of the three children she inoculated on this occasion, one died, one was very ill, and Roger Langdon got off with a mild case of smallpox. The local clergyman then told Langdon's mother about vaccination, and instructed her where to find a charitable doctor who would perform it free of charge.

On one level, Langdon's portrait of Holland fits into the classic stereotype of the ignorant, superstitious, elderly midwife. Holland was clearly a strong figure, who kept the village doing her bidding well into old age. On the other hand, she was not without skill, setting bones, and delivering babies competently. Certainly the unnamed local doctor, too drunk to attend, was not presented as an ideal of medical practice either.

If Nanny Holland represents one stereotyped extreme, Sarah Stone represents another. She was, according to her own reports, a very talented midwife, who practiced in Somerset around Taunton and Bridgewater, and then moved to Bristol in the 1730s.[65] She was trained by her mother, also a midwife. Sarah Stone functioned as a consultant midwife, that is, she was called in by other midwives when things went wrong. She also served as the primary midwife (i.e., the first midwife called in) for some deliveries.[66] Wishing to emphasize her own skills, Stone portrayed ordinary midwives as unlearned and meddlesome. For example, many of them gave their patients a mixture of their husband's urine and the juice of leeks during labor, "which is a notable prescription among Country midwives, but a horrid medicine and as often mischievous as prescribed."[67] But Stone was by no means granted immediate authority over these midwives, even when she had been called in during an emergency. On one occasion, she went to see a woman whose labor was not progressing, but the woman refused to let Stone touch her, Stone "being a stranger to her." Husband and relatives argued with the patient, and persuaded her to let Stone perform an examination. Then Stone decided to give her a glyster, but in this case "some of her friends and the Midwife were entirely against it," and it was two hours before Stone finally convinced them to let her continue.[68]

If on the one hand Stone railed against ignorant country midwives, the Nanny Hollands among her contemporaries, on the other, she criticized man-midwives. For by the 1730s and 1740s in Bristol, the spectrum of midwifery represented by Holland and Stone was complicated by the addition of man-midwives. Stone provides some of the earliest evidence for man-midwifery in the city, saying that she had not encountered it in her earlier rural career.[69] She claimed that men were harsh to their patients, that "dissecting the Dead, and being just and tender to the Living, are vastly different."[70] These man-midwives had two types of clients. "Ladies" created a fashion of bespeaking man-midwives for their confinements, and the men were also called in for emergency cases. The traditional explanation of the replacement of female by male midwives has emphasized men's use of instruments in difficult labors.[71] However, Sarah Stone used instruments, albeit rarely, and intervened in problem labors. It is difficult to know if she were typical of certain female consultant midwives, or extremely unusual, fulfilling a role usually ascribed to men. The apprentice Samuel England's master, for example, functioned as a man-midwife not far from, and contemporaneous with, Sarah Stone's Somerset practice. England echoed Stone's complaints about ignorant local midwives, who caused their patients to catch cold, "to Shew how Dextrous they have performed ye Operation," by letting their patients get up too quickly.[72]

From the 1730s onward, then, both male and female midwives practiced in Bristol, and probably in rural areas as well. Most of the men were surgeons or surgeon-apothecaries who also did midwifery. Women sometimes provided a wider range of functions connected with lying-in. For instance, one woman, who called herself a nurse, "thoroughly skilled in the knowledge of attending Lying-in Women" ran a sort of small maternity home, an apartment for lying-in.[73] Advertisements for places similar to this in London stressed their clients' privacy and even secrecy, suggesting that these were places to have an illegitimate child.[74] Another Bristol midwife advertised that she sent or conveyed babies to the Foundling Hospital in London on a weekly basis.[75]

It is almost impossible to know how women chose among midwives; few advertised, and, as Adrian Wilson has pointed out, "midwives" ranged from highly skilled women like Stone to friends and neighbors with little experience and no training.[76] It does seem that male midwives cost more than female ones. For example, in 1762, an inquest was called on the death of a woman near Bath. The husband had declined to call in a surgeon (supposedly for reasons of cost) although the attending midwife had declared one was necessary. Because the unfortunate wife had concurred with her husband, a verdict of accidental death was reached.[77]

Richard Smith complained that midwifery was unremunerative and that surgeons delivered babies only to install themselves as the practitioner for a growing family.[78] But Smith did not like midwifery; he claimed it "destroys those who practice it."[79] Other Bristol surgeons did not share Smith's views, and specialized in midwifery. For instance, the aforementioned James Ford kept a careful account of his midwifery practice in 1758. He delivered sixty-eight women, earning £201.[80] Thirty years later, Danvers

Ward spent much of his practice in midwifery, delivering at least two or three babies a week, at half a guinea for his standard fee. Delivering twins or triplets seems to have constituted a de facto advertisement; he did not charge in any of these cases.[81] Even practitioners outside of the city occasionally specialized in man-midwifery. For instance, William Jefferies of Mangotsfield was proud to inform Richard Smith in the early nineteenth century that he had attended 2,615 deliveries and never lost a mother; this represented a staggering 150 deliveries a year.[82]

Finally, among the medical practitioners in city and country there were, of course, physicians. But they were few in number and remained insignificant to health care in the city as a whole. Their numbers crept from four or five in the 1720s to over fifteen by the 1770s and 1780s.[83] In this period, many of the physicians in the city were associated with the Infirmary, and enjoyed gentlemanly practices. Richard Smith described them thus:

> The physician, in those days, was distinguished from the common mass by an imposing exterior – He moved in a measured step and affected a meditating abstraction of countenance, with a pomposity of diction and manner which served to keep the vulgar at a respectable distance – The Doctor's Peruke alone was enough in itself to command respect.[84]

Given Smith's nostalgia, this portrait is probably overdrawn, but it does seem that physicians did not always experience the struggles to establish themselves that surgeons did. In the last few decades of the century, the number of physicians increased, although they never amounted to even 20 percent of the total practitioners. In part, this rise was due to the acquisition of M.D. degrees by surgeons already in practice. Several surgeons obtained mid-career Aberdeen M.D.s in attempts to improve their status and, presumably, their practices. But physicians also became a more common type of practitioner overall.

However tidy the occupational titles of physician, surgeon, apothecary, midwife appear retrospectively, the realities of practice were far less well-defined. There were many "occasional" practitioners who had not been trained through the apprenticeship system, and who competed openly for custom. Even those who had been formally trained occasionally adopted the styles and practices of those who had not been. Historians have sometimes made the distinction between "regular" practitioners, such as university or apprenticed-trained, and "quacks," those who set up practice without evidence of formal training. This designation, however, reiterates the early nineteenth-century attempts by people like Richard Smith to disparage mid-eighteenth-century medical and surgical practice. As Roy Porter has said, the early nineteenth century complaints about quackery "were blows in tactical professional infighting; they perhaps tell us more about the politicisation of medicine than the fortunes of quackery itself."[85] Rather, the services of "quacks" should be seen as complementary to, and sometimes competitive with, those of surgeons and apothecaries. Therefore I have described Bristol's medical men and women as either full-time or occasional, apprentice-trained or not, rather than using the word "quack."[86]

In addition, formally-trained surgeons and apothecaries pursued extremely varied careers that could include characteristics of "quackery," making distinction difficult. For example, James Grace, who had been apprenticed to John Hargest, a respectable Bristol surgeon, and who had further trained in Parisian hospitals, opened a druggist's shop in Bristol in 1760. He advertised cheap remedies and offered to prescribe by post.[87] Similarly, James Pidding, an Infirmary pupil, and then assistant surgeon to the Glamorgan Militia, opened a "Quack Medical Warehouse" in London in the 1790s. He then became a broker and ran lotteries.[88] But ten years earlier, Pidding had been on the road to respectable orthodoxy, explicitly comparing his charitable care for the poor to that offered by the Infirmary.[89] Even John Ford, who succeeded his brother as Accoucheur to the Queen, marketed a remedy for indigestion, called Dr. Ford's Pills.[90]

The few instances where a patient's choice of practitioner was recorded suggests that patients did not necessarily make distinctions between occasional and fully-trained practitioners, but used each according to the perceived appropriateness of his or her expertise. Thus, for instance, William Dyer called on Dr. Middleton, a respected former Infirmary physician, in March of 1756. Eighteen months later, he patronized an occasional practitioner: "Father took a walk to Dr. Batters to seek a remedy for my dear Wife, and by viewing her urine the Doctor cou'd describe her complaint: he wrote a prescription for one shilling his customary fee, and 'tis supposed He has about 100 applications dayly."[91] Like elite physicians, Dr. Batters did not dispense, nor did he physically examine the patient. Nevertheless, the practice of uroscopy set him off from the city's M.D.s.

In general, occasional practitioners tended either to deal with a specific range of illnesses, or a specific therapeutic modality. Women were often "occasional" practitioners, barred from formal apprenticeship. As with their male counterparts, calling female practitioners "occasional" does not imply lack of skill or custom. Both male and female occasional practitioners varied tremendously in terms of time spent in practice, therapeutics, and range of clients. For example, William Dyer refers to two women apothecaries. One of them "subsisted on administering some few nostrums." The other, however, had run a successful apothecary's shop for years.[92] Some female practitioners advertised in newspapers, such as Miss Plunkett, the daughter of a doctor, who practiced surgery, especially the excision of cancers.[93] Mrs. Clokowsky advertised a sort of cosmetic practice – she sold hair dye, face cream, hair remover, and cleaned teeth, at five shillings a visit.[94] And a "cunning woman" in Bedminster, a suburb of Bristol, specialized in the removal of charms and in otherwise hopeless cases.[95]

Other women pursued careers as regular barber-surgeons or apothecaries. In the first half of the century, widows routinely assumed their husbands' practices, permitted by the city companies to carry on in their husbands' steads. These women often enjoyed successful careers. Sarah Pye, for instance, widow of the surgeon Samuel Pye, commanded the same £200 apprenticeship premiums that her husband had received. Other women apprenticed the sons of gentlemen and merchants, suggesting that these widows were not at the bottom of the apprentice market. The realization that widows often practiced medicine casts a new light on the domestic economies of medical men. From 1700 to 1750, about half of the surgeons and apothecaries who died in mid-career were succeeded by their widows. This figure implies that many women were practicing alongside their husbands, or had at least acquired rudimentary skills from their husbands, because it is improbable that practitioners with skilled wives suffered a differential death rate. Given the shop-based nature of medical practice, with apprentices and master going out to patients' homes, it is easy to see how women integrated household chores with minding the shop, making medicines and giving advice like any other tradesman's wife.

In the countryside, women pursued at least two kinds of healing careers in addition to midwifery: general medicine, and nursing. Some women provided a wide range of care, the only records of which survive in payments made to them by the local welfare authorities, the Old Poor Law. For example, Sarah Loveless worked as a healer in the Somerset village of Stogursey in the 1790s. Over the course of twelve months she was paid £3.2s.9d for the cure of a number of patients. She healed a felon on a woman's finger, a man's inflamed foot, other injured legs, two scalded children, cuts and bruises, and a range of other ailments. Like any other practitioner, she charged for her ointments and salves as well as her attendance. Loveless was not a nurse, whose careers are further discussed below; some of her patients were being nursed by others.[96] Instead, she was a local practitioner, who happened to be female.

However, by mid-century, fewer urban widows took up their husband's careers, and most female medical practitioners were of the occasional type. Both male and female occasional practitioners often treated specific ailments. Venereal disease, as discussed in the case of patent remedies, was a common specialization. Dr. Goergslenner, resident in posh Queen Square in the 1780s, a doctor and oculist, advertised, "The most profound secrecy is observed to all his patients if desired," a euphemism for venereal disease treatments.[97] So too, Mrs. Speakman, widow of Dr. Speakman, advertised in 1768 that she cured the French disease – and that there was a back door to the house which opened onto a little-frequented alley, an appeal to privacy used by at least one Infirmary surgeon as well. She also offered an "excellent" remedy for the stone. Her husband had practiced in Bristol for at least fifteen years, also treating venereal diseases. He started off practice at a tiler's shop, then moved into premises next to George Whitefield's Tabernacle, frequently advertising his services, and presumably making a living. Other local practitioners and itinerants treated deafness, cut corns, practiced dentistry, and cured eye diseases.[98]

Some occasional practitioners with little claim to any quasi-professional status also plied their trade. For example, in the poor parish of SS. Philip and Jacob, Francis Wickland worked as a "bleeder" for two decades. Presumably, he let blood, either according to a physician's or surgeon's orders, or as requested by his clients.[99] By the 1790s, he functioned as a dentist as well. Such practitioners were even available in the tiny Somerset village of Nether Stowey, where William Holland's servant was able to consult a tooth-drawer and bleeder.[100] Many people seem to have been bled routinely, sometimes in the spring or fall, or as a general tonic. Certainly sources such as Alexander Morgan's casebook often include patients in whom bleeding had gone wrong, resulting in swellings, nicked tendons, bruises, and the like, suggesting that bloodletting was a common therapeutic practice. Francis Wickland is exceptional in appearing in three distinct historical records, and in recording bloodletting as his primary occupation. But he was perhaps typical of many occasional practitioners, who offered specific services to their clients but whose livelihoods went unremarked.

Another widespread type of occasional practitioner ran an institution. Midwives who kept an apartment for lying-in women have already been discussed, but they were not singular examples. For instance, Sarah King, of the Bell Inn, up the Severn river from Bristol, advertised that she had the best establishment for the salt-water cure for the bite of a mad dog. She hired "a person to perform the operation, who has been bred to the practice from his youth," and offered "neat wines, spirituous liquors, and best provisions" to speed recovery.[101] Rabies was much feared in the eighteenth century, and salt water immersion was one of the most frequently recommended cures. No doubt King's service, in offering an institutional alternative to home care, also played upon a fear of people who had been bitten.

Similarly, and more extensively, smallpox inoculation was increasingly carried out in small private nursing homes run by inoculators. These institutions offered the elaborate preparations considered needful, and, more important, isolated the individual recovering from inoculation, ensuring that his or her household would not be exposed to the disease. In Bristol, in the late 1760s and early 1770s, at least two competing smallpox houses claimed to be licensed by the Suttons, the great mass inoculators. One was run by a group of surgeons from the Infirmary; the other by an independent surgeon-apothecary, Mr. Chevasse.[102] Sarah Champion, sister of the Infirmary Treasurer, accompanied her niece and nephew to the Infirmary surgeons' inoculation house on Barton Hill, and found "a very commodious house fitted for the reception of many patients."[103] Another inoculator, John Lancaster, was also licensed by the Suttons, but may not have had a house; he advertised that, "servants may be inoculated with little or no Loss of Time, they being permitted to pursue their daily Employment as usual."[104] For an inoculator, such houses simplified and standardized the process. One Somerset operator inoculated everyone that came to him, and then bled them, purged them twice, kept them on a low diet, and put them two to a bed, three beds per room, until they sweated through the eruptions. He claimed to have inoculated over 1,700 people, and lost only two.[105]

One of the most numerous type of occasional practitioner – the nurse – is also the kind least represented in historical records. The best evidence of these women's activities comes from Poor Law records. Female health care workers, often on relief themselves, provided a number of services. They lodged the sick, fed them, did their laundry, nursed them, sat up at night with the dying, laid out the dead, and cleansed the living of vermin. For example, Anne Langdon lived in a small Gloucestershire village, between Bristol and Bath. She had an illegitimate son in 1767, and received occasional parish aid for him.[106] But she also tended the sick. Sometimes she lodged them as well, as in the case of Betty Gibbons, whom she evidently nursed after childbirth. None of these activities made her any large sums of money; she got sixpence a week for example, for tending to William Strange, although later on this went up to a shilling a week. These fees were paid to her by the Poor Law authorities, for caring for those on relief. There is no reason to doubt that she also earned money nursing individuals privately.

The same kinds of nursing care were provided by the Poor Law authorities and by the Infirmary in Bristol. The Corporation of the Poor, for example, hired various women to delouse workhouse inmates. The Bristol Infirmary paid both regular full-time nurses and occasional nurses who looked after individual patients. For instance, a woman who had had a breast removed in hospital had a special nurse for a month.[107] Others were nursed by family members and fellow patients, as well as staff nurses.

Neither poor relief nor Infirmary, obviously, created the role of the nurse. But both made new opportunities for nurses through institutional provision and payment. The rural Poor Law created niches for women like Ann Langdon to earn a few pence by looking after others. By the late eighteenth century, health care typically accounted for about 8 percent of the annual Poor Law expenditure in Ann Langdon's parish. But in a bad year, the parish could spend as much as 40 percent of its poor-law budget on health care, and the overseer of the poor often provided nursing care as a part of overall medical aid. In the same way, the urban poor-law services and the hospitals also made what had perhaps been an informal female role into a waged, even full-time, occupation.

Doctors like Richard Smith and Thomas Beddoes may have inveighed against occasional practitioners – "quacks" in their terms – but patient choice structured the health-care system in which such practitioners thrived. As Michael Neve has suggested, complaints about quackery can be read as indications of doctors' unhappiness with patient choice as much as dissatisfaction with fellow practitioners.[108] W.F. Bynum and Roy Porter, among others, have pointed out that the historical construction of "quackery" needs to be understood before any conclusions can be drawn about its extent or significance.[109] Calling someone a "quack" had a meaning specific to its historical moment, and reveals the speaker's conception of self far more clearly than the identity of his opponent.

Thus, Bristol's health-care providers were characterized by their diversity. No easy correlations can be made between style of practice and social status, either of practitioner or patient. However, the provision of health care was not without an order and logic of its own. Two features were especially significant. First, patients chose among the wide array of practitioners according to their needs; doctors were not selected at random. Second, the line between patient and practitioner was vague; individuals slipped between the two roles according to inclination and need. Both of these characteristics derived from the marketplace orientation of health care. Patients chose from a bazaar of medical practitioners, and their choices, in the aggregate, shaped that marketplace.

Thus patients, even poor ones, exercised some control over their practitioners, choosing them according to their own criteria, rather than those of medicine per se. William Dyer, for example, sometimes selected his practitioners on the basis of their religious credentials. In referring to his barber, he said "He frequented College early Prayers and likewise St. Werburgh's Early Prayers the latter at 6 o clo[ck] every Monday morning His wife was an awaken'd woman."[110] At another time, Dyer referred to his surgeon as "a serious man, in Mr Westley's connection."[111] Given the importance of the interpretation of illness' meaning, many patients may have made similar decisions, basing their choices of practitioners upon religious issues. Other chains of circumstance leading to the choice of a medical practitioner were equally individual, even fortuitous.[112] For instance, Adam Lowder, a young boy, "will begin to take Physick my wife's mantua-maker's children had it last spring," according to his father.[113]

In the countryside, geography helped to structure patient choice, but it did not dictate absolutely. William Holland, the Somerset parson, refers to almost two dozen different practitioners in his diary. How he actually decided which practitioner to consult on any given occasion is difficult to determine. It seems certain that Holland used the surgeon Forbes because he was so nearby, so convenient. For example, in a frightening moment, when his young son was dragged by a horse and thought gravely injured, Holland sent for Forbes, despite his previous and subsequent disparagement of the surgeon's practice. He also knew that he could call out Forbes in the middle of the night and Forbes would come. Holland managed to get his own way with the surgeon; for example, he negotiated with Forbes that he should take some of a local physician's prescription to help his stomach which would then help alleviate the pain in his face. As Holland put it, "we resolved to try Dr. Dunnings prescription."[114] This Bridgewater physician, Dr. Dunning, often consulted with local surgeons, although Holland's diary does not record who called in whom for consultation, or if patients routinely made use of dual practitioners.[115] Just as in the city, patients like Holland maintained some degree of control over their medical men, in part because they were able to choose from a number of practitioners.

Medical men were well aware of their patients' abilities to make or break medical careers. Samuel England, for example, recorded in his notebook, "The application of Proper Bandages Suited to Every part of ye Body adds much to ye Neatness of ye Dressings and recommends ye Surgeon to ye esteem of ye spectators so it is a Necessary Qualification to a Dextrous Operator."[116] Because bandaging was a common skill, not restricted to surgeons, it was all the more important that practitioners excel at it. England also noted how a disagreement over an alleged fracture between two other surgeons and his master damaged his master's practice, "this case sinking my Master's Reputation among ye Popular part of Mankind."[117] Thus, even in rural Somerset of the 1730s, patients could exercise some measure of choice over their practitioners.

Having found a practitioner, patients were not shy about dictating practice. A woman in rural Gloucestershire "had read in the newspapers that persons once affected with the cowpox could never have smallpox," and so asked the local apothecary to vaccinate her son but not herself, since she'd already had cowpox.[118] Other poorer patients did not hesitate to leave a doctor if they found his treatment unpalatable. Two women cured by the Glastonbury spa waters had refused their surgeons' advice. Honor Powel, for instance, had a cancer on her hand, and after months of treatment, her surgeon said the hand must be amputated. She absolutely refused.[119]

Patients also organized therapeutic episodes themselves, rather than leaving illness management to formal practitioners. Conversely, practitioners sometimes learned from their patients. A patient of Samuel England's master consulted both him and an elderly woman who advised a cataplasm of turnips and hog's lard. This patient continued to consult both of his healers, much to England's master's disgust, "Master check't him for suffering it to be treated as it was."[120] On another occasion, the patient's own inclination saved his life. This man had been burned with lye, and lay dying. But he had a yen for his mother's home-brewed beer (he had been forbidden wine and cider by the surgeon), and downed a pint. He took a turn for the better almost immediately, and England recorded that he drank beer for the next several days, and recovered.[121]

Not only did patients select practitioners and dictate treatment, they might also make use of medical services for reasons quite unknown to their healers. Women used smallpox inoculation to procure abortions, according to two leading inoculators. They would purposely conceal their pregnancies, and apply for inoculation, occasionally as objects of charity, and rely upon the process to cause a miscarriage.[122] In other words, they were using medical practitioners according to their own needs, rather than any medically-defined purpose.

A blurring of the distinction between patient and practitioner was an integral part of this patient-driven health-care system. As already discussed, domestic health care was the norm, and many people prescribed for their friends and neighbors. Two examples of ordinary people assuming the role of practitioner serve to further illustrate the lack of boundaries between "professional" and "amateur." William Dyer, the diarist, and his friend Richard Symes, the vicar of St. Werburgh's, both became practitioners of electrical medicine.

In 1760 Dyer was the first person in Bristol to acquire an electrical machine for medical purposes, which he had ordered from London. Richard Symes used Dyer's machine as a pattern and had a local brightsmith copy it for him.[123] According to Dyer, a few local surgeons also purchased machines, as did the Infirmary, although Dyer claimed that these were little used. During the next few years, Dyer described, "a Multitude of poor People and indeed some few in higher Life, applied at my House and I saw in many cases most wonderful good Effect from Electricity".[124] He electrified people for a number of complaints, and seems rarely to have turned anyone away. Reports of his skill spread, and in the following year, the overseers of the poor from Chew Magna (about ten miles from Bristol) brought a man suffering from rheumatism to Dyer to be electrified.[125] A year later, he was brought a child from Haverfordwest, in Wales, who had been in the Infirmary in Bristol, but had not improved.[126]

Ten years after first acquiring his machine, Dyer was still electrifying people for a variety of complaints. Dyer was not of gentlemanly status like the physicians he was perhaps unconsciously emulating; he was a clerk, whose brother married a servant and whose brother-in-law kept an earthenware shop. What is striking about his electrical practice is how easily he adopted the role of the medical man. Even his choice of words reveals his self-identification as a practitioner. He said that people "applied" to him for treatment, a usage identical with that of charitable doctors or hospital governors. Poor people lined up at his door, while he cheerfully went to visit those who were better off and wished to be electrified.

Dyer's friend Richard Symes carried the emulation of medical practice one step further by publishing a set of his cases in 1771. He explained that he had read a letter of the Abbé Nollet's in the *Gentleman's Magazine* in 1759 that had furthered his interest in electricity. He had been thinking about the balance of opposites in nature, and was then able "to bring forth to open View these hidden secret working Powers, known only to us by their Effects."[127] For Symes electrical machines did not so much create various effects as make visible "what is hidden in Nature."[128] These natural-philosophical interests of Symes' led him to record the effects of electricity on a variety of ailments. He seems to have started at home, electrifying wife and servants, but word of mouth quickly brought him other patients.

For example, Symes saw Joseph Burges, aged twenty-two. Burges had been pressed into the navy two years before, and had then been struck with a paralysis on the right side of his body. He spent three months in a navy hospital at Plymouth, and then his mother managed to get him admitted to the Bath hospital, known for paralysis treatments. He spent seven months there, and a further three in the Bristol Infirmary, all to little avail. Symes gave him thirty to forty shocks for several mornings, and sensation returned to Burges' right side. A few years later, Symes came across his former patient, working as a laborer in a brickyard. As Symes put it, "At this time he earned four shillings per week, but in the Summer Five . . . so that now, instead of being to his Parents or the Parish a heavy Burthen, he had for five years maintained himself."[129] Symes saw many patients such as Burges – shoemakers, masons, sailors, laborers, and their wives. Some of his patients returned for further treatment. For example, Mary Barter, a nurse, had lost the use of an arm, and had been seen by physicians and apothecaries. Symes treated her on three separate occasions, as the arm worsened whenever Barter caught a cold.[130] Although Symes had not trained as a doctor, his interest in natural philosophy, and probably his role as a clergyman, combined to make him a practitioner. His patients seem to have viewed him as they would other occasional practitioners, and his published work on electricity is largely indistinguishable from those of nearby medical writers on electricity.[131]

In summary, England's health-care system was flexible and patient-driven. Men and women took up medical practice when so inclined and abandoned it when interest or patients waned. Patients were neither awed by medical authority nor cowed by high prices; they picked and chose among practitioners until they were satisfied. The ease with which people like Richard Symes adopted a medical framework reveals the close integration of "medical" and "nonmedical" perspectives.

Medicine was consumption, and like other forms of consumer goods and activities, became increasingly commercialized.[132] Any discussion of this phenomenon must address the worlds of the working classes as well as those of middle-class getters and spenders. As Roy Porter has it, "Quackery was the capitalist mode of production in its medical face."[133] Neil McKendrick opened his pioneering discussion of the consumer boom by relating how middle-class and even artisanal household possessions multiplied in quality and quantity in this period. But here is what Isaac Jenkins, the poor man whom Thomas Beddoes visited, had in his home "porringers without handles, a few cracked trenchers, two or three pewter spoons battered and beat in at the sides, a worm-eaten spinning wheel. Above stairs there was nothing but a bed half-stuffed with chaff, and a wad of straw for the children."[134] This was not a participant in the consumer boom in household goods. But Jenkins did make use of an itinerant "quack," that classic product of the medical marketplace. Why did Jenkins spend money the family could ill afford on the quack's white powder? For those who make the medicine-as-consumption argument, emulation is seen as a key motivating factor, but how far down the social scale did emulation operate?

Another way to understand Jenkins is as the victim of a commercialization which had distanced him and his contemporaries from a vernacular herbal medicine, and replaced it with patent nostrums fostered by a corps of professionalizing medical men. Given the problems of documenting orally transmitted vernacular healing practices, this must remain only a suggestion. But a patient-driven health-care system based upon the marketplace obviously privileged those patients able to exercise consumer choice. The structure of such a system made patients, through their roles as consumers, powerful in their encounters with medicine; even practitioners at the lower end of the market needed to attract and please patients. As such a system became increasingly commercialized, those with less economic power were unable to compete. At the same time, as we shall see, certain forms of medicine and types of medical practitioners began to distance themselves from the marketplace, defining their identities around new institutions, such as the Infirmary. As medicine became entwined with poor relief, in certain settings the relationship between doctor and patient was recast from that of client/patron to professional/working class. This process was complex, and owed as much to changing relationships between rich and poor as it did to any internal dynamic of medicine.

4

Charity universal?

In 1736 a group of Bristol's leading men decided to found a voluntary infirmary. Although this institution would become an important one for the city's medical men in years to come, its early years were dominated by lay interests. The new hospital was an emblem of city unity and civic pride; the trigger to its inauguration was probably a similar foundation a year earlier in Winchester, the first such provincial hospital. The Infirmary, as it was known, embodied an understanding of the relationship between rich and poor central to Bristol's male elites' definitions of themselves, as stewards of the poor and paternalistic merchants and manufacturers. The process of admission to the Infirmary served as a rationalization of benefaction, a redefinition of the "deserving" poor. At the annual Infirmary banquets and processions, the lists of subscribers and donors became a part of the provincial city's cultural furniture, such a redefinition became embedded in the social world of the hospital supporter and thus in a developing urban sociability which took organizational, even bureaucratic, forms. The expression of civic unity was also the articulation of social difference.[1]

Many of these themes have been touched upon by other historians of eighteenth-century England, even if they have been overlooked occasionally by medical historians. In Bristol, there was another element to the early hospital which makes that institution's role in disciplining the poor more apparent, and reveals a darker side to the cheery conviviality of urban charity. The Infirmary was in some measure based upon the city workhouse, founded forty years earlier, and it embodied some of that institution's concerns with the behavior and manners of the poor. In this context, medicine was but a supernumerary – just as a charity school required teachers, so too, a hospital required doctors – but

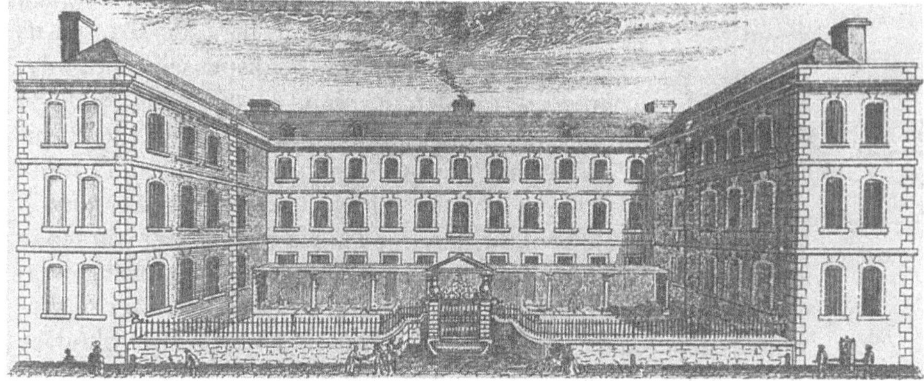

Figure 4.1. The Bristol Infirmary (Bristol Record Office)

neither group was considered fundamental to the reforming nature of the charity.

Leaving aside this moral-reform aspect for the moment, the founding of Bristol's Infirmary can be understood as the intersection of one man's organizational talents with the needs and wishes of the merchant community in the city. Although details of the first few meetings of the committee which created the hospital are scarce, it does seem that John Elbridge had the idea and the initiative to get the hospital underway, and the money and skills to enable it to survive its rocky early years. The newly founded Infirmary committee chose two buildings in St. James's churchyard, which had been a brewery, outfitted the hospital with blankets and beds, and admitted its first inpatient in December 1737; outpatients had been seen since the previous June. Subscribers paid two guineas a year, for which they might recommend one inpatient and two outpatients at a time. John Elbridge served as the hospital's first treasurer and steered it toward financial stability, often by means of his own pocket.[2] Obviously, however, support for the Infirmary came from a substantial body of men in the city and the institution fitted well with their aspirations. To oversimplify, the hospital was made up of equal parts of rationalization, stewardship, and a mercantilist concern with the health of the city. (see Fig. 4.1.)

When Alured Clarke, prebendary of Winchester Cathedral, laid down the rules for the first provincial infirmary, he stressed its rationalizing aspects. Charity would not be dispensed randomly, but would be channeled to where it might do the most good. As Clarke, in promoting his Winchester Infirmary, said of the hospital subscriber, "his bounty *cannot* be misapply'd." Donors could rest assured that, "It is a Charity that is subject to no *Imposture.*"[3] Unlike a charitable bequest, often managed by a churchwarden, a hospital subscription represented a sustained and inquiring relationship with the objects of charity, and a rationalization of untoward benevolence.[4] The structure of the Infirmary – the voluntary organization of subscribers – was characteristic of this reform of charity as it was of many other eighteenth-century foundations. Lending libraries, associations to prosecute felons, tontines, book publishing, and the outfitting of privateers were all organized by subscription, modeled upon the joint-stock company.[5] Such an organization was predicated upon subscribers getting involved with the management of the institution, ensuring that their small subscriptions were put to good use.

What sorts of mismanagement did subscribers fear? Roy Porter has alluded to fears of being duped by impostors, coupled with a distaste for personal mendicancy.[6] Certainly, givers knew that they might be fooled by the undeserving. In the South-West, Bampfylde Moore Carew led a highly publicized career as petty crook who pretended to be the victim of any number of floods, fires, and robberies. In Bristol, he hit upon the ruse of dressing himself like a poor mechanic, and wandering the streets like a religious madman, raving of Wesley and Whitefield – a sight not unfamiliar to Bristolians. On another occasion, he rooked the same donor twice, in the morning as a poor blacksmith whose forge had burned down, and the afternoon as a disabled tinner with a wife and seven children. He conned the well-to-do repeatedly with his heart-rending tales, and the story of his life made a best-selling chapbook.[7] But people continued to give. Local newspapers were full of details of accidents and fires, but also repeatedly listed the large sums of money sent to the distressed from all over the country by the readers of such tales.

Certainly, face-to-face individual charity could backfire. Take, for instance, the case of Lucy Yeats, who aided the Brooks family anonymously in Bristol. Her intermediary's account book survives, and it shows that the brothers Edward and Philip Brooks, and their respective families, were assailed by various disasters in the 1750s. Children had smallpox, the brothers' mother, Widow Brooks, had spotted fever, Philip Brooks left town to avoid debts, the landlady threatened to evict his family, and his wife became dangerously ill with fever. Lucy Yeats, aside from maintaining the family outright through the bad patches, tried to make them self-sufficient, for example, arranging for Philip's wife to be employed in a shop, and placing his daughter Fanny in a hospital as a servant, even giving sixpence "to one of the girles in the Hospitall to Engage her to be kind to littel Fanny."[8]

But then Philip Brooks learned whom his benefactor was, and went out to her house, insulted her, and called her charity a monthly pay (as if it were the Poor Law), demanding it as a right. Brooks may have perceived a unity to charity and relief; not so his patron. Lucy Yeats declared that she would not give his family any further assistance, "Philip Brooks Discharged for being a Silly Fellow & not a Little Impudent."[9] As a hospital subscriber, Lucy Yeats could have relied upon the institution to coerce a patient into a semblance of appropriate and thankful behavior and could have been certain that her charity was well-used. Or so the Infirmary promoters would have argued.

Rationalization, then, was perhaps not only about impostors per se, but also about appropriate relationships between giver and getter. The concern for regulated beneficence shades into another key agenda for the early hospital: a mercantile emphasis upon population. In other words, rationalized charity would go to those for whom it would be most useful in terms of the country's needs overall. The roots of the provincial infirmary, as will be discussed later, lay in Interregnum discussions of political arithmetic; William Petty, for example, was very interested in the relationship between hospitals and urban mortality.[10] But on a simpler level, the Bristol Infirmary helped those people who were crucial to the city's economic functioning. A sermon preached for the hospital governors in 1738, and published by them, expresses their view of Bristol's identity: "We live here in a Place of Great Trade, and Opulence, full of People, by Reason of the vast Numbers of Hands that is required to carry on the extensive Commerce of this City."[11] Unlike charity schools for children, or almshouses for the elderly, an infirmary was targeted on the working man. In this sermon, Carew Reynell pointed out that an entire family would be returned to economic productivity if the head of the family were taken into the Infirmary when ill or injured.[12] Similarly, Alured Clarke painted a sorry picture of the economic strain of nursing a working man at home and emphasized the benefits of hospital admission to the family economy. Clarke moved from this personal aspect of charity to the political, claiming of his hospital, "it is a most certain means of increasing the number of People."[13] In Bristol, as will be discussed, the links to political arithmetic were made through the workhouse and thus indirectly with the hospital.

But the hardheaded calculation of the working man's family economy and its importance to Bristol's commerce represented only a part of the motivations of hospital founders and supporters. The hospital provided an arena for the creation and consolidation of the civic identities of its governors.[14] The public nature of the Infirmary made it an ideal demonstration of appropriate values, as Reynell made clear in his sermon: "Another good Effect of the Benevolence of such Actions, as we are now recommending, is, that they convince Men of the Sincerity of our Religion, and diffuse the Force and Influence of it in the World."[15] On an individual level, participating in the hospital's governance articulated one's social position, defining both privilege and responsibility in the concept of stewardship.

The letters of Richard Champion, an Infirmary treasurer later in the century, elucidate this definition of a role which encompassed commercial success, paternalistic labor relations and a hierarchical vision of social relations. In 1768 he was asked to become the treasurer. He wrote to a friend, "I need not say a principal Inducement was, that from its first Institution this office has always been in our family."[16] He saw himself in a family tradition of stewardship, and thus did not hesitate to take on the extensive duties of treasurer. For him, this role was a natural consequence of his position in Bristol. In another letter he discussed the behavior appropriate to a manufacturer:

> the manufacturer is exercising the Virtues of the Heart by Example. He finds employments for the Poor he cloaths He feeds He protects them. He Encourages the Industerous he rebukes the Sloathful, with the spirit of Charity he relievs the distress of His dependents and teaches them by his conduct to look upon him as a Father and their fellow Workman as their Brethren.[17]

This relationship both sanctified the otherwise godless role of the manufacturer, and served to reiterate the natural divisions among men, "for as our situations are various, duties are annexed to them. Some are taught to govern, others to obey and as long as we act properly in the Situation which is allotted to us, we shall have full enjoyment of them, whether it is in the political, the literary, or the commercial world."[18] In other words, for Champion, the hospital represented the natural outgrowth of his position as an employer – not in the simplistic sense that the Infirmary would patch up his workers for him, but in the larger context of hierarchical social relationships defined by reciprocal obligation.

The origins of the social form of the hospital, characterized by mercantilism and regulation as well as stewardship, lay not merely in Alured Clarke's Winchester Infirmary, but in the city workhouse in Bristol. Indeed, when the Infirmary founders looked for an appropriate site for their hospital, one of the three venues discussed was a set of rooms in the city workhouse.[19] In 1695, John Cary, a Bristol merchant, had started a campaign for a workhouse in the city. He drew upon a tradition of attitudes toward the poor that derived from a mercantilist concern with England's population as well as a utopian vision of the reforming aspect of institutional life. His own interest in the problems of poverty grew out of his economic thought; he gave evidence to the Board of Trade and wrote pamphlets on aspects of political economy. Like many earlier writers, the key to Cary's ideas about the poor was work. He wanted to make "Multitudes of people serviceable who are now useless to the nation."[20] Putting the poor to work would doubly benefit the nation, through the increased creation of wealth, and the reformation of the habits of the idle poor.

As Paul Slack has pointed out, Cary's Bristol initiative was prompted by at least two contingencies.[21] The 1690s saw cold winters, bad harvests and the disruptions of war, all of which contributed to concern about the employment of the poor.[22] Thus, for example, the board of trade began to make inquiries about employment in 1695-6. Second was the relaxation of controls upon dissenters resulting from the Act of Toleration in 1689. As we shall see, dissenters played a key role in the founding of the workhouse as well as the hospital.

Cary aired his scheme for a city workhouse in a public meeting, presented the result to the mayor of Bristol, and lobbied for its

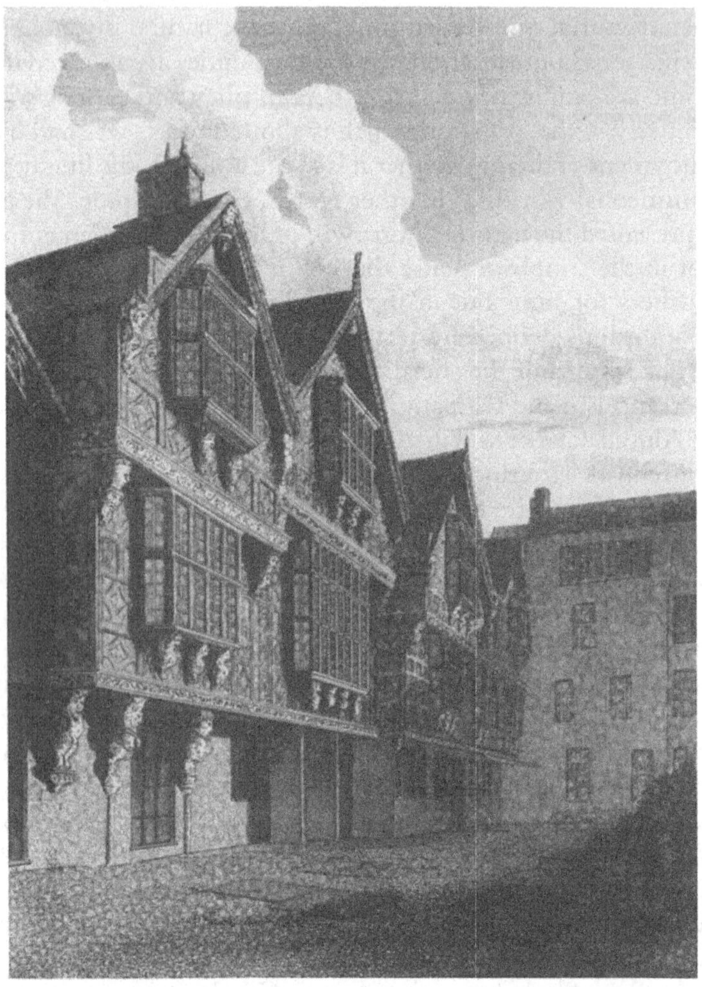

Figure 4.2. The Bristol Mint in the early nineteenth century (Bristol Record Office)

passage through Parliament. In 1696 all seventeen city parishes were unified into a corporation which could collect a poor rate, build a workhouse, and compel the poor to enter it.[23] The Corporation of the Poor borrowed a building from the city council and equipped it for the reception of one hundred girls. Subsequently, it purchased a building which had been a sugar refinery, and then a mint (hence the workhouse was referred to in Bristol as the Mint), which housed the elderly and infirm as well as children (see Fig. 4.2).

Although undoubtedly prompted by the distress of the city's poor, the initiative to found a workhouse had as much to do with their reformation as their survival. Founders of the workhouse had strong ties to the Society for the Reformation of Manners (SRM), the Society for the Promotion of Christian Knowledge (SPCK) and others interested in the morals and manners of the poor. As Sir John Duddlestone, governor of the poor and reform of manners campaigner subsequently wrote about Bristol, "the poor in that city are much reform'd for as none Steal or Starve for lack of Bread, so care is now taken that none shall profane the name of God as they us'd to do."[24] The workhouse thus served to remedy starving and swearing simultaneously.

It had been at Duddlestone's house that the first meeting of a society to reform manners had been held in Bristol in 1699, and this ideology of reform continued to be significant to workhouse and hospital. Initially, the Bristol Society for the Reformation of Manners focused on prosecuting people for swearing and other forms of indecent behavior. It met in the boardroom at the city workhouse, making connections between its own regulation of the poor and that of the workhouse explicit.

Historians have placed the reformation of manners movement in the context of providentialism, which grew from perceptions of the Revolution of 1688, the belief that England somehow had a special connection with divine providence, and that she must live up to this relationship.[25] As the first historian-cum-publicist for the societies, Josiah Woodward, wrote, "National sins deserve national Judgements." England thus needed to "endeavour, by a General Reformation, to appease the Wrath of God."[26] A. G. Craig argues that an obvious focus for these "moral patriots" was the local system of social control centered on the parish.[27] Thus, for example, societies for the reformation of manners paid informers to report on local lapses of conduct and attempted to police neighborhood morals. They emphasized the appearance and outward behavior of the poor.

The Bristol Corporation of the Poor made links between unmannerly appearances, idleness, and immorality similar to those of the SRM. For example, in a sermon preached to the Corporation in 1704, Bristol's poor were referred to as "lousing like swarms of locusts in every corner of the streets."[28] The Corporation used the same imagery, referring to "rooting out swarms of Vagabonds who wander up and down to the danger and indignity of the nation."[29] In other words, the poor were morally contaminating the urban environment by their very appearance.

When the first one hundred girls were brought to Whitehall, (the Corporation of the Poor building leased from the city) they were stripped, washed, and given new clothes, which supposedly so encouraged the children that "they willingly betook themselves to work."[30] These outward changes, of course, led to inner ones as well. The improved mode of living, according to John Cary, led to "a great deal of foulness" being discharged from the girls' bodies, so that twenty or thirty were ill at a time, although, due to God's blessing on the enterprise, only two died.[31] In other words, appearance, behavior and health of the girls were so tightly linked as to be but facets of the same thing – their morality.

The attention to appearance was, of course, becoming something of a preoccupation with Quakers at this time, as manifested in their emphasis upon correct clothing.[32] Appearance, behavior, and moral worth were all the same; one woman was investigated by the Men's Meeting because she had been "walking disorderly" – just the sort of offence of interest to the reformers of manners.[33] Links among reformers and dissenters are discussed below; here it is sufficient to note the same emphasis upon manners and appearance common to both.

Similar attitudes toward inmates of the hospital underline its derivation from the workhouse. Not only would the hospital heal the bodies of its patients, it would reform their manners as well. As Alured Clarke said of his Winchester Infirmary, "It reduces the number of Vagrants by depriving them of one of their most plausible Reasons for begging door to door."[34] Like the workhouse, the hospital would help rid the streets of the idle and disorderly, and England's special relationship to Providence would then be apparent to all.

Emblematic of this concern with the manners of the poor was the Infirmary rule that "no Patient be taken in 'till their Cloaths are well cleansed, and where any of them are so poor they can't pay for it that the visitors of the week do order the Matron to pay for doing it."[35] In other words, only the clean respectable poor, or at least a facsimile thereof, were to enter the institution.

The Infirmary subscriber knew that his funds would go toward moral as well as physical reclamation of the patient. Inside the Infirmary, the poor were removed from the bad influences of their

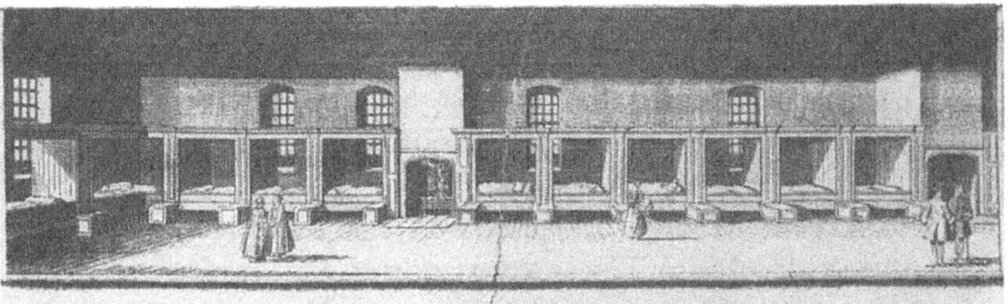

Figure 4.3. The inside of an eighteenth-century infirmary – Guy's Hospital, London (Welcome Library, London)

friends and neighbors, kept in hospital "for so long a time as is necessary to beget contrary habits" in the words of Alured Clarke.[36] In Bristol, patients were exposed to daily prayers, and forbidden to gamble or swear. In many provincial infirmaries, biblical texts were painted on the walls of the wards.[37]

It is difficult to know how the patient perceived his or her hospital stay.[38] An inpatient's day started with servants cleaning the wards at seven in the morning, or, in winter, whenever it got light. The wards were initially furnished with wooden beds, and from illustrations of Guy's Hospital (see Fig. 4.3) and the Northampton Infirmary, we can guess that patients slept in wooden-framed beds behind curtains. Within an hour of the cleaners' appearance, patients could expect breakfast, usually a pint of broth or milk pottage, depending upon the day of the week and whether the patient was on one of three special diets. From nine until ten in the morning seems to have been one of the visiting hours. Every Tuesday morning, patients were read the Infirmary's rules, and on Mondays and Thursdays, patients might see three house visitors, subscribers charged with the day-to-day administration of the hospital.

Patients were not allowed to play cards, dice or any other game, nor were they allowed to smoke. How they passed the time while convalescing is not known. There were sometimes Bibles or prayerbooks on the wards, but not in multiple copies, nor could all patients read. From eleven until two the surgeons or their pupils and apprentices made the rounds and tended to the surgical patients, changing dressings and cleaning wounds. The main meal was in the middle of the day, and alternated between 10 ounces of beef or mutton, and servings of rice in milk. Special diets featured bread puddings or boiled rice. Although food was monotonous, it seems to have been served in generous quantities, washed down by a quart of beer a day.

Visitors seem to have been allowed again between three and seven in the afternoon. The hospital porter was on duty to make sure that no goodies or liquor were smuggled in to the patients by their family and friends. Ambulatory patients seem to have had considerable freedom. On the nod from the porter, they could leave the hospital during the day, only having to return to sleep. Of course, patients who could be of use to the matron or nurses were bound by the rules to assist them, and probably provided a good deal of nursing care, as did family members of the patients.

A patient's day ended with supper in the evening, usually cheese or broth. Night nurses kept watch over seriously ill patients, but most inmates' days were structured by sunrise and sunset. On Sundays, patients who were able could go to church. The hospital's chaplain presumably said prayers and visited with patients, but there are no details of his role, save for his unhappy function in interring those patients who died and were buried in the Infirmary burial ground.

A sermon preached for the Bristol Infirmary by Josiah Tucker in 1746 highlights its disciplinary aspects. Tucker's views on the poor were alarmingly straightforward: "Such brutality and insolence, such debauchery and extravagance, such idleness in religion, cursing, swearing and contempt of all rule and authority, Human and Divine, do not reign so triumphantly among the Poor in any other country as ours."[39] He claimed that the English were so careful of personal freedom that "our People are drunk with the cup of Liberty." The Infirmary might serve as a corrective, instilling the poor with appropriate virtues while not robbing them of liberty, because they were subject only to a set of rules to which they had given consent by seeking admission.[40]

Tucker made the link with the reformation-of-manners campaign explicit in the title of his sermon, "Hospitals and Infirmaries Considered as Schools of Christian Education for the Adult Poor: and as a Means Conducive Towards a National Reformation in the Common Peoples." Just as the workhouse had educated children in morals, so the Infirmary would fulfill the same function for adults, complementing the Mint and the city's growing numbers of charity schools. The hospital was the remedy for debauchery, extravagance, cursing, swearing, and contempt of authority – with no mention of bodily ills. By the mid-1740s, Tucker's message was too explicit; he "could not appear in the streets without being called after and hooted by the boys and rabble."[41] Nevertheless, the sermon was sufficiently consonant with the views of the governors that they had it published.

At the heart of the moral reformers' program of incarceration was the desire to recreate a primitive Christianity. This return to an earlier, purer, past characterized and linked many of their varied interests, from charity schools to church music. This impulse was mediated and shaped by the societies for the reformation of manners, but it was also referred to directly by social reformers and their critics. Thus, for example, the Quaker John Bellers said of his proposed workhouse, "The Poor . . . will be a Community something like the Example of Primitive Christianity."[42] Matthew Tindal, a deist and free thinker who wrote a defense of low-church practices, which included a discussion of the governance of Bristol's workhouse, repeatedly drew upon the example of primitive Christianity. For example, he contested ecclesiastical power by pointing out that the early Christians baptized each other and did not need priests.[43] He wrote, "Christ and his Apostles inculcated nothing so much as Universal Charity."[44]

When the Infirmary was founded, the motto "Charity Universal" was chosen. In his Infirmary sermon, Carew Reynell's stated purpose was, "to excite you to the practice of universal charity."[45] Although to a late twentieth-century reader, the words "universal charity" seem a vague sort of phrase, they were an allusion to these reformers who emphasized the return to the Primitive Church. Sir Richard Bulkeley, associated with the reformers of manners and the SPCK, interested in many of the wilder shores of pietistic religion, founded Universal Charities, utopian communities which bankrupted his estate. "Universal" was also a sort of buzzword in Quaker circles. Friends rejected Calvinist doctrines of election; although not all would be saved, there was universal access to God's grace and potential salvation.[46] In the late 1690s, some of the split between George Keith and the Society of Friends was due to differences about the possibilities of universal salvation. As Melvin Endy has elucidated, Keith maintained that although those who did not know Christ might be saved, the Scriptures were definite that salvation lay through Jesus, and it was arrogant of Quakers to claim otherwise.[47] The Keithian controversy was particularly intense in Bristol, and it seems improbable that the Friends involved in founding the Infirmary a few decades later were deaf to the several resonances of the phrase "Charity Universal."

This group of hospital founders and manners reformers, then, were very much looking backward, seeking a model from the past. Although this model was often drawn from the early days of the Church, these men also harked back to a much more recent, albeit less well-defined past when they discussed social relations. Their vision of society was clearly hierarchical; everyone was to know his or her place and stick to it. And, of course, crucial to the well-being of such a society was work, which defined and proscribed all social life.

Richard Champion's views of the hierarchical nature of social relations noted earlier echoed the pronouncements of reformation-of-manners campaigners. For instance, Arthur Bedford, manners reformer and charity-school supporter, had written, "Parents are obliged to take care of their Children; Masters of the Families of their Household, Apprentices and Servants; the Clergy of their Parishioners; Magistrates and inferior officers of those under their Authority; and princes of their Subjects; that Religion may be propagated and Vice discountenanced and suppressed."[48] God's providence provided for men who were contented with their lot in the hierarchy.

Like any hybrid beast, the hospital embodied certain of its ancestors' characteristics more than others. Although the reform of manners campaign and its expression in the city workhouse were important forbears of the Infirmary, certain of its features were more strongly expressed in the Infirmary than others. Three aspects of hospital life were increasingly significant as the institution became established. First, the hierarchical nature of social relations embedded within the admission process tended to be expressed in terms of the reciprocal aspects of the relationship between rich and poor. Second, the civic function of hospital governorship assumed a life of its own, whereas the Bristol Society for the Reformation of Manners seems to have withered away as fewer and fewer attended meetings, the Infirmary quarterly meetings and annual banquets became a perennial feature of the city's calendar. Finally, the role of dissenters in the Infirmary became institutionalized as the office of treasurer remained within one Quaker family, and the faction which characterized Bristol's political life became expressed through the hospital.

What was becoming a somewhat old-fashioned understanding of the hierarchical nature of society was increasingly restated in terms of reciprocity. For subscribers and supporters, institutions like hospitals and workhouses provided social glue that held together a fragmented society. A hierarchical social structure implied mutual obligations, as Julia Champion, the wife of the Infirmary Treasurer, suggested, "The common people show by their Actions how much they feel a kind Behavior to them and more doubly repay it by an affectionate Conduct in return."[49] John Bellers, Quaker author of a noted essay on hospitals, stated this reciprocal relationship thus, "It's as much the Duty of the Poor to Labour when they are able, as it is for the Rich to Help them when they are sick."[50] He emphasized why the rich should care for the poor, saying that "Duty and Interest are Two as great Obligations as can be laid upon Mortals, and they both as Powerful advocates call upon the Rich to take care of the Poor."[51] In a city riven by faction, in which the poor expressed discontent in frequent riot, hospital subscribers could use their power as benefactors to create and reinforce patterns of deferential behavior while strengthening their own sense of identity.

The structure of the admissions process, in which a prospective patient needed to find a subscriber willing to recommend him or her, emphasized the personal nature of such patronage. It mimicked the politics of the great, and ensured that any petitioner for help could expect to conform to the wishes of his or her patron. Thus, for a hospital governor, a recommendation to the Infirmary was a formalization of an already existing relationship of patronage, a relationship characterized by obligation on both sides.

As the hospital governors shaped their relationship with their clients, so too they created a new relationship among themselves. The hospital, like the assembly rooms, debating societies, lending libraries, and literary and philosophical societies became hallmarks of polite and leisured society. Charities were not so much a reflection of this definition of social boundaries as an arena in which such boundaries were made, tested, and reinforced.[52] The workhouse made social standing very clear: it labeled the poor by forcing them to wear badges. The Infirmary likewise drew specific boundaries; it would only treat those who were too poor to afford an annual subscription, and would not treat the servants of its governors, who should be cared for by their masters. In annual processions to the cathedral, the city's benevolence to its poor was made manifest, and at the Infirmary sermon and banquet, in the lists of subscribers published every year, the individual benefactors were highlighted.

The public quality of charity was significant in the articulation of social difference, but it played a paradoxical role in relationships amongst the givers. On the one hand, charity such as the Infirmary was an attempt to heal the deep divisions in the city, but on the other, charity was always partisan and could not help but illustrate the disunity and faction which characterized Bristol. In part, the prevalence of sectarian religion promoted factional charity, but often benevolence was intended to overwrite such differences. Thus, for example, one meaning of "Charity Universal" was an allusion to the wide range of interests the hospital hoped to attract.

The workhouse had been plagued by faction from its outset, in part because the 1696 Corporation of the Poor in Bristol represented a very new kind of access to city governance. Parishes, after all, were run by select vestries, self-perpetuating small groups who set the poor rate (the tax that provided money for poor relief), chose a churchwarden, and fulfilled a range of other bureaucratic duties. The city itself was run by a sort of select vestry, the city council, which chose its own replacements for vacancies (and did not include dissenters). Although Bristol had one of the largest electorates (5,000 freemen) even the far-from-universal right to vote did not give one a voice in the real running of the city; it merely entitled one to vote for a member of Parliament. The Corporation of the Poor, on the other hand, consisted of four guardians elected from each of the city's twelve wards, plus the mayor and aldermen. Anyone paying more than one penny per week toward the poor rate could vote for the guardians. John Cary's plan, with sufficient taxpaying being the only qualification for voting, meant that electors, and the guardians they chose, need not be freemen, need not even be Anglican.

It is impossible to document the real extent of dissenting involvement in the Corporation, but it seems to have been strong. The only list of members extant is for 1696, and of these men, there are at least six known Quakers.[53] An early treasurer of the incorporation, Thomas Callowhill, who served for two terms, was a Quaker, and later became involved with the Infirmary. Other well-known Friends, such as Richard Champion, Edward Harford, and Nehemiah Champion, also became treasurers.[54] Finally, when the Tory High Church party assumed a temporary ascendancy in 1714, an Act of Parliament was passed barring dissenters from the Corporation (guardians were forced to take a sacramental test). But four years later, it had been found virtually impossible to run the Corporation without the help of dissenters, and a Whig government removed the test.[55]

From its inception, the Corporation feuded with the city council and with the select vestries. For example, the churchwardens, annoyed at being shut out of their former role as Poor Law administrators, refused to collect the poor rate. The mayor, an "unexpected Remora" in John Cary's words, stuck fast to the city's funds and refused to grant his warrants for raising monies.[56] It took amendments to various acts of Parliament to ensure that the Corporation received its funds. Sectarian squabbles over poor relief were a part of its day-to-day administration.

The bitterness with which dissenters battled with High Church Anglicans recurred in many other charities, complicated by political loyalties. For example, Edward Colston, a London merchant, endowed a charity school in Bristol, where he had been born. In 1710 Colston's School, providing for 100 boys, was opened with a procession and special cathedral service. Colston was quite particular about the recipients of his largess; any boy whose parents made the mistake of taking him to a dissenting service was to be expelled forthwith. Similarly, no boy from the school was to be apprenticed to a dissenter. It was not just religion Colston enforced. He had contributed toward the founding of another charity school, in Temple parish. When Temple's vicar voted for a Whig and Low Churchman, Colston was outraged, evidently considering this act an insult to a patron.[57] Charity schools themselves fell afoul of faction, becoming tarred with the brush of Jacobitism, perceived as nurseries of vice.[58] In other words, charity was almost inevitably shaped, for both benefactor and recipient, by considerations of politics and religion.

One of the reasons that the Infirmary was so popular at the outset was because it represented a new form of charity, untainted by charity-school scandals and recriminations surrounding the workhouse. However, the Infirmary soon became largely governed by Quakers, who represented between 22 percent (in 1736) and 4 percent (in 1806) of the hospital's subscribers. The decrease in Quaker representation over the century probably reflects a decline in membership in the Society of Friends in Bristol, and the gradual assimilation of the Friends into mainstream Anglican culture. In the early decades of the Infirmary, the Quaker presence – a fifth of subscribers – must have been very noticeable. Turning the question around and asking how many of Bristol's Quakers were hospital subscribers also emphasizes their disproportionate involvement. In 1750 perhaps a third of all male heads of Quaker households were subscribers.[59] These sorts of figures, combined with the prevalence of Quaker hospital managers, suggests that an ordinary eighteenth-century Bristolian readily perceived the Infirmary's sectarian flavor.

Historians have emphasized the role of charity in uniting urban elites and in creating a new sociability.[60] Again, these developments need to be seen in the light of the recipients of charity as well as the givers, and in the context of the changes in the social meanings of charity. Further examination of other charity in Bristol illustrates that the hospital was not alone in its sectarian composition. Not only was charity factionalized, but new forms tended to outweigh the older, city-based charitable rituals which provided a certain civic unity. These new forms also denied women any active role in benefaction.

Charities proliferated in Bristol, and became increasingly specific over the course of the eighteenth century. Various convivial societies, for example, flourished in the city, based upon regional or political identities. The Gentlemen Natives of Gloucestershire, of Wiltshire, of Somerset, the Dolphin Society, the Anchor Society, and many others, met at annual banquets and collected monies for apprenticing poor boys, for women in childbed, and other life-cycle-specific charities.

So too, individual churches continued to disburse their charitable bequests, creating a sort of nonmunicipal poor law. For example, Lewin's Mead, the Unitarian church strongly associated with the city's councillors, created its own system of poor relief; some people received weekly relief payments, while others got help only in unusual circumstances. For instance, Widow Linging had her rent paid for her and received money for fuel and for medical care. Other people were casual recipients – "a poore woman her husband Kild," or the many Irish who used the port of Bristol to return home. The Committee for Poor Relief was scrupulous in noting when aid was given to members of the group: "gave to a poore Woman of the Sosiatty who Child was in a very sad Condishon." Thus the Unitarians created their own version of the poor law that echoed Anglican responses to poverty while serving to define members of the congregation as a separate group.[61]

Some decades later, a much poorer congregation, George Whitefield's Tabernacle, similarly used charity to define itself and its members.[62] One person, Miss Brain, served as an almoner, dispensing monies as she saw fit. In addition, the committee gave larger sums in special circumstances, such as £1.1s to "Mrs. A in sickness" in 1769. This congregation seems to have been especially concerned with health care, because they hired a nurse on contract for several years.[63] Jonathan Barry has suggested that the Tabernacle was a major impetus in the 1775 founding of the Castle Green Dispensary. The fact that the congregation was paying thirteen shillings annually to an apothecary in 1778, as well as hiring a nurse, tends to support this hypothesis.[64]

As charity was becoming a means of defining a group's corporate identity, a public face, women's roles in such charity were marginalized. Miss Brain was unusual in the extent of her involvement in organized benefaction. Far more typical was Lucy Yeats, giving personal gifts to an individual family anonymously. Donations to lying-in women provide another example of the ways in which charity became a form of social interaction characterized by strong public group identities which denied women active roles.

Women in childbed were perceived as worthy objects of charity throughout the eighteenth century, albeit in different contexts. Three styles of giving characterized this form of charity: the civic pageant, the convivial society, and the women's organization. The first two illustrate the shift toward a particularized form of charity; the third, a development of the late eighteenth century, is discussed in Chapter 6. Two charities, Whitson's and Mary Ann Peloquin's, were created by bequests from people known for their philanthropy. Both of these charities were ritualized civic moments; thirteen women per quarter received one pound each. Peloquin's charity was restricted to the wives or widows of freemen. It was clearly of symbolic as well as actual value; many of its recipients were the wives of skilled artisans rather than laborers.[65] Similarly, Whitson's Gift, distributed by the mayor's wife, was an overt statement of the city's benevolence toward certain of its citizens. These charities also emphasized a personal link; women received Whitson's Gift "by desire of the Mayor" or "by desire of Alderman Smith." Similarly, although any one woman was only supposed to receive the gift three times, the mayoress could bend the rules and provide again for Mary Charles, "very poor and seven children" whose husband was a laborer.[66]

Mary Ann Peloquin was a member of the wealthy group of Huguenot descendants in the city, and when she died, she left one of the largest fortunes in the city to charity. Nineteen thousand pounds, for example, was put into trust to pay yearly doles to 156 poor people.[67] Unlike Whitson, who had founded a charity school and involved himself with other public ventures, Peloquin's giving was of the increasingly old-fashioned, female variety of personal giving and bequests.

Peloquin's charity contrasts with that of the convivial societies. John Latimer, in his annals of Bristol life, describes the newspaper reports of the annual feast of the Wiltshire Society: "The members walked in procession to Christ Church to hear a sermon. 'There was a fine appearance, and a shepherd, with his habit, crook, bottle, and dog attended them.' The proceedings of course concluded with a dinner, which took place in the Merchants' Hall."[68] Here, giving to the poor was constitutive of one's identity in a group, not merely a definition of a certain social standing, but an act which was central to the experiences of a particular group within the city. Needless to add, just as in the case of Lewin's Mead or the Tabernacle, the Wiltshire Society gave its funds to its own, to distressed Wiltshiremen and women.

In sum, charity in Bristol was freighted with political and sectarian meanings. As Stephen MacFarlane has said of similar developments in London, "debates on the poor were as much about *who* ought to govern indigent or able-bodied paupers as *how* they should be governed."[69] In Bristol, the abundance of dissenting groups meant that there were many types of poor relief, each with its own allegiances.[70] Therefore, any portrayal of the emergence of a leisured, mannered class characterized by an urban sociability needs to be tempered by the realization that the governing class was by no means unified.

The Bristol Infirmary's motto, "Charity Universal" can thus be read as wishful thinking. From a more jaded perspective, it looks merely ironic. First, like other charities and like the city workhouse from which it drew much inspiration, the institution was designed to purvey charity to very specific groups whom the benefactors wished to aid, rather than to dispense largess universally. Neither was the charity universal in terms of its appeal. Indeed, given the highly factionalized nature of charity and relief in the city, no organization could hope to be universal. The very word "universal" pointed to a specific interest in the reformation of manners and a harking-back to primitive Christianity not shared by many in the city.

5

The client

The creation of the workhouse and the Infirmary expanded the range of welfare and health-care options for the laboring classes. Obviously, for the poorest of the poor – the vagrant dragged off the street and incarcerated in the Mint, the friendless immigrant who never even made it into an institution – for such a person, speaking of "health-care options" is no more than ironic. These people could not participate in the medical marketplace, could not exercise choice in any but the most limited fashion. The mandates of both workhouse and Infirmary excluded many a needy individual, and historical records rarely if ever express these people's perspectives on the health-care systems they encountered.

However, there was a large group for whom institutional medicine was a new invention, another option in their accustomed marketplace. They are the focus of this chapter. Their choices, in the aggregate, helped to shape these institutions – hospitals, the Old Poor Law, dispensaries – as well as the functions of institutional care in medical practice. To twentieth-century eyes, the hospital looks like a natural locus for medicine, but this was by no means the case in the eighteenth century. Chapter 4, by examining the men and motives that made the Infirmary, showed how the hospital was more closely linked to charity and poor relief than to medicine. The users of these institutions reiterated the connections among medicine, charity and poor relief, but in a different way. Where Infirmary founders connected their benevolence to that of the Corporation of the Poor through sectarian and political agendas such as the reformation of manners, those who utilized such institutions linked them because they offered the same thing: free health care. The same kinds of factors that led one individual to seek free Infirmary care might lead another to the poor-law authorities. Medicine's role in each was shaped by both the wishes of patrons and the needs of clients.

For the patient, an encounter with institutional medicine, be it poor law or infirmary, was often defined by life-cycle crisis. Recourse to such a place was a desperate measure; illness alone did not make a hospital patient. Rather, the loss of a spouse, or the arrival of another child to stretch domestic resources even further, or the inability to keep working in the face of old age or infirmity – these were the circumstances which drove people to hospitals or poor-law overseers. An analysis of two groups of institutional users provides a close-up picture of hospital and poor law from the client's vantage point.[1]

These clients came from Abson and Wick, a small country parish, and from SS. Philip and Jacob, a large one in Bristol. Both parishes were characterized by mixed economies, with some degree of industry. Abson had paper, iron and grist mills, whereas SS. Philip and Jacob housed lead, brass, soap and glass works – manufacturing for the colonies, fueled by local coal. The urban parish extended past the old city walls, and in its greener reaches there were market gardens, although the noisome Frome river added its unhealthy miasmas to the smells of tanning and lime kilns in the outer parts of the parish. Abson, populated in part by industrial laborers, also had farms that afforded work to laborers in dairying and apple-growing. It was a small parish, comprised of three hamlets and overseen by the lords of the manor, the Haynes family, who lived locally. SS. Philip and Jacob dwarfed Abson; for Abson's 500 inhabitants, the urban parish had 10,000. Many lived in cramped accommodations, in tiny courts which opened off crowded and narrow streets. The populations of both parishes grew considerably in the latter half of the century, which added to the numbers relieved by the Old Poor Law.[2]

In neither parish was recourse to poor relief or charity an uncommon event. As Tim Wales and others have shown, although the Old Poor Law may have been relieving only a limited number of people at any given time, such relief was life-cycle-based.[3] In other words, over the course of a laboring person's life, he or she might well resort to poor relief at certain crucial moments. Few working people in city or country could assume that they would never need such aid.

Both Infirmary and poor relief were widely utilized by the laboring classes in Bristol and Abson. By the 1790s, the Infirmary saw around 1,200 inpatients and 3,000 outpatients a year, which represented fourfold and sixfold increases, respectively, since the 1740s.[4] These figures suggest that a sizeable proportion of Bristol's poor came in contact with the Infirmary at some point in their lifetime. For example, in the early 1780s, about 5 percent of the population of the city annually sought medical care from the hospital, either as inpatients or outpatients.[5] Because hospital patients were drawn only from certain groups within the city, 5 percent of the total population is a substantial figure.

In Bristol, as in other provincial centers, the Infirmary was not the only resort. Those who could not get an Infirmary admission ticket, or did not want one, might seek medical help from the Poor Law. Unfortunately, almost no records of the Corporation of the Poor survive. However, estimates of the extent to which the local population relied upon the Poor Law can be made from the burial register of SS. Philip and Jacob, which indicates those who died while receiving relief.[6] A sample of 1,807 interments from seven randomly selected years for the period 1784 to 1814 includes 39 percent who were in receipt of aid when they died. The links between poverty and illness make this figure an unreliable guide to overall levels of dependency. But an analysis of accidental deaths, and deaths due to diseases of sudden onset (making it less likely that illness was a factor in relief) reveals that substantial proportions of the parish were receiving welfare monies; 35 percent of people who died "suddenly," 25 percent of accident victims, 29 percent of smallpox cases were getting poor-law aid at the time they died. Obviously, men and women with chronic and debilitating ailments were even more likely to be on relief; for instance, 42 percent of all consumptives were on the dole when they died. In other words, a substantial proportion of this parish relied upon the Corporation of the Poor for subsistence, and an even greater share of the parish's sick and disabled received some kind of support.

In rural areas, access to medical institutions was very limited; most Bristol Infirmary patients from country villages arrived in hospital because their parish vestry or Poor Law overseer subscribed to the Infirmary. But these individuals accounted for only a small fraction of hospital patients: In Bristol, 84 percent of Infirmary patients came from the city itself. Even rural parishes that were Infirmary subscribers sent a handful of patients to hospital. Most health care was provided by the Poor Law, in payments for individual practitioners, remedies, and the like.[7] As in the city, many people relied upon poor relief for help at some point in their lives. In Abson perhaps a quarter of all late eighteenth-century parish residents benefited from the Poor Law at some point in their lives.[8]

Thus, in city or country, charity and welfare institutions were significant providers of health care to the poor. From the perspective of numbers of users, charitable or welfare provision of health care begins to loom large in the domestic economies and expectations of the poor. Most laboring men and women in Bristol must have known someone who went to the Infirmary; similarly, in Bristol or in Abson, few could have failed to have known someone on poor relief.

The paths by which individuals became clients of the Poor Law or the Infirmary were marked by various crises, by economic hardship, family disruption, and shortages of work, as well as by illness. These precipitants to institutional health care underline medicine's subservience to charity and welfare; health care was a part of larger systems of relief, and illness was a kind of dependency. As a group, the users of such institutional health care were not very different from their neighbors in terms of occupation or age structure. Where they differed seems to have been in the resources available to them in bad times. In the city, many were migrants, or others without strongly developed local ties. In the country, Poor Law users tended to have less well-developed community ties. But these groups cannot be characterized as an underclass, the "residuum" delineated by Victorian analysts of poverty. Rather, they were ordinary working men and women who suddenly found themselves in trouble, without recourse to domestic assistance from kin or neighbors.

In many ways, seeking help from the Poor Law authorities was not that different from seeking hospital admission. The Old Poor Law, based upon Elizabethan statutes designed to crack down on vagrancy, was a very local system. Each parish fixed a rate (a local tax), collected it, and elected an overseer of the poor who disbursed monies to the needy. Although the broad outlines were the same in every parish, local circumstances could vary widely. For instance, it seems that John Skinner's Somerset parish of Camerton was ruled by a vestry made up of farmers who curbed spending in order to keep the rates down.[9] Other parishes, such as Abson and Wick, took a milder stand on neediness and provided a wider range of services to the poor. In any case, a petitioner for relief had to make his or her plea to the overseer, in a manner analogous to a hospital patient's quest for the support of an Infirmary subscriber.

People sought poor relief in Abson for a variety of reasons. Illness was a directly precipitating cause in some cases, and ill health a factor in many others, but there is little reason to distinguish "medical" relief from the rest. And, of course, different types of aid were given to the poor by the overseers. Some people received help only once or twice in their lifetimes, while others were on "Weekly pays" – the dole – for years. Some got standard packages (unwed mothers, for example, were usually given 1s.6d. per week with 25 shillings for their month's lying-in) whereas others were given extensive payments for various needs. As a group, these were not necessarily the down-and-outs of the parish. A third of all relief episodes involved the heads of households and their families, while an additional 13 percent involved aid directly to children, often to apprentice them.

Despite such diversity, certain circumstances characterized many episodes of poor relief. Three groups – broken families, the elderly, and unwed mothers – received the bulk of Poor Law aid in Abson. Disruption of a family unit through death or abandonment of a spouse was a catastrophic event, often requiring help. Although this category accounted for only about 14 percent of all relief recipients, it usually involved a heavy financial commitment for the parish; over 20 percent of all Abson expenditure came under this heading. Much of this disruption was caused by illness or death of the head of a household or spouse. For instance, Hester Dore's husband Henry died in 1767, leaving her with three children after seven years of marriage. The parish paid her rent, and four shillings a week for her children through 1772, when they were given new clothing and apprenticed. Hester Dore had remarried in 1768, but her new husband was not expected to look after her children (nor were most stepparents in this parish). Families also broke up when one of the parents fled, not an uncommon occurrence. Sarah Grant, for example, was deserted by her husband shortly before the birth of their child. The parish paid her two shillings a week, rent, and lying-in money. The baby died when a few months old, and after the burial, Sarah Grant presumably moved on, since she does not appear in Abson parish or Poor Law records again.

Old age and disability was another major category of parish expense. In many cases, it has been impossible to know the exact age of a Poor Law client; this category thus encompasses those who received several years of Poor Law support prior to their death, as well as those known to be elderly. For example, Mary Prewett, a widow, had her rent paid from 1767 until her death in 1778, and was on two shillings per week dole for the last two and a half years of her life.

Unwed mothers were the third major category of poor-relief recipient. The parish tried to track down the fathers of illegitimate children and force them to support their offspring, but these efforts seem to have been fairly unsuccessful. By the turn of the century, unwed motherhood was virtually epidemic in the parish; in 1803, twelve mothers were on the dole, receiving at least 1s.6d each per week for their children. Then as now, single parenthood was one of the surest paths to long-term dependency.

Betty Gibbons, for example, spent most of her life on poor relief, although she was atypical in having borne several children out of wedlock. She first got help from the overseers in 1771 when she had smallpox. Four years later she had a baby, and thereafter Betty Gibbons received regular parish support. The overseers provided at least two more lyings-in for her, and from 1779 she received a minimum of three shillings a week for the rest of her life, even though she married John Hunt in 1788, and had two more children. By the 1790s she was getting five shillings a week and had her rent paid. Betty Gibbons may be unusual in the extent of support she received from the Poor Law, but her circumstances were not unique.

These three groups – broken families, the elderly, and unwed mothers – were the mainstays of poor-relief recipients. Among them they accounted for almost half of all the people who ever got Poor Law help in Abson, and three-quarters of total expenditure. Each of these groups received medical care as an integral part of their welfare support. For example, unwed mothers almost always received payment for a midwife, as did a few poor married women. It seems improbable, however, that either recipient or overseer made clear distinctions between health care and poor relief, since relief encompassed almost all dimensions of dependency. For instance, the combination of food, fuel, lighting, clothing, nursing care, payments to a midwife and to a medical man provided to the Hart family virtually defies separation into "medical" and "welfare" components.

Poor-law medical aid to the Hart family
midwife for attending, 1765
dole, 1s, 2s, 1774–98
rent, 1775–87 (every year)
shirts, 1776, 1782, 1785, 1787
Amy ill, 1781
Joseph ill, 1785
Amy ill, 1788
Joseph ill, burial 1788
Amy ill, 1789, 1792, 1793
shoes, 1792
clothing, 1796, 1797
Amy ill, 1798, including heating and nursing
Amy's funeral

Take also the case of John Bryant, a long-term dole recipient who was ill and lame in 1776–7. The overseers provided him with a doctor for his leg, nursing care, lodging, brandy, new bedclothes, and further unspecified support in addition to his dole money. Again, health care was just one aspect of Bryant's support – illness was subsumed by dependency.

Although such dependency characterized many recipients of Poor Law health care, for some, illness was a clearly defined point of entry to relief and remained a distinctive reason for seeking support. Seventeen percent of all recipients encountered the Poor Law because of illness. Some individuals used the parish solely because of illness. Brice Kains, for example, received aid in the late 1760s when his family was ill, again in 1773 when they had smallpox, in 1780–1 when his wife and son were ill and died, and in his own final illness in 1791–2. In other words, the only instances in which this family required assistance were times of severe illness. Similarly, his son, Brice Kains II, turned to the Poor Law twice, both instances in which his children were fatally ill. Although expenditure on illness, strictly defined, was quite small, it remained an important point of contact for a group of people, many of whom would never else encounter the Poor Law system. And it provided a significant role for rural medical practitioners within the local welfare system.

The final category of poor-relief recipient is the least easy to define. Many people got help from the Poor Law for vaguely recorded reasons, listed in account books as "at sundry times" or "in distress." Like illness, this category was important not so much because of its total cost, but because of its wide reach; a quarter of all Poor Law clients fall into this group. For example, twenty-six year-old Lewis Bryant, a laborer, was given a total of 19s "at sundry times" in 1790. Edward Clark was on the dole (5s per week) off and on, and received rent, and "extra pay," amounting to £4 in one year, intermittently in the late 1790s. Many people who did not otherwise make use of poor relief fall into this category.

Poor-relief recipients were thus characterized by different kinds of dependency. Some needed aid only in rare moments of crisis while others subsisted upon relief for years. The provision of health care within this system was shaped by these different forms of dependency. But common to many recipients was the way in which relief substituted for the care of family and friends. A family's obligations to its members were fairly limited.[10] For instance, stepparents were not expected to be responsible for children from previous marriages. In a time when many children lost a parent, through death or desertion, the Poor Law had a considerable task in looking after them. The responsibilities of siblings to each other were also fairly minimal. For example, Lydia Witcholl was cared for by two different women while her sister was living in Abson. Even if family were available, such care could be transformed from an obligation to a commodity, paid for by the Poor Law. Susannah Hendy, for example, was paid to look after her brother John Hawkins; the parish did not expect her to use her own household's resources to care for her brother. John Skinner, the rector of the nearby parish of Camerton, thought that the Poor Law was a bad influence because it checked the "natural affection which ought to bind a human creature in a more especial manner to his kindred." According to him, families did not offer their members help in times of hardship because they thought that the parish would then be obliged to provide for them.[11] Misanthrope though Skinner may have been, his comments are partially borne out by evidence from Abson.

In the same way that the health care provided by nurses in Bristol became increasingly institutional and commercial – women running lying-in homes, women hired by the Infirmary for cash wages – so too, the Poor Law authorities' willingness to hire nurses began to commercialize home care and to set it off from other types of health care. For the patient, this might mean access to types of practitioners previously unavailable; in Abson, overseers paid for surgeons, midwives, for a prolonged stay at the Bath Infirmary – all forms of health care beyond the means of very poor parishioners. Overseers, however, also created and reinforced distinctions among health-care workers. "Watchers" who sat up with the sick and dying, women who laid out the dead, women who deloused and defleaed people, who nursed and cooked and cleaned for the ill and injured, were increasingly demarcated from male surgeons and apothecaries. Female roles which might have combined cure and care were reduced to care.

Although some Poor Law responsibilities, such as pensions for the elderly and disabled, dealt with groups often considered dependent, others met crises less predictable. Few families in Abson could have considered themselves immune from the kinds of catastrophes that broke up Hester Dore's family, or that struck Brice Kains' family. The death or desertion of a spouse, or an episode of smallpox, could destroy many a precarious family economy. The ability of a family to care for its own was one of the key determinants of Poor Law utilization and of definitions of dependency that shaped the provision of such relief.

In the city, it is more difficult to ascertain the circumstances that led an individual to seek institutional health care. In part, this is a problem of records; Infirmary admission registers do not detail how a patient came to the hospital. However, an analysis of the types of people using the institution and the ways in which they utilized it suggests that paths to the institution were shaped by factors similar to those in the countryside. In the city, of course, there was a range of institutional health-care provision. In addition to the Infirmary, the Corporation of the Poor offered both inpatient and outpatient care through the workhouse, which came to develop its own medical staff. Its role as a second infirmary, to which accident cases were brought and at which local surgeons vied for positions, highlights the connections among health-care institutions in the city, be they Poor Law or voluntary. There is evidence to suggest that the Corporation provided a domiciliary

Table 5.1. *Age structure of Bristol Infirmary patients, 1771–1805*

Age structure England		Bristol Infirmary, % of total			
		Male		Female	
Age	Percent	Inpatients	Outpatients	Inpatients	Outpatients
0–4	13.1–14.7	1.0	9.6	3.3	9.4
5–14	20.6–23.1	13.9	12.0	9.7	8.0
15–24	17.7–18.7	23.2	12.6	30.9	18.5
25–59	37.6–39.1	53.7	55.9	49.6	56.4
60+	7.3–8.5	8.2	9.9	6.5	7.7
Totals		100.00	100.00	100.00	100.00

health-care service, particularly to the elderly, perhaps analogous to both the Infirmary's outpatient department and to the care provided by the rural Poor Law.[12] Because almost nothing remains of the Corporation's records, a set of settlement examinations has been used for comparison with Infirmary patients although individuals so examined cannot be considered representative of urban Poor Law clients.[13]

As in the countryside, city users of health-care institutions are not clearly differentiated from their neighbors; they are not recognizable as a permanently dependent group. For example, hospital patients from the parish of SS. Philip and Jacob had occupations similar to those of their neighbors. Even those who were examined by the Poor Law seem to have held the same kinds of jobs, when in work. The single largest group in each case were laborers, a type of work that ordinarily implied low status, low wages, and intermittent employment. Others were craftsmen, such as cabinet-makers and silversmiths, or unskilled workers in local industries, the glass, brass, lead, and sugar manufactories. Neither Poor Law examinees nor hospital patients were occupationally distinct from the rest of the parish's workforce.[14]

An analysis of age structure and family status suggests why and how people came to seek institutional health care in the hospital.[15] The age structure of England's population (taken from Wrigley and Schofield's reconstruction) and that of the Infirmary's patients differs in a few key areas (see Table 5.1). For example, there were many more young adults in the hospital than would be predicted by the age structure of the country's population. Thus, for example, young people aged fifteen to twenty-four accounted for about 18 percent of the country's population. But 31 percent of all female inpatients were between these ages. Although it is probably true that there were proportionally more young women in Bristol than in the country as a whole, no such overrepresentation characterized outpatient numbers. Only about 19 percent of female outpatients were aged fifteen to twenty-four – a figure in accord with the general population.[16] Men aged fifteen to twenty-four show a similar, although less marked, pattern. These young inpatients were probably unmarried men and women, living in lodging houses, perhaps immigrants to Bristol, perhaps working as servants – those least likely to have household support or domestic care if they became ill.[17]

For example, take the case of the Lackingtons. James Lackington moved to Bristol from southern Somerset with his new wife. Neither knew a soul in the city; they had come seeking employment. When she fell ill, James was able to look after his wife, but their means were slim. Their landlady began to worry, "she seemed very much alarmed at our situation, or rather for her own, I suppose, as thinking we might in some measure become burthensome to her."[18] Lackington spent the family's resources (a total of two shillings and ninepence) on medicines and his wife slowly recovered. Had Mrs. Lackington been single, she might well have been desirous of hospital admission, because she had neither family nor friends in the city, and probably could not have paid the rent while she was ill, let alone afforded medical attention.

By tracing hospital patients back into parish registers, it is possible to determine the probable extent of their local family resources – was a patient single or married, a parent, a widow? However, almost half of the Infirmary patients (42 percent) do not appear in parish registers at all. The most obvious reason for this lack of information is mobility. A person might have lived in the parish for a time that did not include any events likely to be recorded in a register; in other words, neither born nor buried, wed nor a parent, in that parish. Mobility has been shown to be quite high, even in rural districts, in early modern England, and it should be no surprise that relatively few parishioners remained "under observation" for long periods of time.[19] Another explanation is dissent; Bristol had long been known as a city in which various kinds of nonconformity flourished. Anecdotal evidence from nearby rural parishes suggests that a certain proportion of children were never baptized in the Anglican Church because of their parents' beliefs.[20]

However, those who do not show up in the registers were, as a group, more likely to include single, transient individuals who did not have long-term ties to the parish. Although moving across a parish boundary in the city was trivial, SS. Philip and Jacob was large and, in the north and east, did not adjoin any other urban parish, making moving more consequential than in other parishes. In addition, some manufactories in the parish were unique in Bristol, exerting a certain pull on their workers to stay nearby. Many men and women in this sample of patients moved six or seven times, but remained within parish boundaries. Thus, the group who never appear in the registers form a contrast, albeit imperfect, with those who remained longer, married, had children, and presumably developed stronger local ties. In sum, many Infirmary patients did not have local family, suggesting that the hospital played a role similar to that of the rural Poor Law in providing an alternative to domestic care. Although the founders of the institution had emphasized its role in maintaining productive family economies, its clients often used the hospital, not to reinforce family structures, but to substitute for them.

In particular, patients made choices between inpatient and outpatient care based upon family support. The actual route by which an individual became a hospital patient is not entirely clear, but it does seem that he or she had some choice as to whether to seek a bed. First of all, inpatients could be admitted only on Mondays or Thursdays, and were examined by the trustees and house visitors as to their worthiness. Outpatients, on the other hand, were seen on Tuesday, Wednesday, Friday, and Saturday. Clearly, patients probably needed to decide what day to go to the hospital, although the physicians could also switch a patient from outpatient to inpatient status and vice versa. In addition, the recommender might specify inpatient or outpatient status for his client.[21]

As discussed above, young women were especially likely to be inpatients, suggesting that lack of family resources shaped their utilization of the Infirmary. Similarly, old people with family connections were much more likely to remain outpatients than were their counterparts without local kin. For example, in cases of fever, only a third of old people with family became inpatients; 70 percent of those without family did so, relying upon the hospital to provide care that absent families could not. This same pattern holds true for four of the five most common diagnoses.

Although the thrust of this chapter emphasizes the ways in which institutional medicine was embedded within the matrix of charity and poor relief, health and illness were nevertheless significant aspects of that relief. As discussed, 17 percent of all Abson's relief recipients were injured or sick, requiring care and medical attendance as well as support. As Margaret Pelling has recently argued for early modern Norwich, health care was a significant component of poor relief. Ill health was a "worthy" category of poverty.[22] In Abson sickness had a dramatic impact upon the Poor Law in times of epidemics. In the early 1780s, Abson experienced a wave of smallpox cases and probably typhus and ague as well.[23] The proportion of poor relief spent on illness parallels these parish epidemics. The percent of total parish expenditure on illness climbed from 14 percent to a high of 38 percent in 1785, and did not return to "normal" levels until 1789. The knock-on effects of epidemics continued to shape poor relief for years, in terms of aid to disrupted families. In 1788, for example, over a quarter of all expenditure was to families who had lost a parent to disease or desertion. In sum, illness was a significant determinant of overall levels of relief.

Because Infirmary records were largely constructed by physicians and surgeons, the medical aspects of Infirmary utilization are easier to trace than the social or economic ones. Patients came to the hospital with a wide variety of ailments. Although many different diagnostic labels were used to describe what was wrong with patients, the ten most frequent diagnostic categories accounted for 56 percent of all the patients. (see Table 5.2)

The most striking feature of these patients' diagnoses is the large number of fever cases treated by the hospital. Some eighteenth-century hospitals explicitly excluded fever and other so-called contagious diseases from the wards. In Manchester, for instance, a separate fever hospital was created, albeit for political as much as medical reasons.[24] Given the marshy and low-lying land that comprised SS Philip and Jacob, fever could hardly have been uncommon; it seems to have been both endemic and epidemic. In 1774, 1792, 1800, and 1801, atypically large numbers of fever patients came to the hospital. But there were only two years (1776, 1797)

Table 5.2. *The most frequent diagnostic categories of Bristol Infirmary patients*

	Percent of all patients
Fever	16.6
Respiratory	15.1
Trauma	13.9
Abscess, ulcer	13.2
Miscellaneous	10.1
Rheumatism, muscular	7.6
Skin problems	7.6
Digestive	5.7
Reproductive	3.8
Venereal	2.5
Operative conditions	2.4
Dropsy, etc.	1.5

in which no patient in the SS Philip and Jacob sample was diagnosed as suffering from fever. And fever, of course, required the sort of bed rest and domiciliary care that many of the Infirmary's patients could not rely upon family or friends to provide.

The other nine most common diagnoses included trauma (contusions, wounds), symptomatic complaints (cough, itch), and semichronic ailments (rheumatism, abscess, ulcer). I have consistently used the Infirmary's terminology rather than modernizing – retrospectively diagnosing – the hospital's language. Hence "rheumatism" or "ulcer" does not equate with the twentieth-century usage of the same term. Ulcers, for instance, were almost all leg ulcers, probably closer to what twentieth-century doctors would call ulcerations.[25]

All the Infirmary patients had one thing in common: a likelihood of leaving the hospital cured. The outcome of therapy is listed in the register for all inpatients and for the early years of the outpatients. Of this sample, 86.5 percent were discharged as cured. Another 2.1 percent were "relieved." A handful of patients went from inpatient to outpatient status, or vice versa. Of course, the categories of "cured" and "relieved" are problematic. Neither physicians, surgeons, nor patients emphasized rigid categories in their analyses of disease. Perceiving the body as a system that required balance above all, physicians were oriented toward interpreting the meanings of illness and restoring the body to health rather than prescribing specific remedies. Indeed, for the physicians and surgeons, such specific cures might be the hallmark of quackery.[26] Thus, an Infirmary cure should be understood as a return to a balanced state of health rather than as a specific repair of a body part or function.

A more absolute statistic is that only 4.1 percent of all patients died in hospital, mostly of fevers. Previous generations of historians have questioned whether hospitals were "gateways to death."[27] The argument seems pointless in the case of Bristol. There is no way to portray the Infirmary as a last-resort institution where people went to die. It had defined itself as an institution for patients who would recover to lead productive lives. The city workhouse, on the other hand, was more of a nursing home, and greater proportions of its inmates died. In the mid-1790s, there were about four hundred people living in the Mint, many elderly or disabled. Almost 20 percent of the residents died every year. However, for each inmate, there two people who received out-relief on a regular basis, and another four who got on occasional help.[28]

Whatever may have constituted a cure, the Infirmary was purveying something that people wanted or needed. Figure 5.1 indicates the increase in usage the hospital experienced in the latter half of the century. Early voluntary hospitals have been understood as largely insignificant to the local setting of health and disease, irrelevant to patterns of morbidity and mortality by reason of their smallness.[29] For mortality, this is undoubtedly so. But two points need to be emphasized. First, in Bristol the rapid growth of the outpatient sector of the hospital suggests that a significant proportion of the city's population utilized the hospital. Second, this institution was clearly providing something people wanted; however unpleasant hospital treatment may seem to twentieth-century historians, it was much in demand in its own time. Historians of the hospital who have emphasized its impact upon the medical professions have failed to note its crucial function in creating and reforming the role of the patient as well as the status of the doctor.

In other words, patients related to the hospital in a number of ways. For some, it provided cure, for others a mixture of domiciliary care and cure. Just as in the rural Poor Law, the provision of institutional health care varied according to need and circumstance.

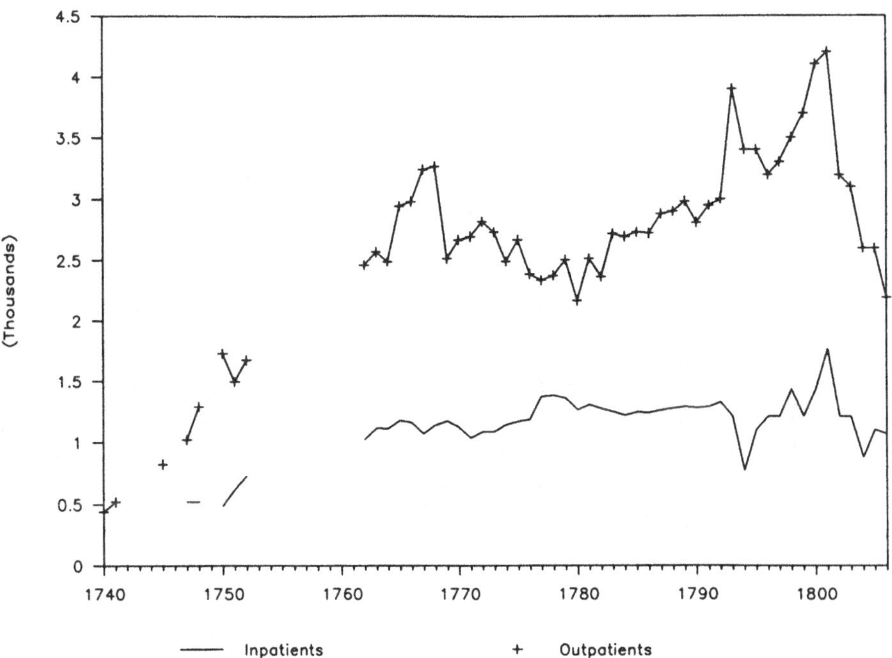

Figure 5.1. Bristol Infirmary patient numbers

No single kind of dependency characterized either institution. Viewed from this perspective, infirmary and Poor Law look quite similar, despite their designers' intent to distinguish between worthy and unworthy poor.

6

The abdication of the governors

Over the course of the century, the infirmary took on a medical character that became increasingly pronounced; the balance shifted slowly from charity to medicine. This process was neither inevitable nor foreordained; it resulted from the intersection of the growth of professional interest with a mutation in charitable impulse. Neither causes nor consequences of this change were solely medical, let alone peculiar to the infirmary. Its effects, often unforseen by participants, extended far beyond hospital gates. However, it was within the infirmary that the changing relationships of rich and poor overlay those of doctor and patient, and it was within the infirmary that a new style of interaction between sufferers and healers was forged from the bonds of charity. Chapters 6, 7, and 8 examine the process of change from the points of view of governor, medical man, and patient in turn. No one group completely controlled events within the hospital; nor were these groups' perspectives wholly consonant with each other.

When the Bristol Infirmary was founded, initial enthusiasm and a commitment to an inquiring and sustained relationship with the objects of charity created an institution closely ruled by its governors. A visiting committee inspected the hospital's household accounts every week, admitted and discharged patients, and generally supervised the day-to-day running of the institution. Those governors who did not take a role in administration nevertheless exercised their privileges to admit patients and elect Infirmary staff. Over the course of the century, however, the close involvement of governors faded, as the role of subscriber became a more ceremonial or symbolic one. The reasons for this abdication were complex; its roots lay in changes in the balance of power in city governance as well as in the burgeoning of a multitude of other medical charities.

For much of the century, however, hospital management was characterized by tight family connections and by highly individualized relationships among donors and recipients. As discussed, the Quaker Champion family provided seven of the Infirmary's treasurers during the eighteenth century. A map of the connections among Quaker hospital subscribers is a virtual blueprint of the family and commercial ties that characterized Bristol's Quaker community. Banking, marriage, manufacturing, and trade made and strengthened the bonds of a shared religious commitment. For example, the Champion family provided hospital supporters in every generation. Nehemiah Champion II founded the Bristol Brass Company in 1702, along with Edward Lloyd, Thomas Coster, and Abraham Elton. Various members of the Harford family soon joined them. All of these men (or their sons), save the Tory member of Parliament Coster, became hospital subscribers. Nehemiah's great-great-grandson Richard Champion III not only had several close family connections with the Infirmary but many of his friends and business associates were involved with the hospital as well. Two of his most faithful correspondents, Alicia Witts and Sukey Rogers, were connected by birth or marriage to hospital governors. In Champion's business dealings, he was associated with Edward Brice, Joseph Harford, Joseph Fry, Abraham Clibborn, and John Peach, all hospital subscribers, and almost all Quakers. Such details could be rehearsed for many of Bristol's leading Quaker families as well as for some Anglican and Unitarian ones.

In other words, this community, knit together by marriage and commerce, existed prior to the creation of the hospital, and the Bristol Infirmary can be seen as one of its products. It would be naive to suggest that the Infirmary solely represented this largely Quaker, progressive, Whig merchant interest. But the people who ran the hospital – the treasurer and committee – were disproportionately drawn from it.[1] And, as discussed, a substantial proportion of the city's Quakers supported the institution.

Simple statistics portray hospital subscribers as an overwhelmingly city-based, nonlanded-gentry group of men.[2] Three points emerge from an analysis of hospital supporters. First, many were merchants, or businessmen associated with manufacturing for the colonial trade, while many others described themselves in pollbooks or directories as "gentlemen" or "Esq."[3] For instance, Isaac

Elton Sr., was an alderman and merchant, whose close relatives swelled the ranks of city governance. Elton himself became Master of the Merchant Venturers, mayor, member of the Tory Steadfast Society, and participated in numerous other civic functions. Or to take a Quaker example, William Fry, distiller and wine merchant, deputy governor of the Corporation of the Poor, was a hospital subscriber from his youth until he died. These merchants and manufacturers, often involved in a range of civic responsibilities and privileges, remained at fairly constant numbers throughout the century. However, as total numbers of subscribers grew, the proportion of these merchants and manufacturers fell.

Second, at the outset the Infirmary had a small following among the "old" professions – medical men and clergymen – but in the 1790s, architects, schoolmasters (mostly unbeneficed clergymen), customs collectors, factors, and surveyors started to patronize the hospital. Men such as John Powell, collector of customs, or the Rev. W. J. Hort, who ran the Ladies Boarding School, began to appear among the Infirmary subscribers. It seems likely that medical men, a few of whom initially supported the hospital, began to fade away when competition became intense for hospital posts and a subscription would have implied supporting one's professional competitors. On the other hand, the "new" professionals, the administrators and public servants, could acquire a certain prestige and social cachet through an Infirmary subscription.

Finally, one of the most notable things about hospital governors was their range of occupations. Although many were merchants and gentlemen, others from more humble backgrounds, such as grocers, carpenters, and mariners, paid their two guineas a year. Slade Baker, a linen draper, who by 1774 styled himself as Esquire, Governor of the Incorporation of the Poor, and member of the elite Steadfast Society, represented one sort of hospital governor. But Nathaniel Ogborne, a Quaker ironmonger, or Nicholas Blanning, a silk dyer, or Messrs. Bulgin and Rosser, booksellers and printers, represented another. These subscribers have tended to be overlooked by historians because biographical data is difficult to obtain for those who led less public and privileged lives than Slade Baker or Isaac Elton. But their rank-and-file support, and their recommendations of individual patients, remained significant to the Infirmary throughout the century.

Bristol's Infirmary thus enjoyed the support of the city's mercantile classes. From what is known of other eighteenth-century voluntary hospitals, it seems that Bristol's character and reputation as a place of trade colored its hospital. Roy Porter has characterized subscribers to provincial infirmaries as a more lordly group than Bristol's seem to have been; other hospitals relied upon aristocratic and gentry support.[4] Such local variation should come as no surprise. As John Pickstone has shown for patterns of development in the North-West, the peculiarities of local social and political structures shaped hospital provision.[5] Although, as Porter argues, emulation was a prod to infirmary foundations, it is also clear that very local political and social factors determined the extent to which such feelings of emulation might be translated into bricks and mortar. For example, it has been argued that party politics determined hospital patronage in the metropolis.[6] But Bristol's allegiances were more complex, made of sectarian loyalties, family ties, and civic ritual rather than the mere bonds of party.

The expression of such allegiances to party, sect, and family translated in a much more personal form in the subscriber's relationship with his patients. For most of the century, admission to the Infirmary was very much an individual affair between subscriber and patient. For example, Richard Symes, vicar of St. Werburgh's, described sending a woman to the Infirmary. Betty Butler, aged thirty, a poor woman, came begging at Symes's door, almost blind from a blow to her eye (someone had thrown a potato at her). Symes, pursuing his avocation as an electrical healer, treated her, and she was healed. The next spring, wrote Symes, "she came to me, begging a Note to the Infirmary, telling me she wanted to take Physic, that it was always her custom every Spring . . . I gave her a Note for an Out-Patient."[7] Betty Butler took her physic, and caught a cold. Then her sight worsened, and she was admitted as an inpatient. But she did not like the hospital treatment, and so left the Infirmary, returning to Symes, who reelectrified her. Fortunately, it worked again, and she was evidently cured. Thus, for Symes and Butler, admission to the Infirmary was only one aspect of an ongoing relationship of patronage. And for Butler, of course, hospital admission was just a part of her own health regimen, integrated into the common custom of purging in the springtime, and interspersed with any number of other therapeutic interludes.

The personal nature of hospital recommendation is supported by an analysis of who recommended whom. About two-thirds of patients came from the same parish as their recommender (64 percent in 1750; 68 percent in 1775). Considering that there were seventeen parishes in Bristol, as well as the parishes of rural Somerset and Gloucestershire, this finding is quite strong, though not unexpected. Given the small size of inner-city parishes, many recipients of Infirmary charity were probably known to their recommenders, at least by sight.

However, even statistics such as these tell only part of the story. Richard Frampton was a most unusual hospital governor; he recommended eighty-two patients in a single year. Clearly, he served as a sort of almoner for a large group of people. He remains an obscure figure, a leather dresser, a Quaker who lived in the parish of St. Peter, probably in King Square. Only 19 percent of his patients came from his own parish. However, another 59 percent came from the two adjoining large poor parishes. In other words, Frampton was known in his neighborhood for his association with the Infirmary, and people relied upon him for admission. So too, Quaker hospital governors counted on Frampton's services in weeding out unacceptable potential patients.

Patients saw their connection to the Infirmary in the light of personal patronage and relied upon one subscriber for multiple admissions. Squire Avery, for instance, was treated for leg ulcers in May 1775, and then returned to Richard Frampton to ask for a second admission in August, for an abscess of his big toe. Similarly, Thomas Shapland, a soap boiler, recommended both Ben and Mary Evans to the Infirmary to be treated for fever and cough. Mary recovered, but Ben Evans came down with peripneumonia a few months later. He returned to Shapland, his patron, for another recommendation to the hospital.

The ties of neighborhood were the strongest and most evident links between patron and client. Probably the connections among churchgoers, especially among sectarian groups, were very strong, but unfortunately they remain difficult to document. A second bond was that between worker and employer, but here evidence is far more mixed. From a sample of patients from the parish of SS. Philip and Jacob, occupations of subscribers and patients whom they recommended can be compared.[8] This data, however, is imperfect; in only thirty-six cases is evidence for the occupations of both worker and recommender complete. Fourteen were recommended by (probable) employers and twenty-two were not.

For example, Elton, Miles & Co. sent Samuel Plaister, a forty-five-year-old glassmaker, to the Infirmary in 1798; he had an ulcerated leg. This firm's use of their subscription extended to sending Rose Evans, the widow of glassman John Evans, to hospital when she had pneumonia. Because this happened eleven years after her husband died, perhaps she had a long-standing relationship of patronage with her husband's employers; this represents a traditional form of charity far more than it constitutes a precursor to any sort of workman's compensation or medical insurance. Similarly, private individuals recommended their workers. Edward Brice, who owned a sugar refinery, sent James Rogers, a forty-one-year-old sugar baker to hospital in 1801 with an abscessed leg. He also arranged for Mary Price, the daughter of a sugar baker, to have her contused leg attended to in 1799. By this point, industrial or workplace accidents would have been sent to the Infirmary as casualties; no patronage of an employer was necessary. Thus, most patronage that appears to be workplace-oriented was more closely tied to older forms of obligation and expectation between master and workman. The same kind of individual connections characterized the patronage of neighborhood and workplace.

This personal context could still shape Bristol charity at the end of the century. For instance, as late as the hard winter of 1814, parishes set up their own committees to provide additional relief for the poor. In the parish of St. James, such a committee evaluated the claims of the poor and then sent on their recommendations to the workhouse, where their appointees would receive bread and soup. Letters to this committee reflect the personal bonds upon which people relied in hard times. Luke Clary declared, "This is to certify that Margaret Green is a Widow & have Two Children she is a sober Wellbehaved Hones Industrious Woman and lives in my house on James Back."[9] Landlords supported their tenants, employers their former workers, a shoemaker his fellow craftsman. By this time, however, these personal ties were becoming rarer, and only a crisis could provoke their assertion.

Strong personal links between patron and client structured rural poor relief as well. Petitioners were usually known to the vestry and overseer to whom they applied, and the local vicar might intervene as well. For example, John Skinner, rector of the Somerset parish of Camerton, was frequently involved in negotiations with a stingy vestry. When a collier had broken his back in the mine, Skinner requested, and paid for, a second doctor's opinion. Skinner threatened the first doctor, who worked for a friendly society, that he "would take minutes of everything that had occurred, and draw up the case, should the man receive any detriment from the delay."[10] When the collier subsequently died, Skinner split the bill for his treatment with the lady of the manor and the vestry, and attended the vestry meeting at which his widow pleaded for support.[11] Clearly, in this case, Skinner saw himself as the patron and advocate of the unfortunate miner.

Often, however, Skinner was on the other side. He made trouble for a woman who attempted bigamy and had borne several children out of wedlock. On another occasion, he took the vestry to task for its support of a "bad" woman.[12] In any case, the recipients of relief in this parish were almost always known to both the vestry and the vicar; relief was neither standardized nor impersonal, but reflected an individual's relationship with the ruling farmers of the community, who managed the vestry, which allocated poor-law monies.

So too, individual charity was structured by deferential social relationships in the countryside. For example, in a fictional narrative of a working man's battle with drink, the man's wife went to beg some ale from the innkeeper, in order to treat her husband's fever. The innkeeper, Martha Pritchard, initially refused, but then relented, saying, "And now I bethink me, Sarah, you always stood back when we were at the church door together, to let me walk out first; and when we meet in the Lane, don't you stop short, and look down upon the ground, and make a curtsey, and say, 'Your servant, Mrs. Pritchard.' "[13] Sarah Jenkins got her ale for her sick husband, because of her previous relationship with the innkeeper. Even on as humble a level as this, charity was a part of appropriate behavior between people of different rank. Just as in the big-city displays of power and patronage, the Infirmary processions and convivial-society banquets, charity provided an arena for the assertion and testing of the fine gradations of a multilayered social hierarchy.[14]

In the latter half of the century, the relationships between patron and patient underwent a dramatic change. No longer were hospital subscribers intimately involved in hospital management; no longer was a recommendation for admission emblematic of the subscriber's and patient's place in society. In 1750 the mean number of patients recommended by a subscriber was 3.8, and fell to .33 by 1806. In other words, the average mid-eighteenth-century subscriber made himself responsible for about four patients per year; fifty years later, only one in three bothered to recommend even a single patient per year. This trend was already underway by 1775; the mean number of patients per subscriber had fallen to 2.5 by this date.

This change was not the simple effect of a growing pool of subscribers; roughly, the number of subscribers tripled, but the number of patients per subscriber fell ninefold. Nor was it the result of hospital overcrowding, because most patients were recommended to be outpatients, on which there was no ceiling. At the same time, many more patients were admitted as casualties: 15 percent of total admissions in 1751, 26 percent in 1805, climbing to 32 percent by 1826. Casualties did not require a recommendation; they were admitted directly by the physician or, more often, by the surgeon, a process detailed further in the next chapter. In other words, surgeons rather than subscribers began to determine who would become an Infirmary patient. Medical rather than social worthiness began to characterize potential patients.

Subscribers' withdrawal from active involvement in the Infirmary was a key factor in the transformation of the hospital from charity to medical workplace. Certainly, it was the surgeons who made the Infirmary their own. But they were able to govern the hospital only as the subscribers abdicated, taking an increasingly detached attitude toward their roles as governors. Such a redefinition of the role and responsibilities of a hospital governor resulted from changes outside the Infirmary. First, on a very local level, medical charity in Bristol was in flux. Medical and other charities became more specialized, and in so doing, created corporate identities for themselves that rivaled that of the Infirmary. Second, the social structure of Bristol changed as the city grew larger. Finally, the shift in patterns of recommendation reflected and embodied a larger process of the distancing of rich and poor, of the retreat of the elite from a social structure that predicated various rights and responsibilities to rich and poor. To put it another way, the formation of class militated against individualized relationships of patronage modeled upon a chain of social relationships stretching from high to low. Charity became the interaction between groups, characterized by economic status, rather than that between individuals based upon personal obligation and expectation.[15]

The shift away from personal styles of benevolence was reflected in expansion and increased specialization of Bristol charities. For instance, a dispensary was founded in 1775, which, unlike earlier ones, flourished for decades.[16] It was designed to complement the Infirmary, by seeing people who could not leave home. The dispensary also inaugurated a midwifery service, for women at home. In its early years, it saw perhaps 500 patients a year, but by 1807 this had risen to 2,000, with an additional 500 midwifery patients.[17] Like the hospital, it had two physicians, at least four surgeons, and one or two apothecaries. Unlike the hospital, it also had four or five midwives, supervised by the surgeons.

The city workhouse also took on an increasingly medical character. From its inception, it had provided basic medical care to its inmates. Its first physician was Thomas Dover, inventor of the eponymous remedy widely used throughout the century. In its early years, the Mint hired women to delouse inmates and sent children suffering from the King's Evil (scrofula) to be touched by the monarch in hopes of cure. By the middle of the century, the workhouse had expanded its medical staff to rival that of the Infirmary. Often surgeons and physicians used a Mint appointment as a stepping-stone to one at the hospital. Probably the workhouse also provided a domiciliary medical service, particularly to the elderly. Although separate medical and surgical wards were not instituted until the early nineteenth century, the Mint was a significant medical institution in Bristol from the middle of the eighteenth century.

Bristol also supported a Sailor's Hospital, although almost no records of its existence survive. It was located at the Hotwells, at the docks, and may have been set up by commercial or merchant interests.[18] Also at the Hotwells, Thomas Beddoes set up his Pneumatic Institute in the 1790s, to investigate the therapeutic effects of gases. Although at the beginning he was forced to bribe patients with payments of sixpence each per day (they were afraid of being experimented upon), Beddoes's experiences changed dramatically when he gave up gases and started to dispense straightforward, nonexperimental health care to the poor.[19] In six months during

Table 6.1. *Medical and related charities in Bristol*

Name	Founded	Object
Bristol Infirmary	1737	Inpatients, outpatients
Dispensary, Wesleyan	1747	Outpatients
Dispensary	1775	Outpatients
Strangers Friend Society	1786	Sick and distressed
Friend-in-Need Society	1789, 1809	Sick and distressed
Female Penitentiary	1800	Wayward girls
Bristol Samaritan	1807	Sick and distressed
Female Misericordia	1809	Lying-in women
Hospital for Diseases of the Eyes	1810	Eye hospital
Dispensary for Eye Complaints	1812	Eye clinic
Prudent Man's Friend	1812	Small loans
Dorcas Society	1813	Lying-in women
Clifton Dispensary	1813	Outpatients
Asylum for Indigent Blind	1813	Home for the blind
Inst. for the Diseased Second Poor	1820	Poor by illness
Bristol Lying-in Society	c. 1820	Lying-in women
SS. Philip & Jacob Lying-in Society	c. 1820	Lying-in women
Refuge Society	?	Distressed women

1803, he saw over 900 patients.[20] Specialized medical institutions were inaugurated in 1810, when William Goldwyer started an Eye Hospital; three years later, he had seen over 2,000 patients.[21] In 1812, a rival eye clinic was opened by another surgeon, J. B. Estlin, in direct if charitable competition with that of Goldwyer.[22] Table 6.1 lists medical and quasimedical charities in the city; the multiplication and diversification of such institutions became significant in the 1780s and 1790s. By 1820, when William Salmon, a surgeon-apothecary, wished to found a medical charity, he had to dream up "Mr. Salmon's Institution for the Relief of the Diseased Second Poor," for those who had been rendered poverty-stricken by illness. Salmon argued that those "who once enjoyed every domestic comfort" should not have to mingle with "the motley group of miserable beings" who attended the Infirmary.[23] In other words, by the second decade of the nineteenth century, Bristol had an abundance, possibly even an overabundance, of medical charities. Thus both philanthropist and patient had an increasingly wide range of institutional choices he or she might choose to patronize, many of which were modeled upon the Infirmary. And, of course, as the Infirmary grew larger, the personal quality of its charity perhaps became less evident.

Many of the new smaller charities were increasingly governed by medical men rather than by subscribers. Such charities were often the purview of one or two medical men, and they saw these institutions as a means of making their name.[24] Perhaps the eleemosynary element of such institutions became less distinct when benefit to the medical man became as apparent as benefit to the sufferer. Offering free care to the poor had long been a gambit of struggling doctors, and many advertisements testify to the popularity of the practice. Contemporaries pointed out that these offers should be examined critically; often they served a dual function. Not only did they enhance the reputation of a practitioner by providing an excuse to advertise; they also provided income. Such "charitable" practitioners might see patients gratuitously, but give them inscrutable prescriptions that could be filled only by one particular druggist or apothecary. Needless to add, the druggist owed the practitioner a large kickback.[25]

But by the early nineteenth century, practitioners who had been trained in hospitals used medical charity to acquire social rather than actual capital. In so doing, they tried to distance themselves from their historical roots in marketplace medicine, drawing instead on the gentlemanly heritage of charity. Thus, for example, many more surgeons than physicians founded and ran medical charities in Bristol; physicians already had the status surgeons were eager to acquire. Recall, for example, Richard Smith's disparagement of "shop" medicine (see Chapter 3) – far better for a medical man to ground himself in the world of urban philanthropy than in the shop.

A sarcastic article in the 1809 *Edinburgh Medical and Surgical Journal* poked fun at the pretensions of medical charity, in the tongue-in-cheek guise of offering advice to the young practitioner. The anonymous author wrote, "Endeavour to establish a hospital or dispensary by the voluntary subscriptions of your friends; for many men have wriggled themselves into notice by professions of charity, and have qualified themselves for genteel practice, by sharpening their wits upon the carcases of the poor."[26] It would seem that this writer's ironic advice was well heeded in Bristol. Thus, the invention of medical charity was the product of the medical marketplace and yet repudiated it, denying the commercial roots of medical enterprise, and adopting instead the demeanor of the gentleman philanthropist. And as charities became the properties of medical men, older style patrons increasingly distanced themselves from such institutions.

At the same time, shifts in benevolence and charity were also a part of larger changes in the structures of Bristol society. In particular, I draw upon the analysis of Elizabeth Baigent, a social geographer who has examined the composition of the city in 1775, using poll books, a directory, and local rates (i.e., taxes). She argues that in the latter half of the eighteenth century, disparities between rich and poor grew. Wealth was concentrated in fewer hands and the gulf between poverty and prosperity increased. The divisions of rich and poor were expressed geographically; a new leisured and professional class established itself in the suburban parishes and in Clifton, distancing itself from the older, crowded inner-city parishes.[27]

This increasing spatial differentiation of rich and poor had two consequences for the Infirmary. First, some of these communities established their own charities, such as the Clifton Dispensary, or the Bedminster-based Bristol Lying-In Society, which provided an alternate means of dispensing patronage and created an identity that was local rather than citywide. The very success of the Infirmary in creating and maintaining a highly defined social group of subscribers perhaps told against it in the longer term. As suburbs like Clifton grew, their elites defined their identities through institutions that mimicked those of the larger city. In this case, emulation spelt diminution for the older institution.

Second, these outer parishes did not have the mixtures of rich and poor, of residence and workplace, that the older inner-city parishes did. In a very real sense, the face-to-face contacts between rich and poor, whether in the context of the workplace (many merchants and manufacturers lived close to, or even next to, their warehouses and manufactories) or just of neighborhood, were no part of Clifton and other suburbs. In 1750, 28 percent of all Infirmary subscribers lived in the small inner-city parishes; by 1806, only 6 percent did so. At the same time, the proportion of suburban hospital supporters tripled, from 4 percent to 13 percent of total subscribers. In other words, patterns of hospital support were in part those of the city's ruling classes; geography and occupational structures tell the same story of growing distance. Patients, on the other hand, continued to be drawn from large, poor city parishes like SS. Philip and Jacob, St. James, and St. Mary Redcliffe.

The patronage of the "new" professions may have also contributed to a separation of patients and subscribers. Like the residents of suburban parishes, these men lacked everyday contact with the poor because they did not manage large workforces. The networks of patronage that sent the daughters and widows of glassmakers to the Infirmary were not constructed by schoolmasters or attorneys, for obvious reasons.

These changes in the Infirmary's role in the social life of the city were also due to subtle changes in the meanings of charity itself. It was not just that individuals wishing to help the poor saw many more institutions clamoring for their support. These institutions were of a much more specialized nature. In part, this specialization was the expression of the highly factional nature of urban charity alluded to in Chapter 4. Thus for example, the roles of the Tabernacle in setting up the Castle Green Dispensary, or the Methodists in establishing the Strangers Friend Society were apparent to all. Where political strife of the 1730s could be momentarily healed by the foundation of the Infirmary, no such easy answers seemed possible in the years of the Napoleonic wars. Even the charities founded as a direct response to the troubles of the war and postwar era, such as the Clifton Dispensary, were resolutely local in character. No longer could a common interest in certain forms of charity be guaranteed to overwrite political difference in the city as a whole.

It was not just that one's sectarian and political alliances were made apparent through charitable giving. The definitions of "worthy" poor were narrowed to specific categories by these smaller charities, and thus they appealed to very particular interests. The Quakers, for example, were instrumental in founding the asylum for blind girls. The convivial Anchor Society relieved over a hundred lying-in mothers every year.[28] New charities focused on wayward girls, reformed prostitutes, travelers, and other specific categories of need. On first glance, the relationships between patron and recipient fostered by these smaller charities resembled those of the early Infirmary subscriber and patient, being based very much on personal knowledge of the recipient.

However, these newer charities inverted the timing and rhythm of the donor-recipient relationship. They represented the working-out of the relationship between middle and working classes rather than the individualized character of the encounters between master and man, or poor and wealthy Quaker. Earlier, a hospital recommendation was a part of a longer-term relationship of patronage, in which the client was already known to the giver, and would probably remain a client of that donor after his or her hospital visit. Not so in new charities, which emphasized visiting and personal inspection in order to assess an individual's merit as a charity case.[29]

For example, Bristol lying-in charities founded in the early nineteenth century represented a very different understanding of the relationship of donor and recipient than had their earlier counterparts, discussed in Chapter 4. The Dorcas, Misericordia, and Bristol Lying-In charities, all founded in the early nineteenth century, were a new type of benevolent institution. Each of these was oriented toward the specific problems of poor mothers. For instance, the Misericordia founded a communal kitchen from which members fed new mothers nourishing meals of meat soups, gruts (a sort of oatmeal), caudle, and puddings, fortified with occasional brandy, rum, or wine. A typical case would be that of Mrs. Mary Edwards, who lived in lodgings in St. Paul's parish. She was loaned a bed-gown, given nine shillings, and ordered food from the kitchen for two months. Often women were loaned baby clothes as well.[30] Similarly, a small group of women, the Dorcas Society, met at each others' houses to sew sheets, childbed linen, and baby clothes, which were then lent to poor married women.[31] Each group managed, on limited funds, to aid about three hundred women a year.

The Bristol Lying-In charity was even more tightly focused; its real agenda was the training of midwives. Like the other two charities, visitors went to inspect the objects of their charity, often leaving small gifts of money, and occasionally a Bible. The midwives were expected to attend for three months gratis, while they were learning, and then were paid half a crown per delivery by the charity.[32]

All three charities relied upon personal inspection to ensure that only the "worthy" poor were aided, because recipients were not usually known to their benefactors. For example, an 1824 visitor found that the Lying-In charity had relieved "a woman of bad character" and a deputation was sent to call on the woman who had erred by suggesting that the charity aid such a person.[33] In a similar manner, the Clifton Dispensary Ladies Committee nominated two Visitors, whose task was "the duty of inspecting and visiting Midwifery Cases, and such other as they may think proper, and ascertaining the claims of the Sick as fit Objects of this Charity."[34] Visiting seems to have been largely a product of women's charities, deriving perhaps from the private aspects of such groups in contrast to the public and civic qualities of the Infirmary.

The minute books of these three lying-in charities reveal how alien donor and recipient were to each other. The Misericordia stipulated monthly visits, so that any individual recipient was probably seen only a handful of times, and by different visitors. About a quarter of the new mothers lived in lodgings, and visitors sometimes did not even know their names; they merely knew that there was a poor woman at a certain address. The Bristol Lying-in charity, more oriented toward medical practitioners, did not even visit those "comfortably provided for," who were presumably sufficiently respectable to avoid inspection.[35] In disagreements between midwives and patients, the lying-in societies did not take the side of their clients. Indeed, it took repeated complaints before a drunken midwife was sacked.[36]

Thus, unlike the earlier lying-in charities discussed in Chapter 4, the objects of such a charity were not known to their benefactors except on an inspection visit. Unlike the earlier ritualized gift of a pound, where a woman's worthiness was certified by her husband's freeman status, or by the personal recommendation of an alderman, these later charities relied upon personal inspection to determine a woman's right to aid. Also, the earlier charities were content to give a gift of money, presuming that the recipient would use it as she saw fit. Later charities were aimed at the symptomatic relief of poverty, or at specifically medical goals;

providing food, clothing and medical care in addition to money, and not incidentally underlining the medical nature of childbirth.

Like many subsequent ventures, these charities also gave a largely middle-class group of women an identity and a purpose; their own respectability was cemented by such gestures, and the monthly sewing circles and kitchen duties provided fellowship.[37] The claim of the Dorcas Society to be "without any partialities in religion" and the Lying-In charity's association with a particular Bedminster church suggest that they may have been the outgrowths of particular congregations.

These tiny lying-in charities indicate larger changes within the relationship of rich and poor. By the early nineteenth century, the personal relationships that had underlain charity and poor relief were beginning to erode; a poor person's worthiness had to be affirmed by inspection and surveillance, rather than by recommendation of his or her patron. As medical charity became increasingly distant and specialized, it came to represent a class-specific demonstration of respectability, as defined against poverty, rather than the perhaps gentler expression of social hierarchy it had been. Within the Infirmary, these changes were to begin to open the door to control of the institution by its surgeons.

7

Surgeons and the medicalization of the hospital

As face-to-face charity came to govern the hospital less, surgeons ruled the institution more. Their interest in the Infirmary derived from its growing role in education; as apprenticeship in the city waned, the hospital assumed a new educational function in the instruction of surgeons and apothecaries. The momentum of this dual change – the decline of apprenticeship and the rise of hospital instruction – had dramatic and largely unintended consequences for the hospital and its patients. In the city, the Infirmary assumed the mantle of corporate authority formerly worn by the city companies of barber-surgeons and apothecaries, and practitioners modeled themselves upon hospital men, rather than identifying themselves with a marketplace of medicine.

The Infirmary was not designed as an educational institution, nor were other early provincial hospitals. For instance, when Alured Clarke, founder of the first provincial voluntary hospital, was promoting his Winchester Infirmary, he barely mentioned medical education. He merely alluded to the fact that hospitals might afford physicians and surgeons a great deal of experience.[1] It should come as no surprise that Clarke did not emphasize teaching. His experience of medical education, like that of his contemporaries, rested upon two quite different institutions: apprenticeships and universities. Barber-surgeons and apothecaries were trained through apprenticeship; physicians through university education.

The first boys to be trained in the Bristol Infirmary were the apothecary's apprentices. In 1740, Joseph Shapland was apprenticed to the hospital apothecary. He was not so much a student as a servant. In the rules of the hospital, its founders had circumscribed the roles of the apothecary and his apprentices. The apothecary was in charge of the day-to-day functioning of the Infirmary; he labeled patients' beds with their names and diets, he visited the wards every morning, he kept the inpatient and outpatient registers, and summoned the physician and surgeons to attend at the hospital. He could not practice outside the hospital, and could not even leave the house for more than two hours without permission from the physicians and surgeons. His apprentices were even more subordinate; they were instructed to obey the physicians, the surgeons, the apothecary, and the matron, and to be polite to the patients. Both apprentices dispensed medicines from the apothecary's "shop," clearly based upon the marketplace model of practice. The junior apprentice also had to clean the surgeons' dressing boxes.[2] In other words, they performed the same sorts of tasks that any other apprentice outside the hospital would have done. As in the rest of the city, a cheaper form of labor can scarcely be imagined: apprentices paid the Infirmary 100 guineas for their maintenance, and made the apothecary an obligatory present of a further twenty guineas.

Joseph Shapland did quite well from this start. He was apprenticed for the usual seven years, and at their close he was appointed apothecary to the Infirmary. He left the hospital in 1752 at the age of twenty-seven to start his own practice. Four years later, he was taking on his own apprentices, sons of gentlemen who paid 100 guinea fees. His practice became so successful that he took one of his former apprentices, William Broderip, into partnership, and lived in fashionable Queen Square. However, even Shapland seems to have desired the cachet of formal medical credentials. In 1783, at the advanced age of fifty-six, he obtained an Aberdeen diploma, and became a physician.[3]

The situation of the Infirmary surgeons was rather different from that of the apothecary. In successful urban practice, as discussed in Chapter 3, apprentices were the usual and necessary accouterments of successful practitioners, providing labor in exchange for training. Surgeons' and apothecaries' apprentices did not experience very different modes of education. But within the Infirmary, surgeons were far more independent than the apothecary, and when surgeons brought apprentices into the institution, those apprentices enjoyed a correspondingly greater freedom than their apothecary counterparts. No longer were apprentices glorified servants; the hospital had its own to sweep and clean. Instead, apprentices constituted their own group within the institution, and when in the 1760s, surgeons started taking on pupils as well as apprentices, this group was greatly expanded. Surgeons had previously taught private pupils, who frequently lodged with them, and functioned like short-term senior apprentices, but Infirmary pupils were centered in the institution, not private practice. These pupils were technically under the direction of all the Infirmary surgeons, and paid each of them a fee. In the first few decades of this innovation, the numbers of pupils and apprentices remained about equal; perhaps a dozen of each were in the Infirmary in any given year. But by the 1780s and 1790s, pupils became the large majority of trainees. Not only were traditional patterns of apprenticeship breaking down citywide (as discussed below) but the Infirmary had, without conscious intent, created a functional replacement for apprenticeship.

Almost all of the information about this educational innovation comes from the memoirs of Richard Smith. In his meticulous attempts to chronicle everyone of merit associated with the hospital, he compiled small biographies of the hospital's pupils. Many of them had studied with him; in the period from 1798 to 1814 he had taught at least twenty-four pupils. But Smith was working largely from memory and hearsay, so his record is probably incomplete, although not necessarily erroneous in detail.

The apothecary's apprentices and the surgeons' apprentices and pupils created their own student subculture within the Infirmary. For instance, in 1776, there was a war between the surgeons' and apothecary's apprentices. Scuffles in the corridors, practical jokes, and hand-to-hand combat disrupted Infirmary routine.[4] In 1790, the matron died, leaving all of her possessions to the Infirmary. At the subsequent auction in the committee room of the hospital, auctioneers and bidders succumbed to fits of sneezing and coughing, and the room had to be cleared; the apprentices had entertained themselves by sprinkling the carpets with hellebore and other drugs.[5]

For surgery pupils and apprentices, training in the Infirmary became an important and recognized phase of their education. Many pupils had already served some sort of apprenticeship, often with a rural practitioner, when they came to the Infirmary. Many went on to spend a year or two in London hospitals, walking the wards to complete their education. Of the 142 recorded pupils and apprentices at the Infirmary from its founding to 1815, at least seventy, or half, went to London for further education. This must remain a conservative estimate, because Smith's memoirs are incomplete. Some attended Hunter's anatomy lectures in Great Windmill Street, others went to lectures at Bart's, Thomas's, Guy's, and the Westminster Lying-In Dispensary. Going up to London had become an established part of a well-to-do Bristolian's medical education by the 1780s and 1790s. For instance, when pupils Brickenden, Hetling, Bowles, Smith Jr., and Lax went to London, each in his turn lodged with Mr Hickmans, a silversmith in the City.[6]

Bristol medical education did not consist solely of hospital experience. Rather, it was a microcosm of London medical education; it followed patterns of metropolitan training.[7] As early as the 1740s, an Infirmary surgeon provided detailed anatomy lectures. There was no formal link between John Page's role as an Infirmary surgeon and his lecture courses, but it seems probable that many hospital apprentices and pupils attended. His first lecture introduced the study of anatomy in general, and the anatomy of animals and humans, particularly regarding the fluid and solid components of the body. Page's subsequent lectures moved into anatomic detail of the human body, providing information for future practitioners, starting with the skeletal structure of the head.[8]

Fragmentary evidence points to an abundance of lecture courses offered by Infirmary men over the second half of the century. Page went on to teach a course with James Ford, and Godfrey Lowe gave a series of anatomical lectures in the 1760s, using cadavers shipped down from London.[9] A Dr. Miller taught anatomy just down the street from the hospital in the 1780s.[10] By the 1790s when Thomas Beddoes arrived in Bristol eager to present his own course of anatomical lectures, he found a crowded market. According to the memoirs of Richard Smith, Beddoes's plan prodded F. C. Bowles to move from instructing "a dozen tyros in a Dead House" to a more formal course of lectures that included specimens from Smith's extensive collection. Beddoes had to join forces with Bowles and Smith, although Bowles had a hard time reading Beddoes's scrawled notes when he had to be a last-minute substitute for the introductory lecture.[11]

The course remained largely Bowles's and Smith's, drawing upon their expertise, and, in the case of Bowles, years of less-formal anatomical teaching. In twenty-five lectures, they covered such anatomical and physiological topics as the pathology of the *prima via,* the functioning of the vascular system and fetal heart, and the physiology of the senses of smell, sight, sound, and taste. Beddoes followed suit with a course in chemistry, and then Bowles and Smith gave their own chemistry course in 1803.[12] Bowles and Smith went on to develop a popular course of lectures for a mixed audience, cleared 100 guineas from it, and claimed it had expanded their private practices.

By the early nineteenth century, courses for pupils and apprentices were so successful that the Infirmary surgeons seem to have been battling to teach them. There were two advertisements in the local press in 1814. One declared that Mr. Hetling would give a course in the principles and practice of surgery, including clinical observations of surgical cases. The second advertisement proclaimed that because Messrs Smith, Lowe, and Daniel could not get the hospital house committee's approval for their rival course, they would be taking it elsewhere.[13]

Thus, a Bristol boy wanting to acquire a medical education need not have ventured across the Channel or even to the metropolis. Between lectures and hospital experience gained as an apprentice or pupil, a young man could have received a fairly comprehensive introduction to the theory and practice of medicine and surgery. The development of this provincial system of medical education is important for two reasons. First, it profoundly affected the hospital. Second, this quiet but productive provincial system suggests a certain reinterpretation of the roles of hospitals in medical education.

Received wisdom points to Paris as the place where hospitals became central to medical education. Ackerknecht's magisterial work on the Paris hospital portrays an institution where physicians and surgeons fulfilled dual roles as clinicians and researchers. These roles hinged upon the new practice of clinico-pathologic correlation, the very performance of which exemplified this duality. Toby Gelfand has emphasized the surgeon's role in creating an anatomically localist tradition in the hospital of the seventeenth and eighteenth centuries as an essential precondition to the creation of "Paris" medicine.[14] The institution of full-time paid positions in medical research and teaching created a new kind of niche in Paris that had no English parallel, and fostered a hospital-based science of medicine. A close look at eighteenth-century England, however, sketches in nuances to this familiar tale, and also suggests why English doctors did not emulate French models.[15] English doctors enjoyed their own institutionally-based system of medical education in which, like their private practices, prestige and income were derived from separate sources. Just as an Infirmary surgeon relied upon the Infirmary's prestige to augment his private practice, so too he relied upon the access to patients and cadavers offered by the hospital to lend technical support and intellectual cachet to his teaching. As the century wore on, some of these external lecture courses were moved into the hospital but they continued to bear the stamp of their proprietors' private enterprise, and were not, as in Paris, made a part of the hospital's formal structure.

Thus, England did not lack hospital-based medical education; rather, its seemingly haphazard assortment of lectures and pupilages has only recently been rediscovered by historians of medicine weaned on the Paris model. Susan Lawrence has emphasized the incorporation of the private enterprise model of medical education into London hospitals (themselves based on private enterprise), and suggests that its ease of fit accounts for London's success over Paris in the English eighteenth-century medical-education market.[16] In the cognitive realm, Othmar Keel has argued that the surgical emphasis on the anatomical localization of disease was not created and institutionalized in Paris, but rather that Morgagni's heirs could be found in several eighteenth-century European cities. For Keel, the Paris clinic was based upon European models, various imperfectly medicalized hospitals that were centers of nonuniversity-based clinical training and medical practice. These arguments have focused upon large cities – London, Dublin, Vienna – as the sites of the alternative development of clinical education.[17] Bristol's parallel development, albeit on a smaller provincial scale, suggests that this process of medicalization was a widespread one. In other words, the clinic was made, not born. It was the product of changes within the professional structures of medicine and surgery, particularly in patterns of apprenticeship, as well as shifts in cognitive style.

The Infirmary's success in appropriating education was due partly to the efforts of its surgeons, who clearly knew a good thing when they saw it, but was also both cause and consequence of

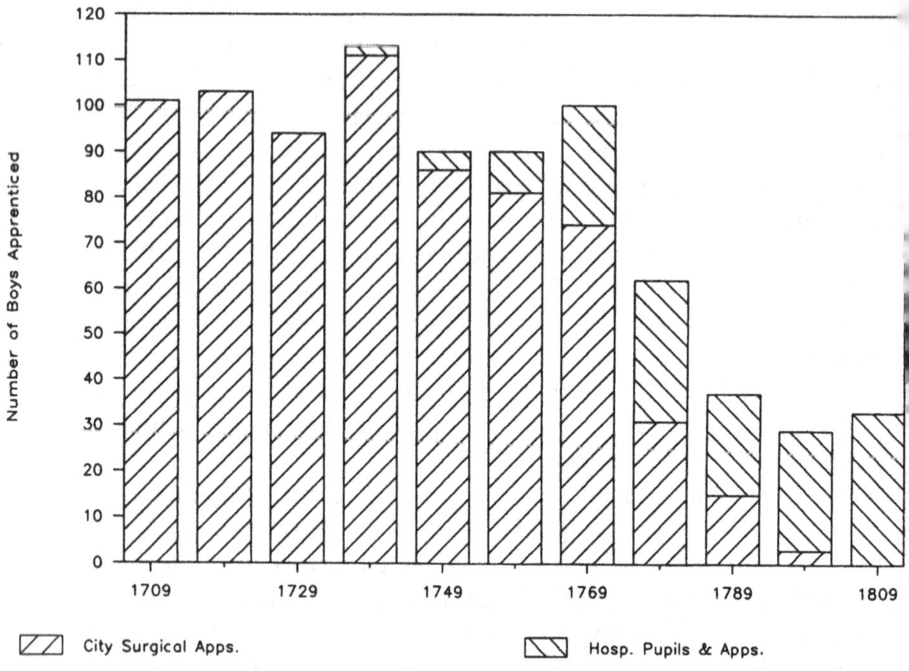

Figure 7.1. The decline in apprenticeship and rise in Infirmary training

changes in apprenticeship. A combination of factors created a situation in which, by the 1770s, the Infirmary had become the de facto center of surgical education in the city. Apothecaries, on the other hand, continued to utilize apprenticeship training, but some young apothecaries also came to the Infirmary for additional surgical education so that they could practice as surgeon-apothecaries.

Figure 7.1 shows the decline of Bristol surgical apprentices in absolute numbers by ten-year increments. In the first four decades of the century, fifty to sixty boys were apprenticed to surgeons in any five-year period.[18] This figure was already declining when the Infirmary took its first surgical pupils in the 1760s, but by the 1770s, numbers of apprentices plummeted, and those of hospital pupils rose appreciably.

The invention of Infirmary-based education accelerated the decline of apprenticeship training by providing an alternative. But the original impetus to that decline was an increase in charity apprenticeship. Since the seventeenth century, various groups had given money to apprentice poor boys. This impulse was similar to John Cary's workhouse scheme: by providing an appropriate education, one could morally redeem a boy, and by teaching him a trade, save him from absolute poverty. But it was in the middle decades of the century that groups like the Gentlemen Natives of Gloucestershire and other convivial societies increasingly took up collections at their annual dinners for the apprenticeship of poor boys, as well as lying-in money for poor mothers.

The increase in charity boys among Bristol surgeons' and apothecaries' apprentices is startling. From a mere one percent of the total in 1725–9, charity apprentices form a third of the surgeons' and apothecaries' apprentices from the 1750s through the 1780s. These charity apprentices were an economic resource for struggling surgeons, and some practices virtually functioned as apprentice mills. For instance, from 1745 to 1769, Thomas Ellis took on seven charity apprentices, whose fathers were gardeners, laborers, and cloth workers, all of whom would have been hard-pressed to find even a £10 apprentice fee. Of course, this intensive style was not peculiar to charity apprenticeship. For example, Peter Wells, a noted barber-surgeon, took on twelve apprentices in twenty years (1746–66) at handsome fees of 100 guineas or more, whose fathers were gentlemen, planters, merchants. But Wells was not typical of the 1750s. Jonathan Whichurch, whose eleven apprentices in eighteen years almost matches Wells' dozen, exemplifies a mid-century style; many of his boys were charity cases, and most of the rest had been turned over when their first masters fled their debts, went bankrupt, or just could not afford to maintain an apprentice. Wells probably made as much money from a single apprenticeship premium as Whichurch did from all of his premiums combined.

Nevertheless, charity apprentices could be a useful source of income and labor for surgeons fallen on hard times. For instance, when Anne Sharp's barber-surgeon husband died in the late 1730s, she kept on her two sons who had been apprenticed to him, and apprenticed a third son to herself in 1741. She attracted one further apprentice, the son of a peruke-maker (wig-maker), also in 1741. By 1748, when her sons had all completed their apprenticeships, she took on two charity boys, the sons of a mariner and of a hair merchant. For Mrs. Sharp, no doubt the £20 of premiums and the labor of the two boys gave her an edge in a market increasingly hostile to women.

Hair merchants? Peruke-makers? It is no accident that Sharp's apprentices came from backgrounds such as these. Although the Barber-Surgeon's Company was broken up in 1745, and subsequently their hall (a room in which John Page had held his first lectures) was sold for a coffee house, the link between the two occupations remained strong.[19] In the middle decades of the century, many marginal barber-surgeons turned to peruke-making to support themselves.

In other words, as the Infirmary began to take the cream of the apprentice market, barber-surgeons both took on increased numbers of charity apprentices, and expanded the barbering side of their trades to include wig-making. This dual relationship is neatly displayed in the career of Richard Allen. From 1733 to 1752, he took on seven apprentices, at least three of whom were charity boys, and a fourth who was his son. Then in 1754 he began to call himself a peruke-maker, and quickly apprenticed three charity boys over the next six years. Other practitioners maintained a flexible outlook; Charles Shearer apprenticed boys as a barber-surgeon in 1771 and 1785, and as a peruke-maker in 1779, 1782, and 1790.

This double devaluation of traditional apprenticeship – surgeons becoming wig-makers, and taking on charity apprentices – did not pass unnoticed by the fathers of apprenticeable boys. Fewer and fewer sons of the elite went into surgery as apprentices; rather, they trained at the Infirmary. The number of gentlemen who apprenticed their sons to surgeons declined, until by the end of the 1760s, a handful had become none.[20] Self-professed gentlemen, however, were only the forerunners of this trend.

The real shift was from apprentices whose backgrounds were in well-off or professional families to those whose origins were more plebian. A majority of surgeons' apprentices began to come from tradesmen's and artisan's families by the 1730s, a trend intensified by the 1750s. At the beginning of the century, surgeons' apprentices tended to come from families headed by clergymen, victuallers, graziers, planters, and other semigenteel, or well-off, occupations, inasmuch as such occupational titles can be relied upon. Although some apprentices had fathers who were nailers, dyers, or laborers, they were not yet in the majority. By the 1760s, 80 percent of apprentices came from such artisanal backgrounds.

Apothecaries' apprentices provide a counterpoint to this tale of decline. Here, too, there was a falling off in apprenticeship, but it was neither as dramatic nor as complex as that in surgery. Throughout the century, the sons of gentlemen, professionals, and artisans became apothecarys' apprentices in roughly equal proportions. There seem to have been fewer who took on charity apprentices; many apothecaries were commanding 100 guinea fees long after their surgeon contemporaries were scrambling for £10 charity fees. Apothecary dynasties like the Grevilles (Charles, Giles, and Brereton) were apprenticing the sons of gentlemen well into the second half of the century. In other words, the experiences of apothecaries make it clear that the collapse of surgical apprenticeship was due both to the influx of charity boys and the development of the Infirmary alternative. Apprenticeship to the Infirmary apothecary never had the cachet that Infirmary surgeon could provide, and thus apothecary training remained in the realm of an older style of marketplace practice.

The breakdown of the civic apparatus of apprenticeship went beyond the mere replacement of surgeons' apprentices by pupils. When Infirmary surgeons did take on apprentices, they did not use the municipal machinery of apprenticeship, but rather struck a private agreement. Godfrey Lowe, for instance, took three apprentices, none of whom are listed in municipal records. In other words, the Infirmary was creating a parallel structure to that of traditional civic authority. There were at least two reasons for this practice. First, many Infirmary men would not have been eligible to take apprentices in Bristol, being neither freemen nor members of the appropriate city company. Ned Bridges, the hospital apothecary, had been apprenticed in rural Sodbury, then studied under William Thornhill at the Infirmary, neither of which gave him the right to apprentice anyone in Bristol. But in his twenty-two year sojourn as Infirmary apothecary, he took sixteen apprentices, none of whom were recorded in the city's rolls. Second, a less rigid apprenticeship could be arranged through the hospital, which was probably an inducement to some students. To be apprenticed through the city usually implied a seven-year commitment. But in the Infirmary, one had a great deal more freedom, and could choose to be apprenticed to a surgeon for four or five years, and then go off to London for further training.[21]

The Infirmary's new role in education had an unintended consequence: surgeons came to have a vested interest in the hospital. Neither the physicians nor the surgeons were paid for their Infirmary work; as aspirant members of the gentler classes, they donated their labor to the charity, in return for the gratitude of their patients and the attention – perhaps patronage – of the subscribers. The apothecary, on the other hand, was a salaried staff member, only a grade above the matron. The development of surgical education created a sort of hybrid role for the surgeon; technically unpaid, he in fact had a very strong interest in the Infirmary because it indirectly provided an important source of revenue in the form of pupils and lecture fees. Initially, pupils were assigned to all the surgeons, and the four guineas a year per surgeon was not princely. But it seems that this system rapidly fell apart, and individual surgeons began to sell their wares in the open educational market. Some surgeons, like Richard Smith, had at least two or three pupils per year, while others contented themselves with the occasional student. The profit to be made from pupils was not inconsiderable; over the period from 1744 to 1757, the surgeon James Ford earned over £700 from private pupils, not including lecture fees.[22]

Professionally, then, the hospital became increasingly central to these surgeons' practices. For the Infirmary, this shift meant that, first, surgeons tried to gain control of the hospital, and, second, that they shaped the institution to serve their needs as surgeons and instructors. Conflicts between hospital subscribers and the surgeons in the latter part of the century serve as markers of this struggle for control.

Admissions constituted a perennial source of discontent. In theory, the subscribers controlled this process through their recommendations. But in practice, surgeons played a large role in deciding who would enter the Infirmary by the latter half of the eighteenth century. In theory, the non-casualty patient was admitted by the physician if a medical case, the surgeon if surgical, and the surgeons' admissions notes were countersigned by a physician. In practice, however, surgeons commandeered the admissions process. Richard Smith, who as a surgeon does not offer an unbiased perspective, wrote "The Physicians never from the first exercised any control or choice over the objects to be admitted but acted, in Signing the Notes under the direction of the Surgeons."[23] Long before Smith became an Infirmary surgeon in the 1790s, the house surgeons had been circumventing the physicians by admitting increased numbers of casualties, as mentioned in the previous chapter. These patients did not require a recommendation; they were admitted on the spot, usually by the surgeons. Virtually all of these patients were surgical.

Moving beyond casualty patients, the increase in the proportions of surgical to medical patients is suggestive of the surgeons' interests in maintaining an appropriate pool of teaching material. In the 1770s, only 28 percent of all inpatient admissions were surgical; this rose to 44 percent by the end of the century. Basically, surgeons packed the Infirmary with patients most likely to provide useful instruction for their pupils.

Once the surgeons had gotten patients admitted, they came into conflict with the governors over the appropriateness of those patients and over their stay in the hospital. For instance, Richard Smith found himself in the council room on the 15th of November 1797, explaining how it was that he had admitted a venereal patient in direct contravention of the rules. Smith claimed that he had not known that the patient had "the pox" when admitted, and that the patient would recover in a few days anyway, and the patient was permitted to remain.[24]

A longer running dispute was that over patients' length of stay in the hospital. Over the years, there had been occasional skirmishes between the surgeons and the committee about one patient or another. But in 1798, the committee went through the Infirmary patient by patient, and found twenty-three men and women who, as they saw it, had stayed in the institution too long.[25] The committee's motives were probably twofold. First, if all of the beds were full, subscribers could not avail themselves of their privilege of admitting worthy cases. Why should surgeons, who were not subscribers, arrogate to themselves admitting privileges? Second, there are hints that "extra" patients were occasionally boarded out in nearby lodging houses at the hospital's not inconsiderable expense.[26]

John Padmore Noble, one of the surgeons, was annoyed by the committee's interference with patients under his care. In particular, he fought for Samuel Stone, who had been in the hospital for many weeks with slow-healing ulcers resulting from a scald. From Stone's point of view, a long Infirmary stay was probably just what he needed; rest, and a good diet, would help to heal his burns while he did not have the worry of supporting himself. Noble threatened the committee, "You are perhaps not aware that the Rule [i.e., that about length of stay] may be rendered nugatory by the Faculty indiscriminantly signing the book – this has been proposed, and is intended to be adopted by some of the surgeons."[27] In other words, if the committee wanted to take it upon themselves to dismiss long-standing patients, the surgeons would respond by declaring that all the patients would benefit by a prolonged hospital stay, and the Infirmary would grind to a halt. Technically, if a surgeon declared that a long-term patient could still receive benefit, the committee had to waive the rules about length of stay. The committee discharged Samuel Stone, who was promptly readmitted by Noble, who was an Infirmary subscriber, unlike most other surgeons. In this case, the surgeons and committee fought to a draw. Stone stayed in the hospital, but the committee drafted a rule that such patients could in future be denied readmission as "improper objects of relief."[28]

These kinds of disputes almost never occurred between physicians and the hospital governors. Perhaps such harmony was due to the closer social relationships between gentlemanly physicians and the city elites who supported the hospital. However, a more significant factor was the importance of the hospital to the surgeons' careers. Surgeons were trying to gain control of the hospital because it provided them with "teaching material" – the drawing card for students. In 1802, Godfrey Lowe was brought before the house committee. He had allowed his son to set the broken arm of a patient who subsequently died. Lowe's son was neither apprentice nor pupil, (although neither of these would have been permitted to perform surgery either), but Lowe argued that his son had done the setting skillfully and while under the direction and supervision of his father. The committee was clearly displeased, but let Lowe off with the promise that it would not happen again.[29] For the surgeon, access to the operating theater was a crucial market advantage, as an essential distinction between Infirmary surgeons and the rest.

The significance of operative surgery to education was made clear in a disciplinary procedure in 1805. The apothecary's apprentice, Benjamin Hawkins, had sworn at an outpatient and refused to make up her medicine properly. By this period, hospital governors were no longer guarding the rights of their patients with assiduity. Hawkins was grounded for a month; he could not leave the hospital premises. He was also barred from the "operation room" for the same period, although his offense had had nothing to do with operations, nor was he a surgical apprentice. This punishment reveals the centrality of the operating theater for the hospital staff, particularly the trainees. To put it crudely, it was where the action was, and Hawkins had to pay for his misconduct by being removed from it.[30]

The issue of access to operative surgery was raised again a few months later. A Bristol surgeon, Thomas Lee, was attending a patient of his, Mary Fiddis, at the Bridewell when an Infirmary surgeon, several pupils, and the jailer burst into the room. Lee and Fiddis had, in fact, been discussing the Infirmary (she had a strangulated rupture that Lee had not been able to reduce) when they were interrupted. The Infirmary group proceeded to rush Mary Fiddis off to the Infirmary; the spectacle of a surgeon and his pupils scouring the city for likely surgical candidates should not pass unnoticed. Not only were the surgeons eagerly admitting casualty patients, they were seeking them out.

Further reduction was attempted at the Infirmary, but to no avail, and everyone agreed that operative surgery was the treatment of choice. But when Lee asked to be present at the operation, he was abruptly refused. Mary Fiddis begged repeatedly that Lee be there when she underwent surgery, saying that she would "submit to it cheerfully" if he were present. The Infirmary surgeons refused; they said it was against the rules. Mary Fiddis held out, and the surgeons threatened her with a speedy return to the Bridewell if she would not comply. For three days there was a stalemate. Then Fiddis had had enough, and left the Infirmary. Thomas Lee performed the necessary surgery in her home, and the resolute Mary Fiddis recovered.[31]

Thomas Lee was outraged at the Infirmary surgeons' behavior. He said "the Bristol Infirmary is in the hands, control, and management of the surgical establishment attached to it; and who use it, as a pedestal on which they stand, to awe and render inefficient those very checks and balances which had originally been supposed adequate to the safety and preservation of the Institution . . ."[32] Lee was right in that the surgeons were using the hospital rule (that no outsiders could attend operations) to defend their privileged position in the educational market. After all, Godfrey Lowe had readily admitted his son, not just to view, but to perform an operation, a few years previous. But to admit an outside surgeon was to threaten the surgeons' monopoly on institutional surgical training.

The surgeons refused to cooperate with the house committee to revise the rule about outside observers. The physicians evidently did not want to be involved; they nominated one of their number to attend meetings and ignored the entire affair.[33] The committee heard testimony about the Fiddis case and one of the surgeons, Morgan Yeatman, denied that Mary Fiddis had ever asked for her doctor. Unfortunately for Yeatman, the day nurse corroborated Fiddis' story. This nurse was then sent on a ninety-mile trip into Devonshire by the surgeons, and when she returned her testimony had changed. Given her dependence upon the institution's surgeons, her about-face should come as little surprise. Meanwhile, another surgeon, the ubiquitous Richard Smith, who had a part interest in the *Mirror* newspaper, had started a smear campaign in the press, attacking Fiddis' character and Lee's professional behavior.[34] The committee found it difficult to proceed, and the surgeons were let off with a reprimand.

It was not just access to the bodies of living patients that surgeons longed to acquire. Cadavers became a very important teaching resource, and questions about the acquisition of such teaching material became a potent source of discord. When Godfrey Lowe gave his surgical lectures in the 1760s, he used bodies shipped down from London. But he was probably the last to do so. Regular body snatching was already a feature of an Infirmary education; anatomical training was a hallmark of the institution, and the dissection of patients' bodies commonplace. As Henry Alford, Infirmary pupil wrote:

> There were frequent operations at the Infirmary of almost every kind. As many acute and fatal cases were admitted, and there was an autopsy in nearly every case of death, there were ample opportunities of getting a practical knowledge of the viscera, and also admitting of superficial dissections of many parts without any apparent injury or disfigurement of the body.[35]

In other words, both dissection and operative surgery were central to educational experience.

Surgeons emphasized anatomy, and anatomical training, because it was the subject that demarcated physic and surgery. Certainly physicians studied anatomy as well, but their focus was on what eighteenth-century doctors would have labeled the fluid constituents of the body, the humours and their precarious balance. Physicians regulated the body like a delicate and idiosyncratic machine, using evacuations to diagnose and rebalance the body. Surgeons cut. They needed both speed and accuracy for the few routinely performed operations – cutting for stone, reducing ruptures, doing amputations – if the patient were to survive blood loss, pain, and shock. As a contemporary description had it:

> The young surgeon must be an accurate Anatomist, not only a speculative but practical Anatomist; without which he must turn out a mere Bungler. It is not sufficient for him to attend Anatomical Lectures, and see two or three Subjects cursorily dissected; but he must put his hand to it himself, and be able to dissect every Part with the Same Accuracy that the Professor performs.[36]

Dissection meant the acquisition of anatomical knowledge, but it also provided lessons in manual dexterity and operative technique. As a London surgeon conflated dissection and surgery in the phrase, "I was performing operations on a dead subject," so too, the practice of anatomical dissection offered practitioners skills and techniques, as well as knowledge.[37] This detailed anatomical experience came to define the surgeon.

For Bristol surgeons, this training seems to have meant a great deal of dissection, although evidence about such practices is difficult to evaluate. Richard Smith frequently alluded to dissections in his memoirs. He is a problematic witness, however, for he created and nourished much of the anatomical subculture in Bristol. His father had started an anatomical museum, furnished with the oddities of many years' worth of anatomical explorations, and Smith continued and expanded on his father's hobby. In his memoirs, Smith presented many body-snatching exploits with glee, eager to show how doctors triumphed over ignorance and superstition in their quest for knowledge. Although Smith may have overemphasized anatomy, other sources, such as newspapers and

Infirmary records, show that dissection was often practiced and discussed. Indeed, Henry Alford recalled many years later that he had done far more dissection at the Infirmary than in his subsequent London training.[38]

As far back as 1728, when an unfortunate shoemaker hanged himself and the body was buried at a crossroads, it did not rest for long before it was unearthed and dissected by surgeons.[39] In this case, obviously, Infirmary surgeons were not the culprits, because the hospital did not yet exist. However, once the Infirmary was established, and in particular once it took on a teaching function, it was repeatedly linked with body snatching and dissection.

In 1761 the son of a collier had been brought to the Infirmary, a casualty with a head injury, who did not long survive. The boy's father stormed up to the home of the hospital surgeon, John Castelman, in the middle of the night. He had opened the coffin containing his son's body, and found the head was missing. The collier threatened to "pull the Furmary down about thy ears!" if Castelman did not return the son's head immediately. Kingswood colliers were a notoriously riotous lot, and Castelman hurried to the hospital, returning with the head in a sack.[40]

According to Richard Smith, such events were not rare. As a student, he had frequently stolen bodies or parts of bodies for anatomy lessons given by F. C. Bowles:

> use makes mastery, and we had reduced this to so regular a system that we practiced it two years without suspicion – we procured a key to the dead house and provided ourselves with screws – hammers – wrenching iron – nails, and everything likely to be wanted . . . whilst the family were at dinner we stole into the Dead House – removed the Extremities, Head, or anything else we wanted, even the whole corps, and then made all fast, and in the same order as before.[41]

Because Bowles was not yet on the Infirmary staff, pupils smuggled him into the deadhouse, "a mere coal-hole lit by a foot-square iron grating" where they "spent hours in the ardent pursuit of anatomical knowledge."[42]

In 1806, a year after the Mary Fiddis controversy, the hospital treasurer received an anonymous letter saying:

> there is scarcely an unfortunate fellow creature who has died in the Infirmary for a considerable time past, whose remains have not been most Shockingly Mutilated by a Mr. Lawrence, Pupil to the Surgeons.

Head, Arms, Legs in short all parts have been taken away from the Dead by him. Some of the nurses through bribery leaving the coffin unclosed.[43]

This letter went on to detail how Lawrence had also stolen a body from the Infirmary burial ground and brought it to Richard Smith's coach house, where Smith had lectured and dissected.

At the inquiry that followed the receipt of the anonymous letter of complaint, the opinions of the various surgeons were sought. The house committee thought that a hard and fast rule concerning dissections should be instituted. Almost all of the surgeons disagreed. Godfrey Lowe said, "I am of the opinion that the bodies are examined with decency and without mutilation and rule of the description proposed is unnecessary." John Padmore Noble used almost identical language, "I have always made the rule of my conduct – to caution the Pupils to leave the Body decent & without mutilation." R. J. Allard referred to "decency and propriety" and Morgan Yeatman said that he would "give my Pupils directions on no account to mutilate any Patient."[44] Surgeons, it was generally agreed, had some rights to examine patients' bodies in unusual cases – in modern parlance, to do autopsies. But it is clear that these surgeons had permitted their pupils extraordinary latitude. Students carrying off arms, legs, heads, were not performing examinations of the cause of death; rather, they were perfecting their manual skills and adding to their anatomical knowledge by dissecting whatever they could obtain. The surgeons were eager to protect their pupils' access to dissections because it was one of the real inducements to an Infirmary education.

The house committee, blocked by the surgeons, was ineffectual. Even ignoring the evidence of dissection-happy Richard Smith, it is clear that patients' bodies were routinely anatomized in the hospital. F. C. Bowles said, "the constant habit of dissections and examination of subjects could not but accumulate a large fund of knowledge respecting the human body both in its morbid and natural state."[45] James Bedingfield, the Infirmary apothecary who subsequently practiced as a surgeon, coolly noted that he had dissected nearly 200 subjects looking for biliary calculi, although he'd almost never found them.[46] He viewed an outbreak of erysipelas as educational, saying "the great fatality of the disease afforded frequent opportunities of ascertaining its nature."[47] Henry Alford, an Infirmary pupil in the 1820s, alleged that almost every patient who died in the hospital was anatomized.[48] Even allowing for exaggeration, it seems that patients had become subjects for anatomic inquiry, what William Hunter called "the passive submission of dead bodies."[49]

Hospital-based training not only reshaped surgical education; it created a new type of surgeon. Richard Smith's disparagement of "shop boys" has already been alluded to, and a part of this change involved surgeons' redefinitions of themselves. No longer men of the marketplace, the new surgeons saw themselves as professionals. On a practical level, these men also experienced rather different career paths than had their apprentice-trained forbears. The hospital was central to both self-image and working lives.

Young men trained in the hospital seem to have entered a rather crowded and competitive field. Very few of them would be able to emulate their teachers and take up lucrative city practices and affiliations with charitable institutions. These men, however, found their niches in other institutions: the army, navy, and militia, the Poor Law, the merchant marine. Individual, fee-for-service practice became a less likely option, particularly at the beginning of a career. Twenty-three percent of Infirmary pupils went on to become army, navy, or militia doctors. Fourteen percent went off to the colonies, usually as a ship's doctor or as a surgeon to the East India Company. Another 20 percent took up rural practices, often with poor-law responsibilities. In other words, well over a third of the hospital's trainees took up some form of institutionally-oriented practice. And of course, there were always the lucky or calculating 6 percent of Infirmary pupils who married heiresses, and gave up medicine to settle into lives of leisure, cases in which medicine functioned perhaps as a means to an end rather than a career.

Often Infirmary pupils followed career paths that included more than one of the options mentioned above. For instance, John Fewster had been apprenticed to Ned Bridges, the Infirmary apothecary, from 1754 to 1761, and was also a dressing pupil to the surgeon John Page. He then went to London, where he did three courses of anatomy lectures at Thomas's and Guy's as well as studying physic and midwifery. When he returned to the West Country, he took a post as a surgeon to the South Gloucestershire Militia, and then started a practice in rural Gloucestershire, including Poor Law work, ultimately sending his own son to be trained at the Bristol Infirmary.

Fewster's career points to another feature of hospital-based training: the blurring of distinctions between the three professions of medicine. Many of the apothecary's apprentices did a year or two of surgical training as well. The career of one of Fewster's contemporaries, Edward Horler, illustrates how flexible any professional boundaries had become. Fewster had been an obedient apprentice; Horler was not, and was discharged for allegedly having an affair with one of the nurses. He then studied in London, obtained a Scottish M.D. (probably by mail) and took up a practice as a physician in Wiltshire. His trial run as a physician was not successful, and he moved to London to work as a surgeon. Evidently private surgical practice enabled him to make but a paltry living since he joined the army as a surgeon, and went to America in 1776. He was subsequently appointed to a hospital in Jamaica, but perhaps the colonies did not suit him, for he returned to England. There he practiced as an apothecary in London for a brief period. Finally he seems to have settled down as a rural general practitioner. Perhaps mere cheek would have enabled Horler to turn his hand to surgery, physic, or pharmacy as economic demand indicated, but his education in the hospital provided the training that enabled him to do so readily.

Richard Smith's memoirs suggest that the lot of the young surgeon was not a happy one. Henry Jeffries studied in London, passed his examination by the College of Surgeons, returned to the South-West but found Somerset too crowded with other practitioners, and had to move to Sussex. Poyntz Adams went bankrupt. John Danvers got a post as assistant surgeon to the Somerset Militia and then took up private practice. But running into debt, and having a large family, he was reduced to becoming a shopman to an apothecary in London. Benjamin Hawkins, the apprentice who had gotten into trouble for swearing at a patient, attained a militia post, but by 1816 he came begging to Richard Smith's door. Not all pupils had careers this disastrous. But many of them evidently struggled to make ends meet by taking on militia or Poor Law posts or going into the army or navy.[50]

The growth of institutional provision shaped careers in another way – it reduced opportunities at the bottom of the market. Substantial numbers were treated by new medical charities. For instance, in the early 1800s, the Dispensary saw over 2,000 patients per year, Beddoes' Institute almost 2,000, and the Infirmary perhaps 4,000 inpatients and outpatients. In other words, out of a city of over 70,000, as many as 8,000 people were treated annually by charities.[51] This increased availability of free care must have been in direct competition with the lower end of the private-practice market. The clients of these charities were not the truly destitute; most such organizations stressed that they were for the "worthy" poor, just those who might have been able to pay a small amount to a surgeon or apothecary for treatment.[52] In other words, the provision of charitable health care by the medical elites of Bristol served to undercut their competition. By the 1810s, newly qualified Infirmary-trained men were competing with each other rather than with the remnants of barber-surgery.

It was not just the career structures that altered in relation to the hospital; surgeons' images of themselves changed as well. As discussed, the rituals that made a surgeon were centered on the operating theater and the dissecting room, on a culture of anatomy and body snatching, rather than on visits to patients' homes and minding the shop. Their roles in the Infirmary helped to confirm their new status, both by emphasizing their charitable functions and by the authority conferred upon them by the city.

This new set of values, in which surgeons became learned gentlemen and stewards of the poor, was lampooned in an article in the 1809 *Edinburgh Medical and Surgical Journal*. The anonymous author makes fun of just such pretensions in an ironic piece entitled "Hints to Young Practitioners." A few examples of his advice illustrate the theme:

> Do something that will make you conspicuous . . . as it is well known no empiric ever reaches any degree of wealth and reputation till after he has been fairly convicted of homicide.
>
> Write a book with a taking title . . . Quote as many cases as the alphabet will furnish initials for.
>
> Write monthly reports of diseases in a newspaper or magazine; swell out the list according to your own fancy.
>
> Hire a chariot, and put a smart livery upon a bill-stick, to ride behind you . . . for nobody in their senses, in London, will send for a walking physician.[53]

In other words, this writer suggested that a practitioner adopt all the signs of learning and erudition that becomes a physician, as well as the status symbols that made it clear that the surgeon was not a tradesman.

Richard Smith paid close attention to these indicators of status in his memoirs. For instance, he noted that John Middleton had been the first physician in Bristol to acquire a carriage. He described William Thornhill, the first surgeon to do likewise, as always attired in a suit of black velvet, with an elegant steel-handled rapier, who lived in "altogether much better style" than other surgeons.[54] Smith noted that the Infirmary men had, for forty years, worn the same "uniform" – wigs, scarlet cloaks, and gold-headed canes – the standard gentlemanly garb of mid-century.[55] It was only when John Padmore Noble was elected surgeon in the late 1770s and refused to wear the "uniform" that the habit died out.[56] In part, of course, these details were recorded because Smith seems to have suffered from regular bouts of status anxiety. But beyond the individual quirks of personality, such signs were markers of surgeons' attempts to move their images of themselves from the world of the shop to that of the hospital.[57]

Thus, by the turn of the century, the hospital had become a medical workplace, run by and for the surgeons who had themselves undergone a transformation. Disputes continued well into the nineteenth century, suggesting that alignments of power within the Infirmary were by no means tidily or permanently arranged. Rather, I want to emphasize the transition from a charity, founded and run by philanthropically-minded laymen, to a medical institution that defined patients by their diagnosed diseases rather than their moral worthiness as objects of charity. This transformation was achieved through the coincidence of two factors: the changing professional interests of the surgeons and the abdication of the governors. The third party – the patient – was an unwitting accomplice to this change. It is to the patient we now turn.

8

The patient's perspective

The coming to power of the surgeons meant a very different kind of hospital experience for patients. First, the increased emphasis on education recast the significances of the patient's own narratives of illness. As discussed in Chapter 2, illness was understood by most people in a deeply historical way; hospital medicine robbed illness of its meaning. Second, in a process that Ruth Richardson has termed the commodification of the body, patients became objects of anatomic inquiry and lost control over the disposition of their own bodies after death. These two processes were facets of the same fundamental shift in authority from patient to medical man. Patients were deskilled, denied interpretative authority over their own bodies as their interpretative roles in illness were contested by surgeons. This denial was accomplished by making patients' bodies speak for them, through the medium of anatomic and pathological enquiry conducted by medical men before and after death. Although it is rare to discern an individual patient's response to these profound changes, resistance to body snatching and dissection provides some indication of patients' points of view.

Some of these developments, such as the rise in postmortem dissection, have been discussed by other historians. What the experiences of Bristolians make clear are the connections among diagnosis, therapy, and medical research, which constituted a powerful denial of the patient's voice. At every step of the patient's progress through the Infirmary – diagnosis, therapy, and in some cases, death and dissection – a new relationship was forged between patient and practitioner.

Diagnosis was probably the most significant moment of a patient's illness where the patient/practitioner relationship changed within the hospital. Three aspects of the diagnostic process altered: Narrative was replaced by physical signs, the language of diagnosis became opaque, and symptoms were replaced by pathology in the causation of illness. The process by which patients ceased to possess interpretive control over their own illnesses can be followed through the writings of medical men, both formal and informal. It is not that these changes were reflected in the writings of medical men; rather, hospital case histories, be they published papers or student notes, were key sites where illness' meanings were reconstructed.

Think, for example, of the barber-surgeon Alexander Morgan, writing in his notebook about the circumstances surrounding a patient's illness: "The third Day after the Wether happened to be very warm he changed his Thick Waistcot for a Linning one & being careless sat a quarter day in a Room that was wett the same evening he found himself not well & a little Feverish & thirsty . . . "[1] This early in the century, in the 1720s, the patient's and the doctor's words are one. It is easy to hear the patient's voice in the doctor's case report. The narrative of illness was the illness, and patient and practitioner alike held the narrative up to the light and examined it for clues as to disease causation.

The most striking examples of the denial of the patient's narrative come from the hospital; it was there that patients' interpretations of illness were made truly redundant. Indeed, in the Bristol Infirmary, the patient was reduced to "a dull contented country lad" with a bladder stone, or "Mary Townsend, aged thirty years, of a dark complexion, disagreeable Mulatto features and emaciated form" who had supposedly "led a very dissipated life."[2] The narrative was replaced by physical diagnosis: patients were evaluated by temperature, pulse, condition of the oft-drawn blood, and respiratory sounds.[3] The body, the disease, began to become the focus of the medical gaze rather than the patient's version of his or her illness.[4] Although a sentence or two about a patient's origins or complaints has long remained a standard introduction to a case history, the site of analysis was changing from story to body.

The transition from the patient's narrative to his or her signs was not immediate, but listen to this 1816 description of a boy in the Bristol Infirmary: "his appearance was florid, his complexion clear. He complained of a slight headache and a sore throat. His pulse was full and rather frequent, the tongue white, the tonsils slightly inflamed, the parotid glands were very much enlarged, the bowels were confined, and there was a little oppression about the chest."[5] The only hint given of the patient's thoughts or interpretations was his "complaint" (already a formulaic usage in such case histories) of a headache. Every other item was derived from physical examination. From such details, James Bedingfield, the Infirmary apothecary, and his co-workers adduced the patient's diagnosis.

It was not just the published case history, such as that of Bedingfield, that overwrote the patient's view. Manuscript case notes, often taken by students in the course of their training, show the same constructions of illness as the printed ones. For Bristol, the student notebooks of Edward Estlin (1820–2) and Alexander Morgan (1720s and 1730s) provide counterpoints to Bedingfield's published case histories. Morgan, as described in Chapter 3, trained as an apprentice and became a successful Bristol surgeon. Edward Estlin, son of a prominent dissenting minister, trained under Richard Smith in the Infirmary, and was set for a promising career when he succumbed to consumption in his student days. The London notebook of Nathaniel Bedford, a Worcestershire student who walked the wards at St. George's, illustrates the ways in which London training resembled and shaped that in Bristol. All three men – Morgan, Estlin, and Bedford – took notes during their training in order to fix details in their memories and to serve as a future reference work. Morgan, for example, compiled an index to his notes, and occasionally annotated them with details of later cases. These student notebooks share a certain family resemblance among them, but the hospital cases – those of Estlin and Bedford – also have features in common with published hospital cases such as Bedingfield's or those published in medical journals like *Medical Observations and Inquiries*. The relationship between manuscript and published genres is a complex one, but it does seem that both were significant in reshaping the definitions and diagnostic approaches to illness.

Nathaniel Bedford's 1776 notebook gives details of the patients he encountered at St. George's, as well as on his subsequent voyage to the West Indies. His experiences were probably analogous to those of Bristol students who went up to London for further training. Like James Bedingfield, Bedford's emphasis upon physical signs denies a role to the patient's own narrative. For example, Bedford wrote of one patient:

John Branscombe, a lad of fifteen, was admitted into St. Georges, supposed to labour under an ascites. His abdomen was very tense & gave the idea of a very deep-seated fluctuation, something like an obscure ovarian case. On examining this more narrowly, a large swelling was found to extend, on both sides, lower than the navel, and below that the feeling of the intestine was very perceptible. On coughing, the abdominal muscles by their action compressed the lower part of the belly very much inwards . . . [6]

The style of this report distances the patient's experience so much that he is not even described as coughing – the body, not the person, coughs. Such elliptical constructions were common in case reports. A surgeon in 1769 wrote a long description of physical signs, adding, "To this oppression of the praecordia were joined a slight cough and laborious respiration."[7] Once again, the patient is written out of the account, present only in a passive voice and passive body.

Two arguments might be made to counter the assertion that case reports indicate a growing distance between hospital patients and practitioners. Perhaps the alienation of the published case report reflects requirements of the genre rather than revealing any emerging differences between hospital and private practice. However, the similarities among manuscript and published cases suggest that the form of the case report was not the sole determinant of its contents. The division between hospital and private patients is more marked than that between manuscript and published cases. Compare this report of a private patient with that of Nathaniel Bedford's hospitalized patient with the same diagnosis:

Mrs. ____, in the 36th year of age, of a slender but healthful constitution, most regular in her *catamenia,* a person of the strictest sobriety and virtue, thro' excess of grief (from the loss of an affectionate husband who died in June 1756) after a long train of nervous complaints, began to find the symptoms of an *ascites* upon her.[8]

Not only are we presented with the lady's life history – the patient is granted an active and participatory role in her own illness; it is she who "finds" the symptoms (not the signs) of her ascites. This nameless patient has her ailments grounded in her own narrative, with attention paid to her conception of significant events, like bereavement. John Branscombe, the named patient in the earlier quotation, has his ascites grounded in physical diagnosis rather than life course. Social differences, expressed in part through the different institutional contexts of patient/practitioner encounters, create alternate narratives.

It might also be argued that case histories are but poor reflections of bedside encounters. The multivalent functions of case histories suggest instead that they were a crucial site of the redefinition of patient/practitioner relationships. As argued in Chapter 2, narratives of illness constructed by sufferers were used by both patients and practitioners as a means of understanding illness. Indeed, illness *was* narrative. Not only were the physical details of the beginnings of an ailment discussed; a much wider range of factors – moral, emotional, spiritual – were open for discussion and interpretation. The narrative was fundamentally the construction and possession of the sufferer and afforded him or her the power to understand and integrate that illness into a larger analysis of his or her life. Thus, for example, Samuel Pye listened to Mrs. ____'s recounting of her grief at her husband's death, and the genesis and experience of her "long train" of nervous ailments. In this instance, illness's meaning was related to life course.

But this type of case history was already under threat in hospital medicine. What were hospital case histories for? A surgeon writing a description of a weaver who died from an aneurysm in the London Hospital tells us, "The great use in publishing histories, as the present one, is to warn surgeons against exposing themselves and their art, by undertaking the cure of cases, where nature will only admit of a little palliating, and being too busy may prove instantly fatal to the patient . . . "[9] In other words, narratives have been supplanted by case histories designed to keep surgeons out of trouble. The instructional feature of case histories extended into nonpublished case notes as well. Edward Estlin, at the Bristol Infirmary, recorded in his notebook, "This case affords a most important lesson: it teaches not to depend on any one sense as to the information it affords & not to think that experience, however great, is able to prevent the commission of mistakes unless with it be joined care and attention . . . "[10] By this point in the 1820s, it is accepted that a case would depend upon physical diagnosis; the function of this case history relates to the dangers of reliance upon such sensory information. In other words, these case histories, as we shall see, reflect the difficulties surgeons experienced with physical signs; the struggles with patients' narratives of illness had long been left behind.

Such physical diagnosis characterized Infirmary cases recorded in Bristol by James Bedingfield. For patients with any sort of respiratory ailments, the sounds of their breathing were noted carefully. Primitive percussion was used, "on striking the diseased side with the hand, it sounded heavily and obscurely."[11] The patient's body seemingly spoke for itself. A patient with hydrothorax was diagnosed by "the symptoms of the disease, together with an attentive examination of the chest in the manner directed by Corvisart."[12] On occasion, physical diagnosis extended to taking patients' temperatures. For instance, Richard Smith, the Infirmary surgeon, noted a rise in temperature in a postsurgical case. In another, the temperature was followed for several days from a high of 102°F down to a near-normal 99.5°F.[13]

Bedingfield and colleagues wanted to break down disease mechanisms into their component parts, manifestations of which could then be perceived upon physical examination. By fragmenting the indicators of illness, Infirmary men not only disregarded the context in which illness events happened, but redefined illness itself as a set of discrete physical events quite unlike the highly integrative versions of illness experienced by patients. These physical manifestations were granted a sort of objective authority by practitioners, which could not help but undermine the more subjective narrative. Simultaneously, the practitioner was assuming authority over the hospital patient.

For example, in a case in which he had recounted the patient's own story, Bedingfield also described the sounds made when the chest was percussed, making an analogy with a half-empty cask with thick oleaginous material inside.[14] He counterbalanced the patient's words with the objective witness of a physical analogy in which the patient became a barrel. Another published surgeon wrote, "the great tension of the parts, accompanied with the other symptoms, seemed loudly to proclaim a tendency towards a universal mortification."[15] Almost all of the "symptoms" alluded to were what we would call signs – black blotches on the legs, blackened gums and tongue, a cadaverous appearance, etc. These signs spoke, proclaimed, for the patient.[16] Such rhetorical techniques echoed actual hospital practice; in both cases, the patient was rendered mute, and authority, textual and technical, resided with the doctor.

Usually James Bedingfield, the Infirmary apothecary, was careful to distinguish himself as narrator from the patient, using phrases like "according to her own account" to demarcate the two points of view.[17] In only two cases did he give his readers extended versions of patients' narratives; both were puzzling and frustrating cases. As Bedingfield put it, "I have found considerable difficulty in compressing this case; and even in its present abridged state, it will perhaps appear tedious."[18] Bedingfield, in his attempts to "compress this case," in his efforts to present himself as an objective narrator, acknowledges some of the tensions inherent in the meeting between working-class patient and middle-class doctor. Hospital practice embodied the changed social realities of the institution. No longer were hospital governors central to the administration of the hospital and no longer were patients treated as their personal objects of charity.

The emphasis upon physical diagnosis recast the significance of the manifestations of illness. Where vernacular medical knowledge looked to the outer surface of the body for the exemplification of health or disease, gradually hospital medicine began to look inward. The surface of the patient's body, like his or her narrative, was open to interpretation. But Bedingfield's taking of the temperature, examination of the blood, percussion of the chest, and attention to the sounds of respiration placed the site of medical interpretation well within the body, accessible only to the trained observer.

However, older styles of explanation did not immediately retreat in response to physical diagnosis. A cooper reported to Bedingfield that "he was first seized with a cold chill since which time he had been labouring under more or less difficulty of breathing." Another man owed his illness to "exposure to great heat in a sugar-house, to which he was not accustomed, and afterwards going into the open air."[19] In both instances, the juxtaposition of hot and cold still lay at the heart of illness, seemingly for doctor and patient alike, just as they had done a century before.

In a similar way, the last hold-outs of the patient's own narratives were descriptions of pain. These were the least amenable, in some ways, to reduction to physical signs. For instance, William

Hey, the Leeds surgeon, wrote of a private patient, "After the healing of the wound, she had complained of an odd sensation, which she described by saying, 'She felt as if blood was trickling down within the skull, opposite the wounded part.' "[20] Here, too, the patient's words are carefully demarcated from those of the practitioner, but they do form part of the history.[21] By comparison, a hospital patient's feelings were described in even more distanced terms, "By what the patient seemed to suffer in the operation [an amputation] there was no apparent diminution in sensibility."[22] Pain is translated from symptom, which the patient himself might describe, to sign, to what he "seemed to suffer." Again, the shift is from patient's to practitioner's authority. So too, such rhetorical moves helped to distance the surgeon himself from the pain he caused and experienced, reiterating the divide between practitioner and patient which the institution emphasized.[23]

The processes that alienated the patient from the hospital practitioner were gradual ones. Like Bedingfield, Estlin does not give extensive details of the patient's life or illness experiences. However, he does preface each case with a sentence or two about the patient, such as, "she has been ill 5 weeks, and the illness came by taking a cold after lying-in. She has been jaundiced a month and had pain in the region of the liver, for which she was bled, blistered & salivated."[24] However, this description of getting ill after lying-in is a far cry from Morgan's discussions of the onset of a chill, in which the patient's own words form the narrative.

Unlike Bedingfield, Estlin does not reveal a tension between the patient's narrative and his own. Of course, he was not responsible for the discipline and order of the patients as was Bedingfield. Nor were his notes intended for publication, so there was no need to make his narrative compelling. Nonetheless, the few sentences about the patient's history were quickly balanced by physical observation and postmortem dissection. For instance, Estlin tried to convey an unusual heartbeat, "His pulse had a very singular feel, which was better felt in the right carotid where the blood seemed to be whizzing or whisking along with great force . . . When the thumb is placed on the carotid artery the pulsation feels like a hammer knocking inside against it . . . "[25] As in this case, Estlin's struggle to convey his physical impressions and sensations in words often outweighed the patient's story. From day to day, Estlin's notes tend to be physical signs rather than the patient's impressions. For instance, a typical entry reads, "*16* Blood inflamed, tongue dry, bowels open, he coughs but does not spit, the inflam: of the skin is gone."[26] Perhaps the best example of Estlin's reliance upon physical signs is in the case of a woman who was brought to the hospital comatose from fever. What is remarkable about Estlin's notes about this woman is their similarity to the rest of his cases; the fact that his patient could not respond to him was not that problematic, because her words were not an essential part of diagnosis or therapy.[27]

These kinds of case notes suggest that the process of diagnosis began to separate patients and doctors by the early years of the nineteenth century. Not only were patients' narratives of illness increasingly overlooked, the very language of diagnosis changed. First, Infirmary physicians and surgeons turned to Latinate diagnoses: "cough" became "tussis," "wound" became "vulnus," "leg ulcers" became "ulcus cruris." Such diagnoses probably reflect surgeons' aping of physicians in attempts to improve their status, but also indicate the hospital's increasing reliance on William Cullen's nosology.[28] By the 1780s and 1790s, many diagnoses in the Infirmary records can be fitted into the Edinburgh professor's scheme of disease classification. Ailments like "cynanche," or "peripneumonia," indicative of Cullen's nosology, appear in the register. The shift from English to Latin diagnosis happened quickly. In the late 1770s, 70 percent of all diagnoses were in English, and 19 percent in Latin (the remainder were diagnoses in one language that lacked any clear equivalent in the other). By the turn of the century, 79 percent of all diagnoses were in Latin; only 1 percent were still in English.

Put in local context, this change is all the more alienating. Somerset dialect was rich in words for illness and disability. For instance, it made distinctions among slow continuous pain ("drimmeling"), continuous aching pain ("nagging") and the restlessness due to illness ("tavering"). Parts of the body had nonstandard names, such as "pook" for stomach. Common minor ailments such as whitlows or pimples had several dialect names each.[29] Thus, even standard English was a step away from ordinary discussions of illness; the use of Latin underscored the social distance between practitioner and patient, emphasizing the former's powerful role within the Infirmary.

In a similar way, case reports began to distance themselves from their patient's words; doctors began to sound like doctors, and patients' voices disappear. A mid-century surgeon, for instance, recorded his interview with a rural West Country farm laborer. Fifteen years prior to the consultation, "he got a surfeit (so the country people call any sudden alteration of the blood and juices, by drinking cold liquors when they are very hot . . .)."[30] Earlier, the distinction between country people's ways of talking about illness might not have needed such a clear demarcation from those of the practitioner. Samuel England, for example, a Somerset surgeon's apprentice in the 1720s, used the same language as his patients, referring to kibs and piles rather than chilblains and hemorrhoids.[31] But in his 1770s manuscript notes, Nathaniel Bedford distances himself from everyday parlance, writing, "If by any means the patient became costive (if I may use the expression)."[32] So too, Edward Estlin underlines the differences in lay and medical uses of words, "About 6 months ago he was taken with (as he says) an attack of pleurisy."[33] In 1771, another West Country practitioner discussed a young man who experienced, "as he expressed it, a fluttering in the precordial region on the least motion."[34] Farm laborers did not refer to their chests as "precordial regions"; the doctor has taken over, commandeered the patient's own words, almost unconsciously interpreting them and replacing them with his own medical equivalents.

Infirmary men were not unaware of the distance language could create. Edward Long Fox, a prominent Infirmary physician, referred to that distance in his 1831 essay on cholera. He used language specifically to protect professional privilege and denigrate quackery. He published antidotes to cholera in English – "to prevent imposition from the vendors of drugs and quack medicines" – but only offered recipes for cures in Latin.[35] He wrote that the cures "are clothed as much as possible in the garb of medical phraseology, to hinder persons when first seized from undertaking the management of their own cases, or committing themselves to the care of ignorant officious neighbours . . . I exhort them to call in the assistance of the most qualified professional person of the place."[36] This was a far cry from every man his own physician. The cholera was to serve as an arena for professional consolidation; never mind whether patients could afford or even find practitioners who would be at home with Fox's Latin prescriptions. Similarly, the power of language was alluded to by Thomas Beddoes, who alleged that patients did not like to go to the Infirmary in Bristol, but instead consulted their neighbors "because they speak to the sick in their own language."[37]

The concepts of disease that underlay these Latinate diagnoses also helped to undermine the conceptual accord between patients and doctors. One of the clearest examples of such divergence is a comparison between causes of death listed in the parish register of SS Philip and Jacob, and Infirmary diagnoses from the same parish.[38] Unlike in London, where elderly semitrained women inspected the dead and recorded causes of death to keep tabs on the plague, in this Bristol parish, causes of death seem to have been obtained by the vicar from family or friends, and recorded because he was interested in political arithmetic. Thus, the parish register indicates laymen's ideas about causes of death, while the hospital register lists causes of illness diagnosed by doctors. Obviously, these two documents had very different functions and recorded diagnoses for different groups of people, but the comparison is suggestive nonetheless.

The burials register clearly incorporates an understanding of social position in its assigned causes of death; illness was defined by social location as well as physical signs or symptoms. This integration of different styles of analysis can be seen in the relationships of four different causes of death. The terms "decline," "debility," "natural decay," and "atrophy" are all used in the register. All referred to a gradual process of some sort of diminution. However, the words debility and atrophy were used only to describe the causes of death of paupers, while decline and natural decay were more often used to describe nonpauper deaths.[39] In other words, encoded within terms such as "debility" or "atrophy" was the designation of an individual's state of poverty or wealth. This kind of multidimensional understanding of illness was not that employed by the hospital. For lay people of the parish, death was not understood as solely the outcome of pathological processes; it encompassed social realities as well as symptoms and signs.

Causes of death listed in the parish register also differed from hospital diagnoses in their continuing emphasis upon symptoms, long after the Infirmary had shifted to a process-oriented style of disease description. Seven percent of all deaths in the parish of SS

Philip and Jacob, for example, were due to "age." Certainly, elderly people were hospitalized, and some died in the Infirmary, but what happened to them there was never attributed to "age." Similarly, causes of death such as decline, debility, natural decay, or "suddenly," were descriptions of how a person had come to die, not why, not analyses of pathological processes that caused life to cease. The most notable examples of this style of discussion were three people (all paupers) who died from "visitation of God." Along similar, but less colorful lines, were designations such as chill, headache, "liver," pain in the bowels, stoppage in the chest, and "delirious." Such descriptions were not inferior medical knowledge; they were a different understanding of death, which incorporated a wider range of factors than did Infirmary diagnosis.

In the hospital, doctors moved away from diagnoses that emphasized the patient's experience of illness. As discussed, narratives of illness became less significant, and doctors came to use Latin rather than English names of diseases. They also focused on pathological processes rather than symptoms. For example, people in the 1750s and 1760s were sometimes diagnosed as having sore throats. By the 1780s and 1790s, this diagnosis disappeared, seemingly replaced by that of "cynanche," or sometimes "angina maligna." But "cynanche," first, was a specialized medical term, unlike "sore throat," which echoed the patient's complaint. Second, it implied a particular sort of pathological process, as defined by William Cullen, rather than any illness known to ordinary people.

Diagnosis was undoubtedly the most important locus of the shift in authority from patient to practitioner, but therapeutics provided the second flank of the attack on lay experience. Increasingly, hospital therapeutics diverged from the collection of plant remedies shared by many practitioners, humble and elite, described in Chapter 2.[40] Bristol hospital medicine was characterized by bleeding, bleeding, and more bleeding. Joseph Metford, an Infirmary surgeon of the 1770s, recounted that Dr. John Paul would ask every hospital patient if he were a Bristol man. If the answer were yes, Paul ordered twenty ounces of blood let. When Metford asked about this unfailing practice, Paul replied, "If he is a Bristol man, I know he sits of an evening smoking tobacco and drinking your abominable fat ale; the first thing to be done is to let some of that run out, and then we shall see what else is the matter."[41] This story may well be apocryphal, but its theme is reiterated in numbers of hospital accounts.

Heroic therapy extended to bleeding patients with hemoptysis, the spitting up of blood from the lungs. James Bedingfield justified this practice in 1816, "We are often reduced to the alternative of taking blood from the arm or of allowing it to rush from the lungs. Which mode I would enquire is attended with the greater hazard and inconvenience to the patient?"[42] And inconvenience to the staff as well; this therapeutic style functioned as a system of management. It enabled a handful of part-time doctors to administer care in a hospital with 180 beds, sometimes filled with two patients each. The surgeons' pupils could, and did, bleed patients. Diet, the other hospital mainstay, was overseen by the matron, and meals were probably served by ambulatory patients. This therapeutic style can be seen as a response to the bureaucratic demands of running a large institution in a period when most practitioners were used to providing their services on a small scale within patients' homes.

As bloodletting became routine hospital practice, performed by students, it acquired a highly bureaucratic mien. Henry Alford, an Infirmary pupil contemporary with Edward Estlin, described how patients were bled, not just from the arm, but by cupping, and from the temporal artery and jugular vein. He said, "all these minor operations were performed by the pupils."[43] He often bled twenty or more patients a day, and reported that the pupils often complained of the expense of having their lancets reground, "I have seen one or two of them strop their lancets on the soles of their boots."[44] Alford described the routine of Infirmary bloodletting:

> On the days of the week when the bleedings were numerous, the pupil . . . would often arrange five or six of these patients in a row, side by side; first fix a bandage around the arm of each, and give them a pewter bleeding-dish to hold in the other hand; then, beginning at one end, open the vein of each in succession, and, when finished with the last, go back to the first, ready to remove the bandage and tie up the arm. It sometimes happened that one of the patients fainted and fell off the bench . . . [45]

In other words, the practice of bloodletting quickly became highly rationalized hospital routine.

By the turn of the century, sanguinary tendencies had hardened into therapeutic ritual. Most patients were put on an antiphlogistic regimen that featured bleeding, purging, blisters, and a bland diet. When patients arrived at the Infirmary, they were routinely bled and given a dose of the standardized house cathartic powder, a potent purgative composed of jalap and calomel.[46] Patients' ailments were quickly categorized as resulting from either inflammatory or diminishing processes. Most patients were evidently suffering from inflammatory diatheses; in Bedingfield's collection of cases, antiphlogistic outweighed phlogistic therapies five to one. In other words, hospital diagnosis and therapy became increasingly rationalized and routinized.

In particular, this style of therapy bypassed the patient's account of him or herself because it relied upon the body's own response; the patient's body served as its own monitor of therapeutic efficacy. For example, in a case of phrenitis, at least twenty ounces of blood were taken from the jugular two or three times a day for four or five days. Bedingfield explained that "No regard was paid to the quantity taken; an abatement in the violence of the phrenetic symptoms formed the criterion by which the flow of sanguineous fluid was regulated."[47] The patient's words were not relevant; his or her body spoke instead.

The body manifested its need for bloodletting in the pulse and in the blood itself. First, the pulse functioned as an indicator of the patient's overstimulated or understimulated state. In apoplexy, for example, if it were full and slow, and the patient's head red, the jugular arteries full, then bleeding was demanded. If, on the other hand, the pulse was "languid" and the body surface cold, it was contraindicated.[48] As for the blood itself, its condition was noted while it was drawn; did it trickle out or flow? Then, it was allowed to sit for a while until it had separated into its constituent parts, which were also examined.

In the same ways that physical symptoms spoke for themselves, so too, the examination of the blood provided direct evidence of the patient's condition. When Arthur Broughton, Bristol physician, studied in London, he recorded in his notes "the buffy coat [i.e., of the blood] however shows the Nature of the Disease and State of the Patient."[49] Or, as Bedingfield put it, "the blood exhibited no inflammatory appearances."[50] Again, it was to physical signs that the hospital men turned for the elucidation of their patients' state of health or illness. Of course, examination of the blood, like uroscopy, was a part of vernacular medical practice as well as hospital treatment. In the hospital, however, such practices made bodily substances speak for the patient, ignoring his or her own perspective. But in the context of vernacular practice, as in the example of William Dyer seeking a uroscopist for his wife (see Chapter 3) the patient maintained greater control over his or her interpretation of illness because he or she had hired the medical man or woman.

Thus, although patients and doctors were becoming distanced in the ways they talked with each other, so too there were growing divisions in the understanding of illness. Practitioners, especially hospital surgeons, abandoned vernacular ideas about the significance of illness – the attention to externals, the focus on illness causation – and turned to systems of medicine devised by their colleagues. Thus, they disparaged or dismissed patients' own accounts of illness and replaced them with signs and symptoms unavailable to the patient, but meaningful within an emergent profession.

At the same time, a growing emphasis on postmortem dissection within the hospital made Infirmary medicine increasingly repugnant to its patients. In Chapter 7, we have seen how a student subculture of anatomy, body snatching, and dissection flourished within the hospital, fostered by surgeons' making of their own identity and by circumstances peculiar to Bristol. However, as other historians have discussed, ordinary people were violently opposed to postmortem examination or dissection. It was not just within the hospital that such issues were significant. The symbolic expression of state authority over the bodies of its people, in the dissection of felons' bodies, placed surgeons and their relation to the human body center stage, and aligned their interests with those of the state rather than the patient.

The possibilities of dissection reshaped the ways in which Infirmary men talked about their patients' bodies. James Bedingfield's quest for a primitive kind of clinico-pathologic correlation (the matching up of premortem and postmortem findings) emphasized the inside of the patient's body and conceptualized the patient's experience of illness as the manifestations of a "deeper" pathological process. The identification of this process was the key to diagnosis. In other words, although external signs were still important, their relationship to the signified changed as the locus of absolute truth began to lie deep inside the body, accessible only to Infirmary men.

Dissection inverted the significance of illness in a second way: where vernacular medicine looked backward to the cause of illness, hospital medicine looked forwards to dissection. Thus, when a woman's puzzling pattern of respiration was made explicable in postmortem examination, Bedingfield could say "the appearances which the parts exhibited upon dissection, afforded a satisfactory elucidation of the symptoms which existed during the life of the patient."[51] The satisfactory resolution of disease was its explication, almost irrelevant to the cure of the patient. So too, Edward Estlin's descriptions of living patients are amplified by long discussions of postmortem dissections. For Estlin, the final arbiter of truth was the examination after death; again and again, he tried to puzzle out what event had caused a patient to die, what signs after death could reveal the progress of disease. Similarly, another surgeon acknowledged his feelings of helplessness in the face of disease and the role of postmortem dissections, "It is some satisfaction to be able to account for morbid symptoms, though the diseases which give rise to them, may be in their own nature, incurable . . . in the present case, every symptom which afflicted this poor man was fully explained by the examination of the body after death."[52] The culture of body snatching and dissection fostered by hospital surgeons such as Richard Smith, in conjunction with Bedingfield's attempts to make clinico-pathologic correlations, ignored the validity of a patient's search for meaning in ultimate causes by counterpoising the truths afforded by dissection.

Patients knew very well what happened if you died in a hospital and your friends did not protect you. A man treated at the Infirmary for heart trouble "was somewhat relieved, but as he was prepossessed with an idea, that in the event of his dying in the house, he would be examined, he insisted upon leaving it."[53] James Bedingfield pointed to the moral of the tale: "He died about three weeks later." In Estlin's 1822 notebook, the only patients mentioned who died in hospital whose bodies were not dissected were those with very careful friends. Dissection could take place in as little as four or five hours after death, and only vigilant relatives could supervene, "His friends remained with him from the time he died until he was taken out 24 hours, and would on no account allow any examination."[54] When an eleven-year-old boy died in the middle of the night, his mother was at the Infirmary very early the next morning to claim the body so it would not be dissected.[55]

Ruth Richardson has shown how the processes of death, laying out, wake, and funeral, allowed both the deceased's relatives and the deceased's spirit to take a gradual leave of the body.[56] Thus the integrity of the newly dead body was particularly important; that is why the collier mentioned in Chapter 7 was so angry about the missing head of his son. The respect due the living was equally due the dead. Even the surgeons made a point of excusing themselves after doing an illicit dissection, saying that the body "was afterwards sewn up, left clean, decent, and not in the least disfigured."[57] They too understood, at least to some extent, the significance of proper respect and attention paid the body of a person who was recently dead. Richard Smith's casual pillaging of body parts from Infirmary coffins was at variance with some medical as well as popular norms. Objections to postmortem dissections were strongly felt by the poor because the cavalier attitude of the surgeons to the body – take a limb here, a limb there – were at such variance with custom and cultural precept.

Details of working people's funerals and ceremonies of death make it very clear that these rituals were extremely important, and underline the cultural importance of appropriate respect for the dead body. For example, friendly societies (mutual benefit clubs that eventually came to serve as primitive unemployment and medical insurance) always provided benefits at the death of a member, and usually at the death of a spouse. Thus, people who could not have afforded the thirty to forty shillings a funeral might cost could ensure that they would be spared the ignominy of a pauper burial by subscribing to such a society. Upper-class benefactors of such societies thought that they were encouraging thrift and other virtues in the lower classes. But benefactors and members clashed on the importance of funerals. For example, in the Somerset village of Shipham, the evangelical reformer Hannah More and her sister set up a women's benefit club. The Mores thought that women should receive benefits when ill, at lying-in and for burial. The members were quite content to do without the first two so as to ensure a really spectacular funeral. As one woman said to a horrified Hannah More, "What did a poor woman work hard for, but in hopes she should be put out of the world in a tidy way?"[58]

These women were delighted when the benefit at death rose to a guinea, and provision was made for smaller payments on the deaths of family members.

William Dyer, the diarist, noted that even a poor washer-woman's funeral could be an elaborate occasion, as when John Wesley made it the centerpiece of a service in Bristol.[59] Funerals were the occasion for an expression of community, of the collective identity of the dead and the mourners, be they Wesleyans or prostitutes, who gathered at the funeral of one of their own in 1762, "The virtuous sisterhood attended the funeral, dressed in a Motley Manner, some with Gowns, some Jackets, but each had such a Profusion of Ribbands, that it was conspicuous that their Heads ran more upon their Dress than the Dead."[60] A local newspaper may have indulged in sarcasm on the occasion, but nonetheless the women were there to see off their comrade, who had been killed by a man in a jealous rage.[61] In other words, funerals were very important social events, even for the poor who could barely afford them, and any disruption, such as dissection, was extremely unpopular.

Evidence of just such disruption was all too apparent. From early in the century, local newspapers frequently noted that graves had been disturbed. For instance, in 1726, *Farley's Bristol Newspaper* recounted the story of a man who had been drinking in a tavern with his sweetheart, making wedding plans. Returning home, he missed his step, fell on his head, and as Farley put it, was "married to Eternity."[62] A week later, the paper reported that this young man was buried by the city (i.e., as a pauper), and that his body "was taken out naked before 3 the next Morning, and the Coffin left in the Grave."[63] Again and again, such reports of disturbed graves featured in the newspapers, to the point where it was not surprising that a coachman would check the coffin of his wife, to ensure that it had not been disturbed.[64] Another young man was less fortunate; when he went to bury his mother, he found that his sister's grave had been disturbed, and his father's body stolen.[65]

The tales of some grave robbings assume almost mythical status, being repeated and embroidered. For example, there is the unfortunate Mrs. Rice, whose body was stolen from St. Augustine's churchyard in 1822. Some versions of the story say that her body was taken to a house in College Street, others have it that the surgeons had obtained a room in the cathedral, and another states that the room was over a greengrocer's shop.[66] (None of these details are inconsistent with this historian's suspicion that the dissection was carried out by Richard Smith at or near his home.) When the irate husband got to the room he needed assistance to see into the second-story room, where he saw "the mangled remains of the late partner of his toils," as a broadside phrased it. A crowd, tipped off by the woman who ran the greengrocer's shop, had assembled and the dissector "was pursued from the scene of action by the mob, and narrowly escaped with his life."[67] This tale went through several different forms: a poster in which the churchwardens offered a reward for information about the surgeons, newspaper stories, and a broadside. By this last, the story included a rerobbing of the same grave and a second rescue and reburial.

The churchyard activities of surgeons, in other words, were common knowledge, and provided an increasingly strident counterpoint to the benevolent image of the Infirmary cultivated by hospital governors. Indeed, a letter to a Bristol newspaper about the Mrs. Rice case quoted the surgeons against themselves, pointing out that if it were "absolutely necessary for the good of society" and "does not hurt the bodies after death," then surgeons, their widows, wives, and daughters should give up their own bodies for dissection.[68]

The role of the Infirmary and its surgeons in body snatching was a curious one. On the one hand, as is indicated by the reward offered by churchwardens for information about the abduction of Mrs. Rice's body, local authority clearly acknowledged the unlawfulness of such activities. On the other hand, surgeons gained authority by their roles in the dissection of felons' bodies and testimony in court. Although surgeons were not supposed to *steal* bodies (although even here, latitude was given them) they were *given* bodies in a highly public display of the power of the law. Surgeons allied themselves with civic authority by conducting such dissections of felons' bodies, reiterating their willingness to transgress popular sanctions. Such public acts symbolized the surgeon's control over the bodies of the poor and criminal and underlined the connections between the surgeon's medical and legal roles.

Surgeons' "rights" to bodies were asserted in two local cases of grave robbing in the 1820s. Although, as mentioned, grave robbing was clearly an unacceptable practice, there could be exceptions. For example, at the Somerset Quarter Sessions of 1823, a bill of indictment was preferred against two surgeons for grave robbing but the grand jury chose to ignore it. Similarly, when five young surgeons battled with a constable after they were discovered digging in a churchyard, they were gotten off with the plea that a conviction would hurt their careers as surgeons.[69] For these surgeons to remain unpunished, not only for robbing graves, but for the far more serious offense of assaulting a constable, was to confirm that surgeons had extraordinary rights and powers over people's bodies.

The courts reinforced this point of view in the most potent display of surgeons' status, namely the dissection of felons' bodies. Nowhere was the theater of the court – the dramatic balance of brute force tempered by occasional mercy – more clearly articulated than in the execution of criminals.[70] The rituals of death, the importance of a proper funeral, the respect accorded a dead body, the emphasis upon an unmarred body, all were stood on their head in the case of executed felons. Other historians have discussed dissection and its perceptions by the public. In particular, Ruth Richardson, in her compelling analysis of the Anatomy Act, describes the links between resurrection men and metropolitan hospital instruction in anatomy. But in Bristol, the connections between dissection and the Infirmary were much more clear-cut than in London; processes within the Infirmary that distanced patient from practitioner were reiterated in the dissection of felons.

Execution was public, and virtually from the moment of his or her conviction and sentencing at the assizes, a man or woman became public property. The last confession, the visits of importuning clerics, the crowd gathered to watch a good death, and its subsequent circulation in ballad form were all widely publicized. This public aspect was maintained and even intensified after death with the invasion of the body, which became the property of the surgeons.[71] Punishment was graded according to the social status of the criminal. Thus, when Captain Goodere, a gentleman, was executed in 1741 for the murder of his brother, his body was not actually anatomized. It was brought to the Bristol Infirmary and "placed in the operation room, and in the presence of as many spectators as the room would hold, a surgeon stuck a scalpel into the breast. In this state it was exposed to the popular gaze until the evening, and then given over to the friends for burial."[72] Social standing protected Goodere from the ultimate degradation of dissection.

In other words, on the same table that hospital patients underwent surgical operations, performed by those same surgeons, bodies of executed criminals were displayed and dissected. The roles of the surgeon and the hospital were central to this dramatic expression of the power of the state over the bodies of its subjects.

In 1802, two young women, Maria Davis and Charlotte Bobbet, were executed in Bristol for the crime of infanticide. They had left Davis's baby out on Brandon Hill to perish. Despite their pleas, and the appeals of their friends and relatives, their bodies were given to the Infirmary to dissect. Such pleas, however, were not made to the court. Rather, they were made to the surgeons, because if the surgeons would have appealed to the court for them, the awful punishment of dissection might have been lifted. But the surgeons refused. The women's bodies were brought to the Infirmary, followed by huge crowds. As in all dissections of felons, the first incisions were made in a dramatic cross shape, as if to atone for the sins of criminal and dissector alike. The women's skeletons allegedly grace the Medical School's collection to this day.[73] Certainly for the friends and relatives who accepted the inevitability of Maria Davis and Charlotte Bobbet's deaths but who wished to spare them the horrors of dissection, the role of the surgeons must have seemed self-seeking and ungenerous, and the allied interests of surgeons and the law made very clear.

The most obvious example of this alliance between surgeons and the law was in their testimony at trials. The ubiquitous Richard Smith testified at the trial of John Horwood. This was a complicated matter; Horwood and Eliza Balsum had quarreled, and he had thrown a stone at her, which glanced off her temple. She did not seem badly hurt, and continued on her way home, where her bruise was treated by her family with cataplasms of dung and other animal matter. Balsum seemed fine, but a month later went into a swift decline, was rushed to the Infirmary and died. Richard Smith was present at the hospital when Horwood was brought in to be identified by the dying woman, and Smith attempted to bring Horwood to a sense of shame by showing him Bobbet and Davis's skeletons as a warning of his own fate. Smith examined Eliza Balsum's body and testified that she had died as a result of the injury.[74] The defense claimed that the injury had been fairly minor and that it was the cataplasms that had caused the death, by promoting an abscess. Horwood was convicted on Smith's evidence, and hanged. His body was used by Richard Smith to illustrate lectures, and then given to his three pupils to dissect.[75] One can only speculate how Horwood and his contemporaries understood the fate that befell him. Smith testified against Horwood. Smith was sufficiently covetous of Horwood's body that he refused to appeal to the judge to remit the sentence of dissection. He even gave the body to his pupils as a privilege. Ultimately, Smith had Horwood's skin tanned to bind up his notes on the case.[76] One can only hope that Horwood's friends and relatives remained unaware of this final indignity. But they could not have overlooked the power over the body granted to the surgeons, nor could they have ignored the curious role of the Infirmary, peopled by healers eager to dissect the bodies of their patients.

The last word on this topic belongs to James Bedingfield, the Infirmary apothecary-turned-surgeon. In 1816 he referred to "a similar appearance in the stomach of two executed patients."[77] This slip of the pen, in which Bedingfield seems to have confused the hospital patient with the executed criminal, reveals that to him they were essentially alike – merely subjects for dissection.

This tale of an Infirmary in which therapeutics became routine and diagnosis obscure, of the dissection of criminals' bodies on the hospital operating table, of the denial of narrative is in contrast to many histories of medicine of the period. My tale is a far more pessimistic one than most. This distinction is not due to authorial melancholy; rather, it is an interpretation based upon an attempt to see the Infirmary from the perspective of patient-practitioner relationships. Obviously, when the only known description by any English infirmary inmate of this period is a laudatory and rather conventional poem by an unknown traveling actor, historians proceed at their hazard to discern any "view from below."[78] Nevertheless, the relationships between patients and their healers can be explored through the healers' records as well as public protests. Here I have found a tale of increasing alienation, of a growing distance between patient and practitioner. Not that the pre-Infirmary medical world represented some idyll in which patients and their doctors always agreed and all was well; any reader of Alexander Morgan's casebook cannot miss the pain and suffering it documents. Rather, a fundamental change in the way practitioners related to patients was underway by 1800.

In part, the emerging gulf between patient and practitioner was one of class structure. In the early eighteenth century in a predominantly market economy, the relationship between patient and practitioner was one of consumer and seller. Patients selected their practitioners and retained a certain freedom in that choice. The hospital was structured by a social world characterized by deference and obligation, a chain of individual connections between high and low. However, the market of medicine changed within the hospital: doctors did not sell their wares to patients. Rather, medical men sold instruction to aspirant medical men, and patients became teaching aids rather than consumers of medicine. Their care was adapted to the needs of running a large institution, and their cure predicated upon surgical technique and a highly routinized therapeutic regime. The social power of surgeons, acquired in part through their Infirmary status, was simultaneously expressed and created through the agency of the bodies of patients and felons. The commodification of patients' bodies was a part of the creation of a hospital peopled by working-class patients who did not even own their own bodies, who served as illustrative material for the education of middle-class medical men. Perhaps the benevolent face of authority was revealed in the care of hospital patients, but its obverse could easily be seen in the disregard for popular convention shown by the toleration of grave robbing and the use of judicial terror in the dissection of felons.

However, the fragmentation of a common understanding held by practitioner and patient was not only a product of hospital medicine or even of surgeons' assertion of social status. This breakdown of accord was a part of a larger process of cultural appropriation and dissociation to which we now turn.

9

The reform of popular medicine

Within the hospital the accord between patient and practitioner was broken as medical men arrogated interpretations of the meanings of illness to themselves. A similar process was underway outside the hospital as the common understanding of health and illness fractured and crumbled until it became the province of working men and women. This aspect of the dissolution of popular and elite cultures was particularly pronounced in the 1750s and again in the 1790s.[1]

The reforms of popular culture of the 1790s – the evangelical attempts to police the manners of the poor, and the state's crackdown on various aspects of political and religious radicalism – are well-known to historians, although their implications for vernacular medicine have not been explored. In contrast, those of the 1750s have not been well-delineated. In part, this lack is due to the amorphous quality of the attack on popular beliefs; it was not centered in institutions or societies. Instead, its traces can be found in sermons, letters to newspapers, and in certain local incidents.

In neither the 1750s nor the 1790s was lay healing at the center of controversy; it was usually just a part of "vulgar" beliefs. Indeed, both of these moments when the differences between popular and elite healing were sharply articulated owe more to religion and politics than to medicine. The connections to medicine were often made through debates over the existence of the supernatural, which provided a topic open to religious and political argument. In the 1790s, the evangelical attack on popular culture was, in part, a response to perceptions of England's ungodliness, a comment on both the unruly lower classes and their decadent betters. The mid-century impulse is more difficult to pin down, but a discourse about polite behavior can be read as the result of anxieties generated by the rebellion of 1745 and the resurgence of popular religion in Wesleyan Methodism.

Of course both of these campaigns were also about social status as well as politics and religion. Clearly, discussions about correct behavior and polite manners suggest a certain need to define social distance. So too, the efforts of the evangelicals centered on the definition of social standing in relation to morality and correctness rather than wealth and ostentation. In many ways, the reformers of the 1750s and 1790s looked back to the reformation of manners movement of the 1690s; where John Duddlestone or John Cary worried about the manners of the poor, Hannah More tried to remedy the vices of the laboring classes.

The links between a critique of "enthusiastic" religion and the creation of polite culture, with a concomitant disparagement of vernacular medicine, are particularly marked. On one level, enthusiastic religion sometimes included a component of healing, usually consonant with and drawn from vernacular practice. But the ties between enthusiastic religion and lay healing were stronger than mere association. The interpretive practices of such dissenting groups, and their focus upon bodily manifestations of divine will, were closely related to the interpretative practices of vernacular medicine.

Both enthusiasm and lay healing relied upon signs and portents. Indeed, one can see these reliances as mediations of the same cultural inclination. Chapter 2 shows how late seventeenth-century everyday medicine often interpreted illness by means of the signs inscribed on the outside of the body. So too, albeit to a lesser extent, did its professional cousin. Medical practitioners lacked interpretative autonomy and professional authority; the meanings of illness were written on the body's surface for all to see and know. The exact relationship between the inside and the outside varied according to styles of healing, but in general, the outside reflected the inside in much the same way that a plant's healing potential was reflected in its shape or color.

The same hermeneutic strategies characterized various forms of dissenting religion.[2] Many of these groups, tarred with the brush of "enthusiasm," were fascinated by signs and portents. These could take several forms – interpretations of the weather, for example, or discussions of manifestations of God's providence in an individual's life were commonplace. More significant for popular healing was enthusiastic religion's preoccupation with bodily signs. Again and again, various groups experienced divine will in dramatic and peculiar bodily manifestations. As Clarke Garrett has pointed out, such sacred theater relied upon a vocabulary of signs that could easily be interpreted by the religious community; even if the convulsions and possessions seem bizarre to us as well as to contemporary onlookers, the group itself made use of a finite repertoire of symbolic expression.[3]

For example, in the 1650s, the Quakers were known for their prayer meetings in which they became possessed by the spirit, manifested in bodily convulsions. The body was both medium and message; Quakers went naked through the streets as a sign, emblematic of Adam and Eve, or of the spiritual poverty of other religious groups. By the early eighteenth century, the Friends had come to a quieter mode of worship; a focus on Inner Light led attention away from the dramatic conversion experiences of earlier decades, and the monthly meeting controlled and policed anarchic interpretation.[4] As the Friends became more inward-looking and socially conservative, other groups assumed the mantle of prophetic knowledge and dramatic revelation. Hillel Schwartz has shown how a range of millenarian groups came together to seek reformation; the Philadelphians, for example, anticipated "divine assistance, effusions of the Spirit, signs and wonders."[5] The French Prophets, Protestant refugees from the Cevennes, also found followers in England in the first decade of the eighteenth century. Reminiscent of other millenarian groups, they experienced revelations through the medium of the body. Prayer meetings were met with instances such as these: "Mr. L is seized with the Agitations, and under the Inspiration is taken with a grievous Consumption-Cough, that makes him groan, and almost faint away. He sits upon the Bed's feet, leans his Head upon a table, and moans and looks pitifully . . . "[6] Such events were mocked by many, but within and without the group the association between enthusiasm and bodily manifestations was cemented.[7]

Recent scholarship has done much to rehabilitate the historical significance and respectability of millenarian groups such as these.[8] Ranging from William Whiston, the successor to Newton at Cambridge, through the French Prophet who disrupted the Yearly Meeting of Bristol Quakers in 1738 by raving and posturing in sackcloth and ashes, different varieties of millenarianism seem to have been a strong and continuous thread in various sets of beliefs in early modern England.[9] The vitality of a millenarian tradition also suggests a reassessment of John Wesley's early ministry.[10] After all, Wesley was preaching in Bristol at about the same time that the French Prophet broke up the Quaker meeting in 1738, and his meetings were the scene of many an expression of the spirit world. Those new to Wesleyanism might experience a battle between good and evil spirits through the medium of their bodies, which were racked by convulsions. Indeed, Wesley was in some measure competing with the French Prophets, and warned that their messages did not stand up to tests of authenticity.[11] In other words, Wesley's ministry, dramatic as it appeared, built upon or referred to extant traditions about interpreting bodily manifestations of divine will and other signs and wonders.

It is tempting to see Wesley's revitalization of popular religion as a key to the repression of lay-healing practices at mid-century. However, other factors, such as the fears of instability generated by the uprising of 1745, expressed in a redefinition of "polite" behavior, also contributed to a disparagement of popular belief. So too, the controversy about miracles generated by David Hume's essay of 1748 and its repercussions in the Royal Society helped to call lay beliefs into question. Often writers linked several of these elements into a denunciation of lay healing and popular religion.

For example, in 1758 John Free, vicar of East Coker, in Somerset, published his *Rules for the Discovery of False Prophets: or the Dangerous Impositions of the People called Methodists. . . .* In the preface, Free claimed that during the events of the Jacobite rebellion of 1745, the king owed his crown, not only to the troops at Culloden, but also to "the steadiness and activity of the well-affected CLERGY of the *Church* of England."[12] For Free, as for many others, an attack on the church was an attack on the state; he argued that "when the *Ignorance* of the Vulgar grows frantick . . . they soon grow weary of *old Rules and Orders . . . Civil* or *Religious.*"[13] His fear of dissenters went to the heart of their hermeneutics, claiming that the controlled interpretation of signs was central to the organized church:

Now these Things are *Visible,* and open alike to our own Observations, and often the Observation of other People, who are Judges in part, as well as we, of every good Word and Work, that is manifest before them: which good *Words* and *Works* are the only kind of *infallible* testimony to this kind of Inspiration. Our saviour says not a Word of any unintelligible *inward* Feelings, distorting *Agonies* or frightful *Convulsions.* For these he knew might proceed from bodily Disorders; and *Enthusiasts* have no Mark to distinguish, when they do not.[14]

Heavy italics or no, in this passage Free presents a standard critique of Methodist enthusiasm. First, the godly can be distinguished by their good works. Not only are works rather than faith the key to salvation; Free argues that the interpretation of those works is to be controlled by the group. He goes on to criticize Methodist emphasis on faith, and belittles their bizarre bodily manifestations of that faith. In other words, central to his attack on Methodism is its enthusiastic and uncontrolled hermeneutics of the body, its focus upon an open and relatively unpoliced reading of bodily manifestations.

William Dodwell, an influential divine, also made the association between superstition, popular modes of interpretation, and dissent. He accused Protestants of having recourse to superstitious ways of foretelling the future, "to pretended Divinations, to magical Arts, to judicial Astrology, to perverse and groundless Constructions of the common Accidents and Events of Life . . . "[15] Such practices were in opposition to God's authority and, by implication, the authority of the church. Dodwell particularly faulted pietists and sectarians for their "neglect of duty" in emphasizing the inner dedication to God, which he portrayed as superstitious.[16] He was alluding to groups such as the Philadelphians, Moravians, French Prophets, and other enthusiastic groups characterized by millenarian tendencies, connections with continental dissenters, and traditions of spirit possession.

John Free was more explicit about the connections between political and religious rebellion, while Dodwell focused on the links between superstition and enthusiasm, but both were fundamentally saying the same thing. As Michael MacDonald pointed out, the argument that enthusiasm and superstition led to sedition was a favorite establishment theme from the Restoration onward.[17] What made Free's and Dodwell's sermons more pointed and topical was, of course, the experiences of 1745. The threat posed by Jacobites, whose ties to Catholicism suggested the same sort of superstitious divinations and prophesies as did Methodism, made the links between popular unbelief and civil unrest all too clear. In part, then, these post-1745 critiques of enthusiasm must be read as more urgent attacks on popular interpretative strategies than their earlier counterparts.

It was not just the fears of instability generated by rebellion that promoted the mid-century disparagement of superstition; a controversy over miracles also made the differences between natural and supernatural an item of public notice. David Hume initiated a debate about miracles and God's general and special providence in his essays of 1748.[18] The details of this dispute are complex, but part of it concerned whether or not God's special providence existed. To put it in an eighteenth-century way, had the age of miracles ceased? Had it ever existed?

James Force argues that the Royal Society, especially after Martin Folkes' ascendancy to the presidency in 1741, took an increasingly Humean perspective on wonders and miracles, denying the credibility of testimony surrounding such supernatural events.[19] If Force is correct – and he admits that this shift seems to have been achieved more through mockery and ridicule than explicit argument – the Royal Society's refusal to exhibit monsters in 1753 makes logical sense. As reported in the *Daily Advertiser,* "it was declar'd inconsistent with the Honour of the Society to admit the Shewing of Monsters there, as the ridiculous Exhibiters made use of their countenance . . . "[20] No longer would the Royal Society resemble the fairs and shows that delighted in manifestations of the bizarre and supernatural. Unlike the instance cited in the Chapter 2 – the woman with a horn growing from her head – the Royal Society would not concern itself with the objects of curiosity upon which popular entertainment thrived.

In Bristol these events and controversies were particularly pointed. Wesley's early ministry was often targeted at the city and its suburbs; so too the city was home to various religious societies as well as efforts to reform the manners of the poor, as discussed in Chapter 4. In addition, Bristol seems to have been particularly susceptible to physical manifestations of religious enthusiasm.[21] Certainly the city was a haven for godly deviance from at least the middle of the seventeenth century, and her residents saw various waves of religious revivalism and enthusiasm take center stage and then fade. Although Bristol's Quakers were a sedate lot by the time they founded the Infirmary in the 1730s, their earlier styles of worship were characterized by dramatic bodily expressions of God's will; they also disrupted other denominations' services dressed in sackcloth and ashes. Even their early eighteenth-century quietist emphasis on Inner Light underlined the importance of the relationship between inside and outside, sign and substance. The Quaker, May Drummond, called her tract *Internal Revelation the Source of Saving Knowledge,* a phrase that stressed the significance of both Inner Light and the means by which one knew of it. She preached in Bristol; her tract was reprinted there in the mid-1730s, and despite her quietism she was known for just the sort of bodily manifestations that would later be seen at Methodist meetings.[22]

Wesley's prayer meetings in Bristol provide some of the best-documented and most dramatic examples of the enthusiastic emphasis upon interpretations of the body. For example, in 1739 a young man experienced "a sharp (though short) agony, both of body and mind" before he "found his soul again filled with peace."[23] Wesley visited a young woman in Kingswood, just outside of Bristol, "I found her on the bed, two or three persons holding her. It was a terrible sight . . . the thousand distortions of her whole body showed how the dogs of hell were gnawing at her heart."[24] These physical manifestations, however frightening, revealed the inner battle for the woman's soul. For both her and the young man, physical agony was an outward sign; significant only in what it indicated about inner spiritual processes.

Wesley repeatedly contrasted "inward" and "outward" in his writings, always to show how the latter revealed the former. For instance, he wrote in his diary about a conversation with George Whitefield, "I had an opportunity to talk with him of those outward signs which had so often accompanied the inward work of God."[25] In *Primitive Physick,* he located illness in the innermost parts of the body, "The Seeds of Weakness and Pain, of Sickness and Death, are now lodged in our inmost Substance: Whence a thousand Disorders continually spring, even without the Aid of External Violence."[26] He added that even when illness was due to outward causes, these too were reflections of man's inner sinful state.

Whereas sermons such as those of Dodwell and Free attacked enthusiasm and sedition at a national level, these themes were articulated in the South-West with particular vigor in the debates about the spa at Glastonbury. From the start this spa was associated with popular divination; the healing properties of the two springs were supposed to have been revealed in a dream. It seems to have been an instant (though short-lived) success with the poor of rural Somerset; huge numbers allegedly made use of the waters.

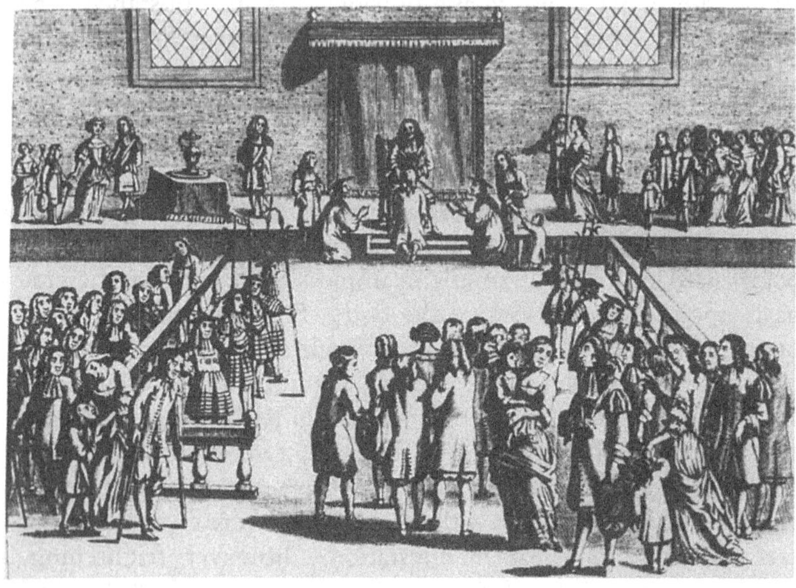

Figure 9.1. Stuart thaumaturgy in action. Charles II touching for the Evil (Wellcome Library)

Polite society's response, as expressed in that arbiter of manners, the *Gentleman's Magazine,* was almost uniformly negative, albeit spiced with curiosity. The first piece on the Glastonbury waters, in 1751, distanced itself from its own report, "This is fact, and inserted here to shew the capriciousness of popular taste."[27]

Later that year, a subsequent letter from Bristol to the *Gentleman's Magazine* made the connections between popular belief and political threat much clearer. It cited two recent instances of popular belief, one of the Glastonbury waters and the other of touching for the King's Evil. The writer disparaged the spa users, claiming that "the ignorant vulgar are ever fond of miracles."[28] This Bristolian also dealt with the Birmingham incident in which a person was cured by an angel who used the language of the ceremony of royal touching for the Evil. Queen Anne had been the last British monarch to touch, and the practice was subsequently linked to Jacobitism (see Fig. 9.1). The Birmingham cure had taken place on the 29th of May, the anniversary of the Stuart Restoration, and the writer emphasized that this story had been spread to give support to the Pretender. The Bristol writer went on to say "every honest and sensible man of the town despised his story," and emphasized the distinctions between believers and nonbelievers:

> Can any man of sense believe, that the bare touch of a man's hand, with three or four serious words spoken, can penetrate the whole mass of human blood, tainted and contaminated for many years before with such a stubborn, chronical malady as the Evil is known to be and communicate an instantaneous cure?[29]

This writer was not just attacking Jacobite practices; in doing so, he was denying the validity of lay interpretations of illness and healing associated with popular religion. For this writer, the connection between the inside and the outside of the body was more problematic than the ceremony of touching would admit.

Touching for the King's Evil, because of its links with Jacobitism, remained a favorite target of abuse. As J. C. D. Clark has pointed out, thaumaturgic powers and the legitimacy of the Hanoverian succession were addressed by competing Tory and Whig histories in the late 1740s. Christopher Lovell, a Bristol laborer, had been sent to Avignon in 1717, financed by a group of Bristol Jacobites eager to see the legitimate kingship of James III verified by a cure of the Evil. And it seemed that their faith was justified; Lovell returned cured, and his story was republicized decades later in the Jacobite Thomas Carte's *History of England*. Unfortunately for Carte, many Bristolians knew differently. Lovell's cure had been of but brief duration, and his patrons had paid for a second trip to France, but the unfortunate Lovell died en route. Josiah Tucker, critic of Wesleyan Methodism, manners-reformer and preacher of the vituperative sermon mentioned in Chapter 4, exposed Carte's error in the London press.[30] Tucker, of course, was known for his vehement opposition to many forms of popular recreation and amusement, and his involvement in the history controversy illustrates the connections made among vernacular healing, Jacobitism, and the emerging definitions of "politeness" which made "popular" into "vulgar."[31]

In a similar manner, the Swiss writer Samuel Werenfels's work on superstition was translated and republished in England in 1748. It attacked popular belief in healing practices such as wound-salves, astrologically significant herbs, numerical superstitions, and the transference of illness to animate and inanimate objects.

Appended to this work was a condemnation of touching for the King's Evil, in which Werenfels or his translator compared the Pretender to Sally Mapp, the noted English bonesetter.[32] Mapp was well-respected, even in the pages of the *Gentleman's Magazine;* Werenfels's attack shows how even "acceptable" lay healers could be rhetorically placed on the slippery slope to sedition.

A few months after the Glastonbury spa correspondence, another letter to the *Gentleman's Magazine* played upon a favorite threat to political stability, linking a miracle cure to the Jesuits, a veiled dig at Jacobite links to popery. This writer considered such a cure "a glaring proof of the superstitious credulity of the lower class of people."[33] Again and again, it was in letters such as these that the very idea of a "popular" culture (distinct from that of the "polite") was created, and the divisions between professional and lay healing made significant.[34] For instance, the *Bristol Weekly Intelligencer* published a brief essay "On Credulity" in 1750. It argued that people who listened to astrologers denied divine revelation, and then gave an instance known to the author:

> I met lately with an odd Fellow in the country, who is remarkable for Credulity and incredulity, as well as for several other Particularities in his Character. He does not believe one Word of the Old or New Testament, and with him Angels and Devils are equally Non-Entities; and yet this aged Infidel receives for the profoundest and most infallible Truth, whatever an Astrological Weaver in the Neighborhood tells him . . . If you talk to him of a Future State, he laughs at you; but if the weaver tells him of a future broken Skin, he trembles and looks pale.[35]

It was probably no accident that the writer situated this person (fictional or real) in the country; the opposition city/country paralleled those of sense/credulity and polite/vulgar. Such dichotomies were often repeated; the upper classes were described as "honest," "sensible," and "man of sense," while the lower classes made do with "vulgar," "credulity," "ignorant," "miracles," and "superstitious." Such "descriptions" were really prescriptions, guidelines for boundary maintenance between popular and polite. More important than these tropes, however, is the threat to social order implicit in this credulous individual's beliefs. The afterlife meant nothing; neither campaigns to reform manners nor evangelical sermons promising hell fire would have coerced this individual into behavior deemed appropriate by his betters. Worse yet, his source of authority, the person with access to truth, was a weaver, one of the most rebellious of trades.

Despite their occasional involvement with the Royal Society, doctors did not play a significant role in this mid-century denunciation of popular error. One of the few medical men to allude to superstition devoted himself not to the troubling aspects of healing but to the maintenance of health. William Cadogan, who had been a physician at the Bristol Infirmary, published his essay on infant care in 1747, and asserted the supremacy of medical modes of interpretation over those of lay individuals. He said that nurses lacked proper knowledge, "What I mean is a philosophic knowledge of Nature, to be acquir'd only by learned Observation and Experience, and which therefore the Unlearned must be incapable of."[36] Cadogan continued by disparaging the vernacular practices to which nurses were given, "I know not what strange unaccountable Powers in certain Herbs, Roots, and Drugs; and also in some superstitious Practices and Ceremonies; for all which Notions, there being no real Foundation in Nature, they ought to be looked upon as the Effects of Ignorance, or the Artifices of designing Quacks . . . "[37] For Cadogan, superstition's harm derived from its lack of connections with science rather than its religious or political implications. Nevertheless, his attack on lay practice was in accord with the more general assertion of politeness and its distinction from vernacular medicine, and the rhetoric of science was an appeal to authority paralleling those of Dodwell or Free.

In the 1750s, then, popular medicine was called into disrepute because of its associations with forms of popular culture under attack. Dissent, particularly Methodism, was linked to Jacobitism; the attack on church was an attack on state, and the "superstitious" practices of Methodists were easy to compare with those of papists, making the connections between political and religious threats to stability very clear. Practices of divination and prophecy were labeled superstition and tied to enthusiastic religion, which, of course, itself drew upon traditions of popular theodicy, making the equation of enthusiasm and superstition particularly easy. Lay-healing practices were peripheral to the spearhead of these attacks, but were easily included under the rubric superstition. More fundamentally, the interpretative practices that underlay both popular healing and religion were denounced from pulpits and attacked in the press.

At the end of the century, the condemnation of vernacular healing became more pronounced and was increasingly cast in a quasi-medical light. Once again, lay practices were linked with unacceptable, deviant forms of popular religion and with political threat. As J. F. C. Harrison documented, popular millenarianism came to be associated with popular radicalism in the troubled 1790s and was closely observed by the state as well as the church. Various forms of healing practices were associated with leading millenarian prophets, and their imprisonment or public exposure as frauds reflected upon vernacular healing. Harrison argues that millenarian beliefs embodied many of the same concepts and beliefs as popular literature and what he terms "folk culture."[38] The equation ran the other way as well: the "vulgar" beliefs tainted by millenarianism were made increasingly unacceptable to the middle and upper classes. For instance, forms of popular divination often employed in diagnosing illness were similar to those employed by millenarians, and were severely criticized. The anti-millenarianism of the mid-1790s was particularly pronounced, and it was recalled and reinvigorated by Joanna Southcott's claim to be pregnant with the child of Revelation in 1814.

In the 1790s ministers were again concerning themselves with the political divisiveness of sectarian religion, and making links between enthusiasm and sedition. What makes these late-century denunciations of superstition and enthusiasm particularly pointed is their willingness to make connections with the sectarian strife of the previous century. Unlike writers in the 1750s, who looked back to the Jacobite rebellion and thence argued that enthusiasm, sedition, and superstition were all-too-cozy bedfellows, these later writers dared to raise the specter of regicide and revolution in order to criticize lay belief systems.

M. J. Naylor, for example, published four linked sermons under the title *The Inanity and Mischief of Vulgar Superstitions* in 1795. He opened with a standard critique of Wesleyan Methodists, saying that superstitions had been yielding to "the progress of science" until Wesley "nourished and revivified" them.[39] Naylor then used the old gibe of comparing Methodists to papists, saying that Wesley's followers granted him "an almost Papal infallibility."[40] The connection between religious and political deviance is made when Naylor says that superstition leads to wars of religion, which "deluged the earth with blood" – an almost millenarian turn of phrase.[41] Because Naylor never specified which wars of religion he was alluding to, the reference remains capable of multiple interpretation. Not so in the case of another pamphlet on "Methodism and Popery Dissected." The anonymous writer makes an analogy between Methodism and some kind of monstrous growth, "were this all, such monsters are undoubtedly the objects of horror and detestation: but to go no farther than the Annals of our own Country, the hatred and bloodshed which the differences in religion have caused in society, are sufficient to make us execrate the designing, malevolent authors of such misery . . . "[42] Methodism, then, could be attacked from both ends – faulted on the grounds that it was too close to popery and thus Jacobitism or, as in this case, all too reminiscent of sectarian excesses of the previous century.[43] As Michael MacDonald argued, although it would be far too simplistic to suggest that the elite's abandonment of supernaturalism was solely due to the turmoils of the seventeenth century, it would be perverse to overlook any connections between the two.[44] In this case, one can certainly argue that the horrors of the seventeenth century provided a rhetorical stick with which to beat superstition, whether or not the hand that held the stick was motivated by such visions or by revolutions closer in time.

In his four sermons, M. J. Naylor pointed to the counterweight to superstition available to the modern age: experimental philosophy. One sermon is centered on the scriptural episode in which the Pharaoh of Egypt required miracles of Moses and Aaron and then commanded his own necromancers to duplicate these events. The sorcerers were successful in carrying out the first few of these miracles – problematic for interpreters of scripture because obviously these were not divinely ordained miracles as were those of God's chosen people. Naylor asked "Was there really any occult science, any hidden powers of nature" that the Pharaoh's magicians might have employed? He replied, "In an age like the present, when experimental philosophy is so accurately and extensively cultivated, no one can for a moment withhold his negative to this question." Earlier he had alluded to the "wonderful operations of nature" displayed by experimental philosophy.

The fact that Naylor consistently refers to *experimental* rather than *natural* philosophy is significant. As Simon Schaffer showed, natural philosophy became increasingly problematic in the second half of the eighteenth century. To oversimplify, it represented a form of uncontrolled interpretation that emphasized the wonders and miracles of nature, often performed by itinerant lecturers who had dubious political or religious connections. Schaffer shows how this system of representation became increasingly controlled – as he says, "the merely spectacular was an insufficient guarantee of moral effect."[45] Thus direct experience, often tainted by superstition, had to be replaced by controlled and progressive experience characterized by rationality.[46] Although the kinds of popular healing addressed here were not necessarily associated with natural philosophy, its downfall had severe repercussions for lay healing based on signs and wonders.[47] Once appearance and spectacle were utterly discredited, the hermeneutics of lay healing were denied any validity. Worse yet, as in the case of enthusiasm, such hermeneutics were again associated with the causes of political instability. Thus when Naylor refers to experimental philosophy, he underlines the interpretative control that characterized the management of nature's wonders at the end of the century. It is no accident that one of the evangelical Hannah More's Cheap Repository Tracts featured Mr. Fantom (the name perhaps a play on deceptions connected to the production of natural philosophy), the philosopher who led a servant astray; natural philosophy represented a threat to stability of all kinds.

Millenarian prophets were subject to close scrutiny as well as public ridicule in the 1790s. Richard Brothers, for example, who thought he was the nephew of God, captured the attention of London in the mid-1790s with his interpretations and visions of the coming of the end.[48] Like others, he combined healing and prophetic roles; he attempted to heal the blind through touching, and also performed various acts of divination and prophecy for individuals. According to *The Times*, God had revealed to his nephew that all sovereigns would be destroyed during the next three years.[49] In 1795, in a country in the midst of serious unrest caused by a terrible harvest, and which had only to look across the Channel to see what the end of monarchy might look like, this prophecy was too much. Brothers was taken into custody, examined by the Privy Council, and ultimately incarcerated in a private asylum. Obviously, the end of Brothers' prophetic career did not singlehandedly demolish the forms of vernacular divination and healing practices he had employed. But the publicity granted to Brothers' prophecies (many Londoners fled the capital on the evening he predicted an earthquake) meant that maximum public attention was focused on certain kinds of popular cultural phenomena. When polite society laughed at Brothers' pretensions – even while they may have feared his political implications – the divide between popular and elite culture was made very apparent.

In Bristol, one of Brothers' disciples, William Bryan, had a smoother career as a healer. Bryan was a copper-plate printer in London, a seeker after religious enlightenment who relied upon many popular practices of divination. For instance, when he was seeking a good place of worship he'd let his walking stick fall to the ground just outside his door, and set off in whatever direction it pointed.[50] He traveled to Avignon under divine guidance to visit a group of seekers there, and when he returned his former employers would not hire him because they were afraid he might go crazy again.

So Bryan moved to Bristol and became a druggist and apothecary. His autobiographical testimony relates his critique of local styles of dubious practice: "I could not crowd in draught after draught to enlarge my bill."[51] His healing practices were unorthodox, but not alien to some forms of religious or vernacular healing: Through the love of God, Bryan entered into a sympathy of feeling with his patients and felt the symptoms of their diseases himself. Bryan thought that knowledge was open to all who cared to seek; "I am confident that the true knowledge is not withheld from any man by the Lord."[52]

In early 1795 Bryan took his healing role a step further. A friend of his opened a dispensary for soldiers in Bristol, and Bryan ministered to them.[53] These soldiers had been pressed into service in County Mayo, and allegedly through the collusion of the local justice of the peace and the colonel of the regiment had even been denied their signing-on money. The conditions under which they had been housed had led to fever, and two of the men were discovered near death in the streets of Bristol after crossing the Irish Sea in an open boat. For Bryan, the political implications of his healing role were apparent. He criticized the "vile, unjust and diabolical" means used to raise these new regiments, as well as the government policy that encouraged such tactics.[54]

William Bryan, while looking back to various kinds of enthusiastic healers of the previous century and a half, was also looking forward to a sort of countercultural form of alternative medicine.[55]

In the nineteenth century, various unorthodox and fringe medical activities can be read as critiques of the orthodox profession. In the eighteenth century, such explicit political commentary on the profession was well nigh impossible, if only because 'the profession' was inchoate and contained within its capacious reaches virtually all forms of healing. Bryan, whom contemporaries always noted was sweet-natured and bore a strong resemblance to contemporary representations of Christ, enjoyed a long career as a healer, finally earning the orthodox-flavored epithet of "the Galen of Hoddesen" in his old age.

The incarceration of Bryan's prophet, Richard Brothers, and the discrediting of his millenarian prophecies, took place against a backdrop of a more generalized attack on popular culture. In a style analogous to the reform-of-manners campaigns of the 1690s discussed in earlier chapters, the group which came to be called "the evangelicals" initiated various campaigns from the 1780s onward. Indeed, specific allusions to earlier reforms were made; their leader William Wilberforce wrote in his journal that "God has set before me as my object the reformation of manners."[56] Despite Ford K. Brown's detailed analysis of this group, and their predilection for founding institutions, many of their activities on the local level remain shadowy.[57] What is clear is that this group, guided by William Wilberforce and Hannah More, launched an attack on many aspects of popular culture and recreation. In general, one can summarize their campaigns as an attempt to make England a godly society by abolishing irreligion in many forms. Brown has made much of their skills in utilizing ends to means; whether or not one concurs with his assessment of their success, their subsequent management of many medical institutions made their views on vernacular healing significant to medical professionals.

Two areas of the evangelicals' reforms of manners were important for lay medical practices. First was the activities of the Society for the Suppression of Vice (henceforth the SSV). The extent of this group's identity with the evangelicals has been debated, but however loose or tight the association, the SSV was engaged, albeit often unsuccessfully, in putting down various kinds of popular cultural expressions, such as fortune-telling and lotteries, which were related to healing in a manner analogous to the efforts of the evangelicals.[58] Second was Hannah More's attack on popular culture contained in her Cheap Repository Tracts. Again and again these little stories denigrate forms of vernacular diagnosis and hermeneutics, linking lay healing with other unacceptable practices of astrology, fortune-telling and divination.

Letters to newspapers made links between quackery and the discipline of the poor since at least the 1770s, but the SSV went one step further by utilizing an obscure portion of the Elizabethan vagrancy laws to prosecute fortune-tellers, physiognomists, and astrologers. A 1777 letter to the *Morning Post,* for instance, poked fun at a dentist who extracted teeth with the point of his sword, while on horseback. (It is not recorded if the patient were also on horseback.) This letter writer had no hesitation in linking the dentist with "prophets of various denominations" – i.e., enthusiastic religion – and with lotteries. What was wrong with this practitioner, according to the letter writer, was that he reaped "the benefits which ought to attend the efforts of honest industry."[59] In other words, such quackery, associated with popular divination and lotteries, undermined honest labor and the discipline of the poor.

The SSV made explicit the links between fortune-telling and the discipline of the poor in their prosecution of Joseph Powell, who was brought to court at least twice with the help of the SSV. In 1807 Powell fell into a trap prepared by a surgeon, Mr. Blair. Blair's servant had received one of Powell's handbills.[60] Blair sent one of his servants to Powell with a request for the nativity of another servant. The astrological predictions for the servant were detailed – even Blair had to admit that Powell provided a certain value for money. For half a crown, there was information about health, riches, marriage, children, and travel, along with guidelines about avoiding certain hazards – the servant should never travel toward the North-East, for example.[61] But Blair had scratched his initials into the half-crown fee, and once the sale was complete, a constable was at the ready to arrest Powell. In a pamphlet published by the SSV about the case, Powell was castigated for his role in luring servants to spend money on lotteries, for predicting the deaths of various individuals, and for dream interpretation. More important, he was linked to millenarian prophecy: among his collection of astrological texts (which the court impounded) was a pamphlet of the prophet Richard Brothers.[62] Thus, for the SSV, all the links were made between irregular healing, popular astrology and divination, radical religion and sedition. In the popular press, opinion was more mixed, and much fun was had at the SSV's expense. Nor was Mr. Blair well-received.[63]

A year later, Powell was again set up by the SSV. This time an SSV stooge purchased a headache remedy from Powell, and once again the constable was just around the corner and arrested Powell, who got six months in jail.[64] Powell seems to have attracted many servants and laborers among his clientele. Part of the threat he posed to the social order was related to these clients' wishes to spend their small wages on lotteries, prophecy, and other practices that denied God's providence.

More generally, the all-out attack by the evangelicals on various forms of popular cultural expression helped to widen the gulf between polite and plebian cultures. Hannah More, the chief polemicist of the evangelical movement, was born in Gloucestershire, taught school in Bristol, and spent most of her life in the South-West. Hence her reform activities were of particular weight in Bristol. At seventeen she published her first lengthy work, a pastoral drama. As an adult she turned her literary talents to reforming the manners of the lowly and the great. In 1784 she and her sisters moved to a small village in the Mendips, and it was there that More, under the guidance of Wilberforce, found a mission in educating the locals in morals and religion. Her contacts with the working classes, coupled with a ready pen, produced a series of popular chapbooks, intended as proper reading for the working classes, with an omnipresent moral message.

Her story of Tawny Rachel, presumably of gypsy heritage, who scrapes together a living as a cunning woman and healer on the Somerset wastes, illustrates the links More and others made between fortune-telling, quackery, and interpreting the outside of the body. Rachel, "was continually practicing on the credulity of silly girls."[65] Her success was due to her ability to read the significance of physical characteristics: "Rachel was also a famous interpreter of dreams, and could distinguish exactly between the fate of any two persons who happened to have a mole on the right or left cheek."[66] In the story, she takes advantage of a superstitious dairy-maid, who ultimately dies of a broken heart after being abandoned by the husband Rachel selected for her. More pointed to the moral: "God never reveals to weak and wicked women those secret designs of his Providence which no human wisdom is able to foresee."[67] Compare this assertion with William Bryan's assured statement that God's knowledge was open to all, and the epistemological differences between millenarians and evangelical reformers become clear.

In a companion story, about Rachel's husband Black Giles the Poacher, More links Rachel's fortune-telling abilities to quack remedies. She sells distilled waters; but appearances are deceptive. Rachel tops up bottles of water with a peppermint liquor, and offers prospective customers tiny sample vials of the peppermint. They taste the samples, sniff at the larger bottles, and unwittingly buy mostly water.[68] Once again, things are not what they seem, and More manages to deny the significance of appearances while denigrating the practices of lay diviners and healers.

As Susan Pedersen has shown, More's tales cunningly used many of the devices of popular culture in order to subvert it.[69] Tawny Rachel can be seen as the mirror image of Mother Bunch, or any other of the number of women who authored chapbooks that told the reader how to interpret dreams, practice simple physiognomy, manipulate charms, and other elements of popular prophecy and divination. Hannah More's attacks were launched at contemporary cultural forms, even if those forms were at least a century old.

It was probably no accident that More made her fortune-telling character female. Women seem to have been particularly involved with forms of healing that combined astrology and fortune-telling with attention to the outside of the body. In a sense these women were the commercial exemplification of the Mother Bunches of chapbook fame – they provided a very similar service to their customers to that of Bunch to her readers. For example, the astrological healer Mrs. Williams treated women only and was presumably successful – in addition to her London practice she traveled the South-West circuit, to Bath, the Bristol Hotwells, and Wells. She sold cosmetics, such as Persian Cream and Armenian Tooth Powder, as well as ministering to women's unspecified nervous complaints by retailing her Nervous Batavian Tincture.[70] Many astrological healers in the 1780s and 1790s appear to have been women, particularly in the metropolis.[71]

Female healing and its denouncement by the evangelicals may also have been related to female prophecy, particularly of the millenarian kind.[72] Enthusiastic and millenarian women prophets were often referred to as "Mother," as were the alleged authors of such popular works of prophecy such as Mother Bunch. Indeed, the divisions between "cunning women" like Tawny Rachel, and prophets like Joanna Southcott were more of degree than kind.[73] Southcott was known locally as a wise woman, as was her fraudulent associate Mary Bateman, whose hen produced miraculous eggs marked "Crist is Coming" (no one said the Almighty was a good speller). Although Southcott tried to emphasize the differences between thaumaturgy and prophecy, for many observers, the similarities, especially regarding women's practices, were marked.[74]

Thus the conceptual framework of vernacular healing was shaken, and shaken again by the storms of enthusiastic religion and the repressions associated with it. What made such denunciations so powerful was the intersection of various causes and consequences of what Keith Thomas called the decline of magic, the complicated untangling of the worlds of the natural and supernatural. The dissolution of great and small cultures was not the gradual ebbing away of accord but was the focus of specific battles about political and religious stability. The vehemence, indeed the cruelty, of the attacks on vernacular culture that characterize the works of Hannah More suggest that the evangelicals enjoyed an uneasy and uncertain tenancy of the moral high ground. Nevertheless, the bell had already tolled for the respectability of vernacular medicine, not merely because of associations with "unacceptable" religious practices but because the very basis of lay diagnostic procedures became untenable in an era that knew miracles had ceased.

But what of the doctors? How did organized medicine perceive and respond to the divergence of popular and elite cultures? The answers to such questions remain unclear, in part because professional medical men tended not to make many pronouncements on the subject of lay healing. There were exceptions, of course – the Leeds surgeon William Hey, known for his evangelical activities, did not hesitate to denigrate lay healing in his medical articles.[75] Nor was Thomas Beddoes ever silent for long about the dangers of quackery. But in general medical men kept their heads down and avoided controversies over lay beliefs. Two instances in which medical men did get involved with disputes about popular interpretation show how problematic such activities could be and reveal that medical men experienced many of the same tensions between signs and things signified. Both instances were also direct confrontations by medical men of enthusiastic religion.

The first controversy is concerned with the Yatton demoniac, George Lukins. Lukins, a Somerset lad, suddenly became subject to fits in 1787, in which he seemed to lose his sanity, declaring himself to be the devil.[76] The controversy lay in whether or not he was faking these fits, and it was played out in a series of letters to Bristol newspapers. Samuel Norman, a local surgeon, claimed that Lukins was not possessed by the devil in any way, that he was an impostor. Others disagreed. This controversy did not center around Lukins's actual condition or Norman's diagnostic skills, but the plausibility of demoniac possession and the characters of the opponents. The elements of possession, miracles, enthusiastic religion, and the credibility of witnesses were at the heart of the controversy.

At one point Lukins alleged that he was possessed by seven devils and that only seven ministers could cure him. Joseph Easterbrook, the vicar of Temple parish in Bristol, tried to recruit local clergymen "most cordial in the belief of supernatural influences," but those he approached, although sympathetic, avoided his invitation to conduct an exorcism. So Easterbrook relied on local itinerant Methodist preachers. These men must have seen some familiar aspects to Lukins' fits which resembled the convulsions some Methodists underwent as the devil struggled for their souls. Lukins was probably more dramatic than many: he barked like a dog, and the spirits conducted a multivoiced rendition of the *Te Deum*. Nevertheless, the kinds of spirit possession familiar to enthusiastic religious activities were similar to those Lukins evidently experienced.

For Samuel Norman and his correspondents in the Bristol newspapers, the questions about the possibility of worlds of the spirit were refracted in questions concerning the credibility of witnesses, in a manner analogous to David Hume's denial of miracles. Were these letter-writers gentlemen and therefore trustworthy observers? What was deception? Norman ultimately published a collection of these letters in a pamphlet, probably hoping to justify his claims. In the introduction, he referred to the "insolence, prevarication, and personal abuse" to which he had been subject, which "are at all times unbecoming the character of a gentleman."[77] His purpose, he later reiterated, was to "prevent the honest and well meaning" from deception.[78] *Justiciae Vindex,* the pseudonymous author of letters supporting Lukins, also made character the central issue. He began by pointing out Lukins' respectable character – a young man in a decent trade, reputable family, religiously educated – what would he have to gain by such trickery?[79] He then reminded his readers that Norman was not without such mercenary agendas, "who no doubt has undertaken this enquiry from the purest of motives, and not from any pique that the parish never thought it *worthwhile to ask his opinion,* nor employ *him* for the recovery."[80] *Vindex* goes on to rhetorically place Norman among the credulous, advising him to "rise superior to the little vulgar tales and silly anecdotes in a village."[81]

Norman quickly retorted that his account of Lukins' behavior "was very lately repeated to me by a gentleman of this parish" – in other words, allying himself with a gentleman rather than the credulous vulgar. He also pointed out that he had been hired by the parish overseers to treat Lukins but that he "quickly gave his case up as unworthy of my notice."[82]

In subsequent letters *Justiciae Vindex* reclaimed the authority of class and social position for his side of the argument. He criticized Norman's literary style, "surely I have the right to expect common sense and intelligible language."[83] Finally, he reminded the reader again of the central problem of the debate – the relationship between appearance and reality. He writes that he "cannot help suspecting, when I see such pompous declamations on the beauty of virtue, that they are calculated to cover the deformity of vice." Nothing is as it seems. The problem of appearance and reality shaped Norman's assessment of his patient and the world's assessment of Norman.

This instance reveals how arguments about the world of spirits and the possibility of miracles might be couched in a discourse about politeness and gentlemanly behavior. The connections between Methodism and supernaturalism were very clear to contemporaries, and the discussions of "polite" behavior in the Lukins case makes clear references to these links. Norman, not surprisingly, took the opportunity to deny the possibility of supernatural forces and attempted to assert the authority of medicine through social class. But his failure indicates that social standing, rather than science, was the key to local esteem and, perhaps, a successful practice. No wonder few others engaged in conflict with the worlds of the spirit.

The second instance in which a medical man intervened in a case of lay beliefs bore many of the hallmarks of the Yatton case. This was the controversy that surrounded Joanna Southcott's alleged pregnancy. Joanna Southcott, born in Devon in 1750, spent most of her life in the South-West, finding work as a domestic servant when she grew up. She began to prophesy during the difficult years of the 1790s. As several historians have pointed out, prophesying represented an exaggeration of common elements of West Country popular culture, known for its predilection for the supernatural.[84] Southcott's initial prophecies were of local, practical things – good or bad harvests, the death of nearby worthies. She moved beyond local celebrity in 1801 when she took her writings to an Exeter printer and used her savings to publish them. Soon her followers numbered in the thousands, and Southcott moved to London. After a few years, some of the furor calmed, but in 1814 Southcott was again national news. She was supposedly pregnant with the child Shiloh, predicted in an obscure passage of Revelations.

Richard Reece, the author of works on domestic medicine, which often served to remind their readers of the authority of medical men, was asked to see Southcott and pronounce on her pregnancy. His account must rank as one of the clearest about-faces in medical literature; he initially thought she was pregnant, and his change of heart took some time.[85]

Despite Reece's public exposure as, at best, gullible, he published his pamphlet as a warning "to the weak, ignorant, and deluded; and it will serve also as a guard to every professional character, in trusting to no appearances of candor or veracity, in circumstances where he has an opportunity of forming a correct judgement."[86] At the outset, Reece stated that he saw no evidence of imposture, and was impressed by Mrs. Southcott's mien and simplicity. Despite a letter to *The Times* which reminded the public that doctors had also been deceived in the case of Mary Tofts – the woman who had given birth to rabbits (also interpreted in a millenarian context) – Reece continued to maintain that Southcott might be pregnant.[87]

Not so the surgeon and apothecary P. Mathias, who found the idea of an elderly virgin birth ludicrous. Joanna Southcott asked

Mathias if he would believe her when he saw the infant at her breast. Mathias's response was revealing:

> I thought it high time to give a firm and decisive answer to questions, evidently to my comprehension, so revolting to common sense, and to enter my protest against opinions so blasphemous and profane. I said *seeing was believing*, and that I must be present and have ocular demonstration of the fact.[88]

But the key to this case was the problem engendered by the equation of seeing and believing. Just as with the Yatton demoniac, when authorities could not agree on the meaning of what they saw, chaos ensued, and the basis of authority was called into question.

To take just one example, Reece and another surgeon, J. S. Sims, disagreed over the signs of pregnancy exhibited by Southcott. They argued about her breasts – Reece said that their fullness was due to pregnancy, whereas Sims averred that it was just plumpness. Reece argued that the shape of the nipples, the ratio of length to width, showed that he was correct, whereas Sims maintained that this effect was merely the accumulation of fatty tissue.[89] When Southcott died, a post-mortem examination was carried out, and Sims' arguments were vindicated. Reece was forced to reassess, and attempted to save the phenomenon by claiming that some accomplice had repeatedly enlarged Southcott's breasts by suction, making Reece the victim of deliberate deception.

No, seeing could not be believing; the relationship between sign and substance was too precarious to support the scaffolding of professional authority. As the Society for the Suppression of Vice emphasized, nothing was what it seemed – "Vice asserts the name of Virtue, assumes her form and challenges her rights."[90] The truth lay hidden from the gaze of the vulgar, where only the trained observer could find it. James Gillray, in his cartoon of Southcott and the doctors made the point very clearly; Joanna is represented as saying "Seeing is believing." For medical men the lesson implicit in Reece's comeuppance was exactly the reverse – seeing could not be believing. The fissure between professional and lay beliefs about healing had become a gulf, and medical men were well-served by ignoring lay beliefs.

The purpose of my exploration has been to suggest, first, how vernacular medicine came to be abandoned by all but the working class. Through the construction of "politeness" and the denigration of superstition, middle- and upper-class people came to rely upon new professionally-oriented forms of illness-interpretation and healing. Obviously, this shift was related to the commercialization of domestic remedies discussed in Chapter 3; but this was not the full answer.

Second, I have tried to formulate some analysis of the formation of a distinctively working-class "popular" medicine. This seems neither to be merely hand-me-downs of elite wisdom nor the politically articulated creation of alternative medicine. The model of great and small, popular and elite, folk and literate cultures has received much deserved criticism, and I have hesitated to use a version of it here. Nevertheless, the case of nonprofessional health care seems to be well portrayed as a sort of gradually but inexorably increasing segregation; ideas and practices acceptable to many groups in 1690 were acceptable to fewer by 1790. It should come as no surprise that the body was subject to the same cultural policing as other forms of popular culture. Earlier chapters have shown what a potent site for the reform of manners the body proved itself to be. In this light, the discipline of the workhouse and the discipline of the doctor were once again united, outside the hospital as well as inside.

10

Conclusions

This book originated as an examination of the health care provided by the Old Poor Law, an attempt to understand the influences of welfare and social policy on medicine. It expanded to include other forms of institutional provision, and then, to put these in perspective, all of health care, save that for the very wealthy. The reconstruction of health-care options in one early modern city has created, as always, more questions than it has answered. Nevertheless, some conclusions can be drawn, some agendas for further work sketched in.

First, an understanding of health-care institutions and practices indicates the multiform ways in which the body served as a site of cultural policing, rarely initiated by medicine itself, but often abetted by it. This theme can be restated in a different way: local health-care patterns reveal how social policy served to mediate the interests of the great. In this period such policy was often intimately bound up with religion; the bricks and mortar of health-care institutions represented an intersection of different religious and civic interests. The second group of conclusions, then, relates to the ways in which medical institutions were not very medical; they embodied all kinds of local and national interests quite outside the realm of the profession. The medicalization of these nonmedical institutions remains to be explained.

"The body" has become the focus of considerable historical attention in recent years, due to the legacy of Foucault as well as trends within social history and the history of science and medicine. My own interest derived from questions of medical authority and how it was created in a context of the seeming domination of vernacular medicine. Control of the body however, was as much a political and religious issue as a medical or domestic one. Although it is no more than a truism to point out that bodies are always freighted with cultural significances, the ways in which this is so are specific to historical moments. Two meanings of the body seem particularly important for the eighteenth century.

First is the body in relation to work. As Michel Foucault has shown, institutions like prisons, hospitals, and asylums are, on one level, about work discipline. Thus, for example, lines of filiation can be drawn from the two workhouses in Bristol to the Infirmary. The workhouse, or Mint, was designed to discipline those who would not work, while the Infirmary mended those who could not work; infirmaries can be understood as expressions of mercantile interest, places where, on a very local level, the creation of health was the creation of wealth.

But a closer examination of the workhouse and the Infirmary reveals another layer of meaning about the body. It was the mirror of godliness, an emblem of society's sanctity. Thus, for example, John Cary noted that the early inmates of the Mint got sick, and their bodies threw off a good deal of foul material, as they became accustomed to a regulated, well-mannered, structured life. So too, the imposition of godly habits would reform the soul through the medium of the body – or at least, create the appearance of reform so crucial to England's providential role. In a similar fashion, the Infirmary simultaneously mended the sick and corrected their behavior, while ridding the city of beggars by eliminating a plausible reason for mendicancy. Of course, beggars were more likely to end up incarcerated in the workhouse, but nevertheless the rationales for making a clean and godly city, rid of beggars and frauds, were the same.

But this style of policing the body changed as the bodies of the poor became a repository for different kinds of anxieties. Reforms of popular culture made what had been a shared understanding of the body, held by rich and poor, patients and doctors, into "superstitions," fit only for the lower classes. The reasons for this abandonment were tied up with the interpretive practices central to vernacular medicine of the later seventeenth century, commonplaces which could be found in any number of types of cultural expressions, from proverbs and chapbooks to domestic remedies for common ailments. Put most basically, the significances of illness were inscribed on the outside of the body, where they were open to interpretation by all. Of course, it was not just illness that could be read off the body's surface; as in the case of vagabonds incarcerated in the workhouse, moral worth, integrity, and personality were all apparent.

But interpretive strategies that focused on the outside of the body were attacked in mid-eighteenth century and at its end. In neither case was medicine central to this process. Rather, vernacular hermeneutics became linked with Jacobitism and enthusiastic religion at mid-century, and were thus a part of a campaign to distinguish between polite and vulgar behaviors. In the 1790s vernacular medicine again became linked with deviant religion, this time in the shape of radical millenarianism. At the same time, lay healing fell afoul of the evangelical campaign to reform the manners of the poor, which stressed the unreliability of appearances. Again and again, a range of reformers emphasized this point: appearances were deceptive, not to be trusted. This attempt to break the links between appearance and reality was a part of the destruction of supernatural beliefs, which rested upon the assumption that there were connections between the worlds of matter and spirit, the seen and unseen.

Just as religious dissension shaped the cultural body, so too it influenced the social disposition of the bodies of the poor. The creation of the hospital and the workhouse owed much to the factional nature of city life in the early eighteenth century. Such institutions served as theaters for the negotiation of local interests, as arenas for power and privilege. In Bristol, both hospital and workhouse were a means of wresting power from the select vestries and the city corporation who controlled the city and blocked access to dissenters. The Corporation of the Poor and the Infirmary offered a very wide access to city governance and, not surprisingly, were soon controlled by a dissenting counterweight to civic authority. Of course, such a picture is too simplistic. Both institutions simultaneously afforded moments of civic unity, allowing various interests to bury their hatchets. But these moments of coalition were brief and charity remained highly politicized and sectarian throughout the century.

Indeed, in the era that raised clientage to a high art, how could such instruments of patronage be otherwise? For admission of a patient was very much a form of charitable patronage, an assertion of obligation on the one hand and deference on the other. It was only with the withdrawal of the governors from their tight control of the institution – probably a reflection of changing relations of neighborhood and workplace – that medical men came to reshape the Infirmary in their own interest.

As governors abandoned their hands-on style of running the hospital, surgeons, through their new utilization of the hospital as training ground, came to have a vital interest in the institution. Medical men of all kinds had long been eager to serve in hospitals because it gave them opportunities to make lucrative contacts with potential patients – the governors – and served as a form of advertisement. But with the advent of Infirmary training, there were richer pickings in the guise of student fees. Surgeons began to see their patients in a new light, as clinical material, both before and after death.

While these developments were, in all likelihood, going on in other English provincial infirmaries, some aspects of Bristol's tale seem exceptional. The historiography of eighteenth-century English medicine has been strongly weighted toward the metropolis, and when writing about Bristol medicine one frequently feels that Bristol and London were on different planets. Certainly, many a Bristol lad went off to London and walked the wards for a year or two before returning to practice in the South-West. But the familiar names and themes of eighteenth-century medicine – Lettsom, Fothergill, the Hunters, discussions of sensibility, or of theories of fever – all are lacking for eighteenth-century Bristol.

Indeed, about the only nationally-known medical figure in the city (Cadogan, Cheyne, and Farr all left Bristol before making names for themselves) was Thomas Beddoes. However, within the context of Bristol medicine, Beddoes was, at best, deviant. He put patients in cowsheds and experimented with gases; he ran a free clinic that was a blatant critique of Infirmary medicine, and thus of the city's medical elite. He was associated with all sorts of dangerous Jacobin ideas and he published pamphlets, articles, and books constantly. No one could have been more different from the dean of Bristol medicine, Richard Smith, whose few publications included one on good methods of whitening bones for display. It is Beddoes who must be considered eccentric in this provincial context.

Indeed, this close examination of Bristol medicine reveals how strong were local traditions and professional habits. As described, entry into the culture of Bristol Infirmary medicine meant student years filled with anatomy, dissection, and grave robbing on a scale seemingly unequalled by other educational institutions. Without doubt, among the foundations of this ghoulish subculture were the Smiths, *père et fils,* their passion for dissection, their styles of lecturing, and their museum. While other hospitals practiced anatomy and dissection I doubt that it was inevitably such a strong interest and rite of passage for students. Thus despite exposure to metropolitan ways, local medical culture seems to have remained strong into the nineteenth century, and viewed from the perspective of the provinces, developments in Edinburgh and London seem less significant.

I have tried to understand both the cultural and the social roles of the bodies of the poor from the patient's perspective, arrogant though such an attempt may be on the part of a late twentieth-century historian. From such a vantage point, the reform of manners that reduced vernacular concepts and practices about the body to "superstition" and the processes by which hospital patients lost the ability to interpret their own illnesses look the same. Both derived from the transformation of social relations, from the process by which inequalities of rich and poor became those of nascent class relationships. Not that the modern body/hospital is the crude product of class formation. Instead, to use E. P. Thompson's terms, class struggle, not class, describes the interactions of rich and poor which denied the poor ownership of their bodies. In a manner parallel to the enclosure of common land, or the denial of use rights, the poor lost the right to construct their own bodies in the public realm. Certainly, individuals long continued to interpret illness in "early-modern" terms for themselves, but only the well-to-do could expect those definitions to be accepted by their medical men.[1] Where the city workhouse appropriated the labor of its inmates, its descendant – the infirmary – took something more fundamental from its patients. Not only did it steal the bodies of those who died in hospital, it also denied meaning to those who lived.

Appendix: Medical practitioners in Bristol and Somerset

Given the open market for medical care in the eighteenth century, it is very difficult to estimate how many practitioners there were at any given time. Compounding the problem of definition – who counts as a practitioner? – is that of sources. My analysis of city practitioners comes from a list of over a thousand medical men and women who practiced in the city during the eighteenth century, compiled from a number of sources. First is a typescript in the Bristol Medical School Library, which lists all the medical men who became freemen of the city, and some other names acquired from a variety of sources. Because one's freedom was taken up at the completion of apprenticeship, and seems to have been done by those who wished to practice in the city (rather than those who went elsewhere, or returned to their home towns), this seemed a better guide than indenture registers. This list was amplified by including all men who apprenticed anyone for medical training, by references to medical men gleaned from newspapers, by all medical men in the 1775 and 1793 city directories, by those in the Bristol Biographical Memoirs who practiced in the city, as well as a number of medical men mentioned incidentally in other records.

This list reveals certain biases in those used by other historians. For example, Samuel Foart Simmons's Medical Register of 1783 has been used to reconstruct patterns of medical practice in eighteenth-century Britain. Simmons collected his names for his registers (this was his third, and best) largely by word of mouth, personal acquaintance, and through institutional connections. His list of medical practitioners is biased accordingly, and might be understood as a rhetorical plea for a particular kind of medical practitioner rather than an innocuous attempt to list doctors.

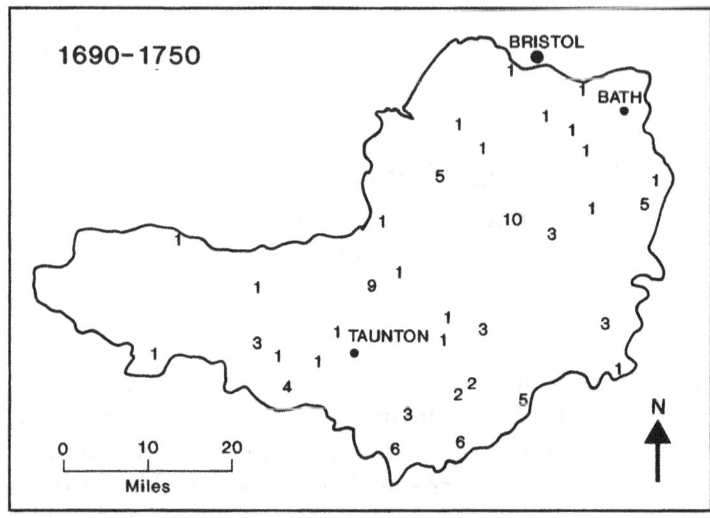

Map 3. Somerset practitioners, 1690–1750

A comparison of his register with my compilation of practitioners in Bristol illustrates Simmons' predilections. He was most accurate in his recording of M.D.s and apothecaries, only missing 3 of the 11 M.D.s then in Bristol, and 2 of them may well have been semiretired. Apothecaries (perhaps because of their shops) were also well-represented; only 7 of 34 were overlooked by Simmons. It is in surgery that Simmons's list is particularly inadequate. He recorded only 16 of the 29 surgeons practicing in Bristol in 1783. In addition, none of the 13 practicing barber-surgeons appear on his list. It is of course, not surprising that these were the practitioners of whom Simmons never heard; they were the least likely to have the institutional and associational ties he so valued.

Recently Wallis and Wallis compiled a valuable and massive list of eighteenth-century practitioners, including well over 35,000 individuals. Even here, however, there are inevitably problems of completeness. For example, I include more widows who took over their husbands' practices in Bristol than do the Wallises. But these problems of definition do not obscure the basic point that most Bristolians had an abundance of health-care practitioners available to them throughout the century. Most of the changes in urban health-care provision were those of kind rather than degree. Thus, for example, by the 1790s, many more Bristol med-

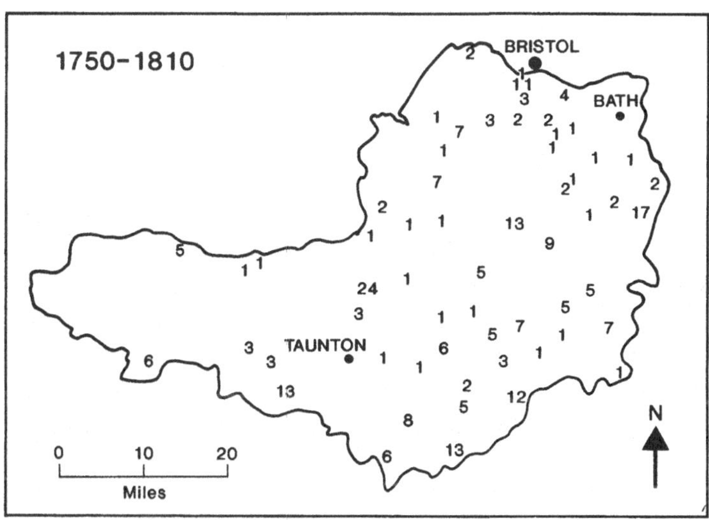

Map 4. Somerset practitioners, 1751–1810

ical men described themselves as surgeon-apothecaries, although the barber-surgeon was much less common than a generation earlier. So too, as the city became spatially segregated by social standing, medical men followed suit. By the 1790s, medical men with aspirations often lived and worked on Park Street; those ministering to the poor of SS. Philip and Jacob would be found in its main trading thoroughfare, the Old Market.

In rural areas, changes were of degree as well as kind. I have compiled a list of eighteenth-century Somerset practitioners, although such a list will always be more incomplete than that for the city in the absence of early directories and urban civic structures, such as apprenticeship. In both absolute and relative terms, numbers of Somerset medical men grew during the eighteenth century. Maps 3 and 4 show where practitioners were in the first and second halves of the century. Figures indicate the number of practitioners. Because this analysis focuses on rural areas, the large towns and cities of Bath, Bristol, Taunton, and Wells have not been plotted on the maps, although smaller towns like Bridgewater have been.

Not only did the numbers of medical men increase, the types of rural practitioners changed. Surgeons remain at about 40 percent of the total Somerset medics throughout the century. Apothecaries, however, disappear, replaced by surgeon-apothecaries. Thus, in the first quarter of the century, only about 5 percent of practitioners used the double title to describe themselves, while apothecaries were half the total practitioners. By the end of the century, the picture is the other way around: 45 percent are surgeon-apothecaries and only 5 percent call themselves apothecaries only. Physicians were always few in the countryside, but as many as 10 percent of all Somerset practitioners were physicians. Not surprisingly, they were usually in the larger towns, like the diarist William Holland's Dr. Dunning in Bridgewater. Finally, by the last quarter of the century, about 10 percent of medics call themselves druggists. They were not confined to very large towns, either; John Periam was selling drugs in Wellington, James Toomer in South Brent, William Curtis in Shepton Mallet.

In the first half of the century, there were 91 practitioners in Somerset; this rose to 238 in the second half of the century, although obviously not all these men were practicing simultaneously. This increase is in contrast to the urban situation. In Bristol, although absolute numbers of practitioners rose, relative to the population they declined. Thus, in the first decade of the eighteenth century, there was one practitioner to every 163 people in the city. By the last decade, this had declined to one practitioner for every 468 individuals – still quite a healthy ratio. In rural Somerset, by comparison, there was one practitioner to every 1,300 people at the end of the century. Larger towns, however, were beginning to show practitioner-to-patients ratios similar to those of Bristol; Bridgewater had 1 practitioner to 484 people at the turn of the century. And, of course, the catchment area for such provincial practitioners was larger than just their town of residence.

Medical practitioners were not evenly distributed about the countryside. They were clumped in towns – hence, for instance, the preponderance of medics in the South-East of the county. Of course, potential patients were also clumped in towns. I've used the 1801 census, with all of its inaccuracies, to try to characterize the distribution of medics across the county in relation to population. Although bigger towns had more medics, they didn't necessarily have them out of all proportion to their populations. Thus, for example, Yeovil had about as many medics per 1,000 population – 1.8 – as did Porlock or Quantoxhead, towns a quarter of Yeovil's size.

The 1801 census also classifies the populations of each parish according to agricultural workers, and those engaged in trade, manufacturing, or handicraft. Unfortunately, as is well known, the basis for these categories varied from parish to parish, so any subtle analysis is impossible. However, the most significant aspect of these occupational groupings as they relate to medicine has to do with agricultural parishes. The ten hundreds with the highest percentages of agricultural workers differed significantly from the ten lowest. The agricultural hundreds averaged just 0.1 medics per 1,000 population; the nonagricultural hundreds did nine times better with 0.9 per 1,000, which is slightly above the county-wide average of 0.7. Obviously, part of the explanation for this discrepancy lies in population density – practitioners were more likely to be in towns, which had higher concentrations of potential patients than did rural areas. But perhaps agricultural workers also had less money to spend on formal medical care, or were less inclined to seek professional advice.

In sum, city and country became increasingly similar by the end of the century. In rural towns, as in the city, patients could choose among a group of practitioners. Even in the countryside, many had access to a practitioner, although access was constrained by cost. Both rural and urban practitioners were often engaged in dual practice as surgeons and apothecaries, although the advent of the druggist altered patterns of consumption.

Notes

CHAPTER 1

1 Pioneering work on the patient's view has understandably focused on those literate enough to leave narrative records of their experiences of illness and medicine. Roy Porter, ed., *Patients and Practitioners* (Cambridge University Press 1985); Lucinda Beier, *Sufferers and Healers: The Experience of Illness in Seventeenth-Century England* (London: Routledge & Kegan Paul, 1987). Michael MacDonald has used a practitioner's records to analyze a variety of patients' experiences of mental illness in his *Mystical Bedlam: Madness, Anxiety, and Healing in Seventeenth-Century England* (Cambridge University Press, 1981).

2 See, for example, J. E. Janzen, *The Quest for Therapy in Lower Zaire* (Berkeley and Los Angeles: University of California Press, 1978); G. L. Chavunduka, *Traditional Healers and the Shona Patient* (Gwelo: Mambo Press, 1978); Z. A. Ademuwagun et al., eds., *African Therapeutic Systems* (Waltham, Mass.: Crossroads Press, 1979); P. Stanley Yoder, ed., *African Health and Healing Systems: Proceedings of a Symposium* (Los Angeles: Crossroads Press, 1982); or, more generally, Steven Feierman, "Struggles for Control: The Social Roots of Health and Healing in Modern Africa," *African Studies Review* 28 (1985): 73–147.

3 Some examples include, K. D. M. Snell, *Annals of the Labouring Poor, Social Change and Agrarian England 1660–1900* (Cambridge University Press, 1985); Paul Slack, "Poverty and Politics in Salisbury 1597–1600," in Peter Clark and Paul Slack, eds., *Crisis and Order in English Towns* (London: Routledge & Kegan Paul, 1972).

4 See, for instance, Olwen Hufton's *The Poor of Eighteenth Century France 1750–1789* (Oxford: Oxford University Press [Clarendon Press], 1974).

5 Tim Wales, "Poverty, Poor Relief, and the Life-Cycle: Some Evidence from Seventeenth-Century Norfolk," in Richard M. Smith, ed., *Land, Kinship and Life-Cycle* (Cambridge University Press, 1984), pp. 351–404; Richard M. Smith, "The Structured Dependence of the Elderly as a Recent Development: Some Skeptical Historical Thoughts," *Ageing and Society* 4 (1984): 413–15; David Thomson, "I Am Not My Father's Keeper: Families and the Elderly in Nineteenth-Century England," *Law and History Review* 2 (1984): 265–86.

6 On the social roles of eighteenth-century city elites, see particularly Peter Borsay, "The English Urban Renaissance: the Development of Provincial Urban Culture c. 1680–1760," *Social History* 5 (1977) 581–603; idem, " 'All the Town's a Stage': Urban Ritual and Ceremony 1660–1800," in Peter Clark, ed., *The Transformation of English Provincial Towns 1600–1800* (London: Hutchinson, 1984), pp. 228–58; idem, *The English Urban Renaissance* (Oxford University Press, 1989). See also P. J. Corfield, *The Impact of English Towns 1700–1800* (Oxford University Press, 1982), esp. ch. 8 and 9.

7 See E. P. Thompson, "Eighteenth-Century English Society: Class Struggle Without Class?" *Social History* 3 (1978): 133–165; idem, "Patrician Society, Plebian Culture," *Journal of Social History* 7 (1974): 382–405.

8 For sources of this brief survey of Bristol history, see John Latimer, *Annals of Bristol in the Eighteenth Century* (Bristol: printed for the author, 1893); Patrick McGrath, ed., *Bristol in the Eighteenth Century* (Newton Abbot: David Charles, 1972); Jonathan Barry, "The Cultural Life of Bristol, 1640–1775," (D.Phil. diss., Oxford University, 1985); Michael Neve, "Natural Philosophy, Medicine and the Culture of Science in Provincial England: The Cases of Bristol 1790–1850, and Bath 1750–1820," (Ph.D. diss., University College, London, 1984).

9 Nicholas Rogers, "Money, Land and Lineage: The Big Bourgeoisie of Hanoverian London," *Social History* 4 (1979): 437–54; Henry Horwitz, " 'The Mess of the Middle Class' Revisited: The Case of the 'Big Bourgeoisie' of Augustan London," *Continuity and Change* 2 (1987): 263–96; Peter Earle, *The Making of the English Middle Class* (London: Methuen & Co., 1989). On Bristol's middling sorts, see Barry, "Cultural Life of Bristol."

10 On English hospitals, see Roy Porter, "The Gift Relation: Philanthropy and Provincial Hospitals in Eighteenth-Century England," in Lindsay Granshaw and Roy Porter, eds., *The Hospital in History* (London: Routledge, 1989), pp. 149–78. Craig Rose discusses the London hospitals in terms of power struggles, but unfortunately he limits his analysis to political difference and ignores religion. Craig Rose, "Politics and the London Royal Hospitals, 1683–92," in Granshaw and Porter, *Hospital in History*, pp. 123–48. For the Continent, see especially Kathryn Norberg, *Rich and Poor in Grenoble 1600–1814* (Berkeley and Los Angeles: University of California Press, 1985); Sandra Cavallo, "Charity, Power, and Patronage in Eighteenth-Century Italian Hospitals: the Case of Turin," in Granshaw and Porter, *Hospital in History*, pp. 93–122.

11 For a similar interpretation of American hospitals in a later period, see Charles E. Rosenberg, *The Care of Strangers: The Rise of America's Hospital System* (New York: Basic, 1988). Many parallels can be drawn between the situation of British hospitals in the latter half of the eighteenth century and their American counterparts in the middle of the nineteenth century.

12 See, for a nonmedical example of such an analysis, T. V. Hitchcock, "The English Workhouse: A Study in Institutional Poor Relief in

Selected Counties 1696–1750," (D.Phil. diss., Oxford University, 1985).

13 Toby Gelfand, "Hospital Teaching as Private Enterprise," in W. F. Bynum and Roy Porter, eds., *William Hunter and the Eighteenth-Century Medical World* (Cambridge University Press, 1985); Othmar Keel, "The Politics of Health and the Institutionalization of Clinical Practice in Europe in the Second Half of the Eighteenth Century," in Bynum and Porter, *William Hunter;* Russell C. Maulitz, *Morbid Appearances: The Anatomy of Pathology in the Early Nineteenth Century* (Cambridge University Press, 1987); Guenter B. Risse, *Hospital Life in Enlightenment Scotland. Care and Teaching at the Royal Infirmary of Edinburgh* (Cambridge University Press, 1986).

14 For works that avoid the trap of the Continental model, see especially the work of Irvine Loudon and of Dorothy and Roy Porter. Irvine Loudon, *Medical Care and the General Practitioner, 1750–1850* (Oxford: Oxford University Press [Clarendon Press], 1986); Roy Porter and Dorothy Porter, *In Sickness and in Health: The British Experience, 1650–1850* (London: Fourth Estate, 1988). For an earlier period, Margaret Pelling's work provides a model of a local focus on medical practitioners: Margaret Pelling, "Occupational Diversity: Barber-surgeons and the Trades of Norwich, 1550–1640," *Bull. Hist. Med.* 56 (1982): 484–511; Margaret Pelling and Charles Webster, "Medical Practitioners," in Charles Webster, ed., *Health, Medicine and Mortality in the Sixteenth Century* (Cambridge University Press, 1979), pp. 165–235.

15 Loudon, *General Practitioner;* Roy Porter, *Health For Sale: Quackery in England, 1650–1850* (Manchester University Press, 1989).

16 N. D. Jewson, "Medical Knowledge and the Patronage System in Eighteenth Century England," *Sociology* 8 (1974): 369–85; idem, "The Disappearance of the Sick-man from Medical Cosmology, 1770–1870," *Sociology* 10 (1976): 225–44.

17 Peter Burke, *Popular Culture in Early Modern Europe* (London: Temple Smith, 1978); Bob Bushaway, *By Rite: Custom, Ceremony, and Community in England, 1700-1880* (London: Junction Books, 1982); Robert W. Malcolmson, *Popular Recreations in English Society 1700–1850* (Cambridge University Press, 1973).

18 Keith Thomas, *Religion and the Decline of Magic* (New York: Scribner, 1981), is the classic statement of the position that supernatural beliefs were on the wane by the end of the seventeenth century. Those who trace their survival include Jonathan Barry, "Piety and the Patient," in Porter, *Patients and Practitioners,* pp. 145–76; Charles Phythian-Adams, "Rural Culture," in G. E. Mingay, ed., *The Victorian Countryside* (London: Routledge & Kegan Paul, 1981), pp. 616–25; James Obelkevich, *Religion and Rural Society: South Lindsey, 1825–1875* (Oxford: Oxford University Press [Clarendon Press], 1976).

19 See, for instance, Risse's rather ambivalent reading of Foucault in the Scottish setting in *Hospital Life.*

20 Michel Foucault, *The Birth of the Clinic,* trans. Alan Sheridan (New York: Pantheon, 1973); idem, *Discipline and Punish. The Birth of the Prison,* trans. Alan Sheridan (Harmondsworth: Penguin Books, 1979).

21 Quoted in Colin Jones, *Charity and Bienfaisance: The Treatment of the Poor in the Montpellier Region, 1740–1815* (Cambridge University Press, 1982), p. 62.

22 On Philadelphia, see Gary B. Nash, "Poverty and Poor Relief in Pre-Revolutionary Philadelphia," *William and Mary Quarterly* 33 (1976): 3–30; idem, "Urban Wealth and Poverty in Pre-Revolutionary America," *Journal of Interdisciplinary History* 6 (1976): 545–84; John K. Alexander, *Render Them Submissive: Responses to Poverty in Philadelphia, 1760–1800* (Amherst: University of Massachusetts Press, 1980).

23 Cavallo, "Charity, Power, and Patronage"; idem, "Patterns of Poor Relief and Patterns of Poverty in Eighteenth-Century Italy: The Evidence of the Turin Ospedale di Carità," *Continuity and Change* 5 (1990): 1–33; idem, "The Motivations of Benefactors: An Overview of Approaches to the Study of Charity," in Colin Jones and Jonathan Barry, eds., *Charity and Medicine before the Welfare State* (London: Routledge, in press).

24 Jones, *Charity and Bienfaisance,* p. 129.

CHAPTER 2

1 On an earlier period, see Paul Slack, "Mirrors of Health and Treasures of Poor Men: The Uses of the Vernacular Medical Literature of Tudor England," in Charles Webster, ed., *Health, Medicine and Mortality in the Sixteenth Century* (Cambridge University Press, 1979), pp. 237–73. The term "vernacular" seems the most appropriate for this type of lay healing. "Domestic" medicine alludes to William Buchan's work of a later period, when lay healing was beginning to lose its status, slowly becoming a form of knowledge limited to plebeians. See Chapter 9.

2 Ginnie Smith, "Prescribing the Rules of Health: Self-help and Advice in the Late Eighteenth Century," in Roy Porter, ed., *Patients and Practitioners* (Cambridge University Press, 1985), pp. 249–82.

3 Keith Thomas, *Religion and the Decline of Magic* (New York: Scribner, 1971), p. 107. See also Chapters 10 through 12 on astrology.

4 Charles E. Rosenberg, "The Therapeutic Revolution," *Perspectives in Biology and Medicine* 20 (1977): 485–506. For a modern example, see Cecil Helman, " 'Feed a Cold, Starve a Fever' – Folk Models of Infection in an English Suburban Community, and Their Relation to Medical Treatments," *Culture, Medicine and Psychiatry* 2 (1978): 107–37. For just one example of this concept in other cultures, see Katherine Gould-Martin, "Hot Cold Clean Poison and Dirt: Chinese Folk Medical Categories," *Social Science & Medicine* 12 (1978): 39–46.

5 James Lackington, *Memoirs of the First Forty-five Years of the Life of J. L . . .* (London: printed for the author, 1792), 2d ed., p. 130.

6 John Bennett, MS. autobiography, Bristol Record Office (henceforth BRO) 36097, p. 8.

7 *'Wilt Thou Be Made Whole'* . . . (London: Benjamin Matthews, 1751), pp. 21–2.

8 Charles Manby Smith, *The Working Man's Way in the World* . . . (London: William and Frederick Gash, n.d.), p. 11.

9 Richard Wiseman, *Severall Chirurgical Treatises* (London: E. Flesher and J. Macock, for R. Royston, 1676), p. 17.

10 Alexander Morgan, Casebook, Wellcome Institute for the History of Medicine Library, London, MS. 3631, p. ii.

11 Thomas Willis, *The London Practice of Physick, or the Whole Practical Part of Physick Contained in the Works of Dr. Willis* (London: Thomas Basset and William Crooke, 1685), p. 73. In Willis's own practice, as indicated in the casebook that he kept in the early 1650s, he used hot/cold explanations, such as in his discussion of a woman two days after the birth of her child, "The clothes applied around the pudenda were changed, not being properly arranged. Because of this she caught cold in that spot; and then the lochia, previously flowing copiously, were at once suppressed" (Kenneth Dewhurst, ed., *Willis's Oxford Case Book (1650–52)* [Oxford: Sanford Publications, 1981], p. 96; see also pp. 99, 102).

12 Nicholas Culpeper, *Culpeper's Last Legacy* (London: Nathaniel Brooke, 1671), p. 161.

13 Dewhurst, *Willis's Case Book,* p. 82.

14 Thomas, *Religion and the Decline of Magic.*

15 Nicholas Culpeper, *The English Physician Enlarged* (London: J. Churchill, 1714), p. 117.

16 Henry Bourne, *Observations on Popular Antiquities . . . John Brand* (London: William Baynes, 1810), v.2, p. 596. See also *Gentleman's Magazine* 57 (1787): 719.

17 *Gentleman's Magazine*

18 Culpeper, *Last Legacy.*

19 John Cannon diary, Somerset Record Office, DD/SAS C/1193/4, p. 24. This custom has been recorded from all over the South-West of England. See *Gloucestershire Notes and Queries* 3 (1885–1887): 672; *Somersetshire Archaeological and Natural History Society Proceedings xxxviii* (1892), pp. 362–9.

20 Wiseman, *Chirurgical Treatises,* p. 96. Wiseman does say that he prefers to treat warts with caustic and ligatures, but he does not disparage the beef-burying technique.

21 Willis, *London Practice,* p. 144.

22 Ibid., p. 141.

23 Culpeper, *Last Legacy.*

24 John Wesley, *Primitive Physick* (London: printed and sold by Thomas Trye, 1747).

25 Culpeper, *Last Legacy,* p. 73.

26 Thomas Beddoes, *Observations on the Nature and Cure of Calculus, Sea Scurvy, Consumption, Catarrh and Fever* . . . (London: J. Murray, 1793), p. 2.
27 Culpeper, *Last Legacy*, p. 266.
28 William Falconer, *An Account of the Efficacy of the Aqua Mephitica Alkalina* (London: T. Cadell, 1792).
29 On astrology in this period, see Patrick Curry, *Prophecy and Power, Astrology in Early Modern England* (London: Polity Press, 1989).
30 "Aristotle," *Complete Works* (London: L. Hanes, 1772), p. 4 of Aristotle's Problems. On Aristotle's Masterpiece, see Roy Porter, " 'The Secrets of Generation Display'd': *Aristotle's Master-piece* in Eighteenth-Century England," in Robert Purks Maccubbin, ed., *'Tis Nature's Fault: Unauthorized Sexuality During the Enlightenment* (Cambridge University Press, 1987), pp. 1–21.
31 British Library, Wing Almanac, 1710.
32 *Vox Stellarum* 1701 (British Library, hereafter BL, PP 2465). Bernard Capp, in *English Almanacs, 1500–1800*, (Ithaca, N. Y.: Cornell University Press, 1979), p. 263, suggests that the *Vox* was the most popular. Over two hundred thousand copies per year were published in the late eighteenth century. This phrase was, of course, a restatement of the old maxim that had been associated with the astrologer William Lilly. See Curry, *Prophecy and Power*, pp. 30–1, 36–7.
33 *Vox Stellarum* 1740 (BL, PP 2465).
34 William Davis, *A New Almanack Made in Wiltshire* (London: n.p., 1692).
35 See Curry, *Prophecy and Power*, pp. 99–100.
36 William Salmon, *Synopsis Medicinae, or a Compendium of Astrological, Galenical and Chymical Physick* . . . (London: William Godbird for Richard Jones, 1671). It is notable how many of this school of antimonopolists writing in English gave Latin or Greek titles to their works. Perhaps, despite their demystification efforts, buyers and readers liked the professional cachet of learned languages.
37 Willis, *London Practice*, p. 186.
38 Ibid.
39 Curry, *Prophecy and Power*.
40 For instance, see Jonathan Barry, "Piety and the Patient: Medicine and Religion in Eighteenth-Century Bristol," in Porter, *Patients and Practitioners*, pp. 145–76.
41 Barry has shown how complicated religious faction and sect were in shaping ideas about nature. It is impossible to overstate the importance of local political and sectarian debates in the reporting of "supernatural" events. For instance, a broadside temptingly titled "Strange and Wonderful News from Bristol," detailing peculiar happenings in which the bodies of mutilated sheep were found in the fields, seems upon first glance to be a standard "strange omens" broadside. But a closer look reveals that it was actually an electioneering device, designed to turn voters away from the (unnamed) papist candidates and towards the

(equally unnamed) righteous ones. (*Strange and Wonderful News . . .* [n.p., 1678?]). Similarly, it is impossible to distinguish between anti-Quaker rhetoric and actual belief in the tale of a Chard (Somerset) bookseller who conjured up small devils in *A Strange and Wonderful (Yet True) Relation of. . . Abraham Moon: A Pretended Quaker* (London: R. Lee, n.d.).

42 *Letter to the Bishop of Gloucester from a Bristol Clergyman* (London: H. Hills, 1704). This was evidently written by Arthur Bedford, a Bristol clergyman with interest and expertise in matters supernatural.

43 Cannon diary, p. 48.

44 Ibid.

45 Gloucestershire Record Office, MS. receipt book. P 218 MI 1. Internal evidence suggests mid- or late-eighteenth-century origins.

46 *Gentleman's Magazine* 21 (1751): 295.

47 Champion family letter-book, BRO, 3803 (1) 20 June 1761. On the death of "superstition," see Chapter 9.

48 See John Latimer, *Annals of Bristol in the Eighteenth Century* (Bristol: printed for the author, 1893), p. 28. Also, Stephen Pole, "Crime, Society and Law Enforcement in Hanoverian Somerset" (Ph.D. diss., Cambridge University, 1983), ch. 2.

49 See Rosenberg, "Therapeutic Revolution," on this point.

50 Culpeper, *English Physician,* p. 259.

51 Wesley, *Primitive Physick,* p. 65.

52 Salmon, *Synopsis Medicinae,* p. 419.

53 Willis, *London Practice,* p. 98.

54 Arthur Broughton, MS. lecture notes, Bristol University Medical School Library, DM 1H.

55 Arthur Broughton, MS. lecture notes, Bristol University Medical School Library, DM 1C7.

56 The links among various remedies for stone are complex. For example, both Thomas Page, a Bristol surgeon, and Culpeper suggest preparations of filipendula, or dropwort, for the stone. For Page, see BRO, Bristol Biographical Memoirs (hereafter BBM) 1, between pp. 49–50. Both Culpeper and an anonymous author of a manuscript remedy book, which seems to have been from Bristol, include nettles as a remedy for the stone (Wellcome Institute for the History of Medicine, London, MS. 3576).

57 Letter, *Gentleman's Magazine* 1 (1731): 314. I am indebted to Dr. Roy Porter for this reference.

58 Salmon, *Synopsis Medicinae,* pp. 383, 416; Willis, *London Practice,* p. 22.

59 Willis, *London Practice,* p. 24.

60 Salmon, *Synopsis Medicinae,* pp. 391, 398, 417.

61 W. P. Williams and W. A. Jones, "A List of Somerset Dialect," *Somerset Archaeological and Natural History Society Proceedings* 18 (1878).

62 Falconer, *Aqua Mephitica Alkalina.*

63 Gloucestershire Record Office, P218 MI 1.

64 Margaret Pelling, "Appearance and Reality: Barber-Surgeons, the Body, and Disease," in A. L. Beier and Roger Finlay, eds., *London 1500–1700 The Making of the Metropolis* (London: Longman, 1985), p. 89.

65 Pelling, "Appearance and Reality," pp. 94–5.

66 There is little of quality written on monsters and prodigies in the early modern period. In this brief analysis of monsters' roles in elite and humble culture, I follow the work of Lorraine Daston and Katherine Park, "Unnatural Conceptions: The Study of Monsters in Sixteenth and Seventeenth Century France and England," *Past and Present* 92 (1981): 20–54. They somewhat overstate the extent to which popular and elite traditions had diverged by the end of the seventeenth century, although they do say that both wonder books and the Royal Society shared "a taste for the rare and singular for its own sake" (p. 48). In 1727, for instance, John Maubray was still saying that unnatural births were due to parents' sin. (John Maubray, *The Female Physician Containing All the Diseases Incident to That Sex, in Virgins, Wives, and Widows . . .* [London: 1727]). Although Blondel published his analysis of the influences upon unborn babies a few years later, "scientific" arguments replaced theological or supernatural ones in a slow and complex process (James Blondel, *The Power of the Mother's Imagination over the Fetus Examin'd . . .* [London: John Brotherton, 1729]). See also, Herman W. Roodenburg, "The Maternal Imagination. The Fears of Pregnant Women in Seventeenth-Century Holland," *Journal of Social History* 21 (1988): 701–16; Paul-Gabriel Boucé, "Imagination, Pregnant Women, and Monsters in Eighteenth-Century England and France," in G. S. Rousseau and Roy Porter, eds., *Sexual Underworlds of the Enlightenment* (Manchester University Press, 1987), pp. 86–100.

67 "Aristotle," *Complete Works,* pp. 91–2.

68 *The Miracle of Miracles,* reprinted in John Ashton, *Chapbooks of the Eighteenth Century* (Welwyn Garden City, England: Seven Dials Press, 1969).

69 John Johnson Collection, Bodleian Library, Oxford, Human Freaks, Box 2. There is no date on this sheet, but the claim that this woman was examined by Sir Hans Sloane strongly suggests that it was prior to his retirement from the Royal Society presidentship in 1741.

70 Daston and Park claim in "Unnatural Conceptions" that monsters served a dual function in the Baconian system, offering insight into normal processes of development and inspiration for human invention, emphasizing the role of the craftsman.

71 "Aristotle," *Complete Works,* p. 101.

72 Salmon, *Synopsis Medicinae,* p. 310.

73 Ashton, *Chapbooks.*

74 *A Warning to Married Women* (London: Printed for A. M. W. D. and T. Thackray, n.d.). Bodily marks were also, of course, the sign of a witch.

75 *The Five Strange Wonders of the World, or A New Merry Book of All Fives* (Tewkesbury: Printed and sold by S. Harwood, n.d.), p. 7.

76 Cannon diary, p. 89.

77 William Dyer diary, Bristol Central Library (hereafter BCL) 20095.

78 Rice Charlton, *Cases of Persons Admitted into the Hospital at Bath under the Care of the Late Dr. Oliver* (Bath: R. Cruttwell, 1774).

79 Samuel Sholl, *A Short Historical Account of the Silk Manufacture in England . . .* (London: n.p., 1811), p. 43.

80 On narratives of illness, see Gareth Williams, "The Genesis of Chronic Illness: Narrative Reconstruction," *Sociology of Health and Illness* 6 (1984): 175–200. Given the chronic nature of many early modern experiences of illness, Williams's model is particularly useful. Where Williams sees chronic illness as a process of remaking the story of one's life, so as to make sense of prolonged episodes of disability, I would emphasize the centrality of illness experience to the construction of early modern autobiographical narratives, although this difference derives in part from the genres of our sources. See also Barbara Duden, *Geschichte unter der Haut: Ein Einsacher Artz und seine Patientinnen um 1730* (Stuttgart: Klett-Cotta, 1987); Harold Brody, *Stories of Sickness* (New Haven, Conn.: Yale University Press, 1987); Thomas Laqueur, "Bodies, Details, and the Humanitarian Narrative," in Lynn Hunt, ed., *The New Cultural History* (Berkeley and Los Angeles: University of California Press, 1989), pp. 176–204; C. Herzlich and J. Pierret, *Illness and Self in Society*, trans. E. Forster (Baltimore: Johns Hopkins University Press, 1987); Dorothy Porter and Roy Porter, *Patient's Progress: Doctors and Doctoring in Eighteenth-Century England* (Oxford: Polity Press in association with Basil Blackwell, 1989); Roy Porter and Dorothy Porter, *In Sickness and in Health: The British Experience, 1650–1850* (London: Fourth Estate, 1988); A. Kleinman, *Illness Narratives: Suffering, Healing, and the Human Condition* (New York: Basic, 1988); Charles E. Rosenberg, "Disease in History: Frames and Framers," *Milbank Quarterly* 67 supp. 1 (1989): 1–15.

81 David Vincent, *Bread, Knowledge and Freedom, A Study of Nineteenth-Century Working Class Autobiography* (London: Methuen & Co., 1981), pp. 14–19. Margaret Spufford, "First Steps in Literacy; the Reading and Writing Experiences of the Humblest Seventeenth-Century Spiritual Autobiographers," *Social History* 4 (1979): 407–35.

82 Andrew Wear, "Puritan Perceptions of Illness in Seventeenth Century England," in Porter, *Patients and Practitioners*, pp. 55–99.

83 Sholl, *Historical Account*.

84 Of course, professional medical men claimed forms of knowledge peculiar to themselves, but I have tried to suggest that such claims were problematic, that most professional medicine was consonant with lay practices. Even seemingly exclusive humoral and chemical theories could be related to hot/cold wet/dry schema and astrological medicine, respectively. But such an argument does not imply that early modern individuals did not seek out and rely upon professionals; it merely suggests that such a reliance needs to be explained in a context of medical pluralism.

CHAPTER 3

1 "Coughs and Colds," Bristol University Medical School MS.

2 Thomas Beddoes, *Hygiea, or Essays Moral and Medical . . .* (Bristol: J. Mills, 1802), p. 16.

3 See Roy Porter and Dorothy Porter, *In Sickness and in Health: The English Experience, 1650–1850* (London: Fourth Estate, 1988), pp. 258–72.

4 My discussion is indebted to Jonathan Barry, "Piety and the Patient: Medicine and Religion in Eighteenth-Century Bristol," in Roy Porter, ed., *Patients and Practitioners* (Cambridge University Press, 1985), pp. 145–76. On the more general point, about the interpenetration of lay and medical culture, see Roy Porter, "Lay Medical Knowledge in the Eighteenth Century: The Evidence of the *Gentleman's Magazine,*" *Medical History* 29 (1985): 138–68. See also Charles E. Rosenberg, "Medical Text and Social Context: William Buchan's *Domestic Medicine,*" *Bull. Hist. Med.* 57 (1983): 22–42.

5 William Dyer diary, Bristol Central Library (hereafter BCL) 20095, 22 Feb. 1764.

6 Dyer diary, BCL 20096, 17 May, 21 May, 12 June, 1762.

7 Most likely, Dyer read Anton Stoerck, *An Essay on the Medical Nature of Hemlock* . . . , trans. from the Latin, (London: J. Nourse, 1760).

8 Dyer diary, BCL 20096, Peglar 6 Sept. 1762, Roe 9 Sept. 1762.

9 Ibid., 15 Oct. 1762 et seq.

10 Ibid., 30 Sept. 1762.

11 Porter, "*Gentleman's Magazine.*"

12 James Lackington, *Memoirs of the First Forty-five Years of the Life of J. L.* . . . (London: printed for the author, 1792), 2d ed.

13 John Cannon diary, Somerset Record Office, DD/SAS C/1193/4, p. 41.

14 Cannon diary, p. 42. This diary is actually a memoir combined with a diary – hence we are given details of Cannon's lustful youth (his spying on the maidservant led to masturbation, for example), as a warning from a man in his fifties looking back. It is difficult to know how Cannon's perceptions of these events changed in the interim.

15 Nicholas Culpeper, *The English Physician Enlarged* (London: A. & J. Churchill, 1698), p. 149.

16 Remedy book, Gloucestershire Record Office, P218 MI1.

17 See also remedy books in the Bristol Record Office (hereafter BRO) 24759 (14) and HB/X/4 for further examples of commercial measures and ingredients. Both date from the later eighteenth century.

18 Ephemera collection, Patent Remedies, Wellcome Institute for the History of Medicine, London.

19 Roy Porter, *Health For Sale: Quackery in England, 1650–1850* (Manchester University Press, 1989).

20 Thomas Beddoes, *The History of Isaac Jenkins* (Bristol: J. Mills, 1804), p. 7.

21 Hugh Smythson, *The Compleat Family Physician* (London: Harrison, 1781), p. 279.

22 BRO, HB/X/4.

23 My thanks to David Allen for this and many other points about herbal remedies.

24 William Holland, *Paupers and Pig Killers, The Diary of William Holland*, ed. Jack Ayres (Harmondsworth: Penguin Books, 1986), p. 49.

25 John Addington, "Cases of Gonorrhea Treated with Muriate of Quicksilver," in Thomas Beddoes, ed., *Contributions to Physical and Medical Knowledge, Principally from the West Country* (Bristol: Biggs and Cottle, 1799).
26 Porter, *Health for Sale*, pp. 43–55.
27 See Irvine Loudon, *Medical Care and the General Practitioner, 1750–1850* (Oxford: Oxford University Press [Clarendon Press], 1987), pp. 54–62.
28 See W. F. Bynum, "Treating the Wages of Sin: Venereal Disease and Specialism in Eighteenth Century Britain," in W. F. Bynum and Roy Porter, eds., *Medical Fringe and Medical Orthodoxy 1750–1850* (London: Croom Helm, 1987), pp. 5–28.
29 *Felix Farley's Bristol Journal* (hereafter FFBJ), 7 Sept. 1782.
30 See Arthur Young, *A Six Weeks' Tour through the Southern Counties of England and Wales* (London: W. Nicoll, 1768), for estimates of working men's wages. Young's comments are borne out by Bristol evidence.
31 Loudon, *General Practitioner,* pp. 65 et seq., and pp. 209–214; Porter, *Health for Sale,* p. 142.
32 Margaret Pelling, "Occupational Diversity: Barber-surgeons and the Trades of Norwich, 1550–1640," *Bull. Hist. Med.* 56 (1982): 484–511. Margaret Pelling and Charles Webster, "Medical Practitioners," in Charles Webster, ed., *Health, Medicine and Mortality in the Sixteenth Century* (Cambridge University Press, 1979), pp. 165–236.
33 See the Appendix for information about sources for this reconstruction of medical practice in Bristol.
34 To see apprenticeship as the cut-rate alternative to a university education, as Geoffrey Holmes comes close to implying, misses its structural importance in the provision of health care. Geoffrey Holmes, *Augustan England: Professions, State and Society 1680–1730* (London: Routledge & Kegan Paul, 1982), pp. 17–18.
35 This discussion of apprenticeship is based upon a compilation of all medical apprenticeships in eighteenth-century Bristol, from the indentures register in the BRO. Obviously, this register becomes less and less useful as a guide to patterns of medical education in the city over the course of the century; see Chapter 7 for details.
36 Because Samuel Pye had a surgeon son by the same name (in fact, there was a dynasty of five Samuel Pyes, all surgeons, in Bristol), it is quite possible that the second half of this set were actually the son's apprentices.
37 BRO, Bristol Biographical Memoirs (hereafter BBM) 2, 253v.
38 Holmes, *Augustan England.*
39 Loudon, *General Practitioner.*
40 N. D. Jewson, "Medical Knowledge and the Patronage System in Eighteenth Century England," *Sociology* 8 (1974): 369–85; idem, "The Disappearance of the Sick-man from Medical Cosmology, 1770–1870," *Sociology* 10 (1976): 225–44.
41 It has been assumed that apothecaries outnumbered surgeons, but the basis for this assumption is not clear. Joan Lane has used Samuel Foart

Simmons's 1783 Medical Register to construct a picture of the medical professions in the late eighteenth century, and others have relied upon her work. (Joan Lane, "The Medical Practitioners of Provincial England in 1783," *Medical History* 28 (1984): 353–71.) Although Lane is quite straightforward about the limitations of her data, a close examination of Bristol's entries in Simmons's Register makes it a very problematic source. See the Appendix for details.

42 *FFBJ*, 9 Mar. 1754.

43 For bills, BRO, BBM 1, p. 74. For Barber Surgeon's Company, BRO, 04435 (3) fo 37, 39 Tolzey Court Recognizances.

44 BRO, BBM 1, p. 59.

45 Alexander Morgan, Casebook, Wellcome Institute for the History of Medicine Library, London. Morgan's further career can be traced in the apprenticeship registers in the BRO.

46 Morgan, Casebook, p. 17. For a discussion of an earlier surgeon, whose practice sounds much like that of Deverell, see Lucinda Beier, *Sufferers and Healers: The Experience of Illness in Seventeenth-Century England* (London: Routledge & Kegan Paul, 1987), pp. 51–96.

47 See in particular, Loudon, *General Practitioner,* chs. 3 and 4.

48 BRO, BBM 2, pp. 152–64. The oft-quoted phrase, "the golden age of physic," is on p. 154.

49 BRO, BBM 1, p. 22.

50 See Loudon, *General Practitioner,* pp. 65–72, 209–14.

51 BRO, BBM 2, pp. 159–64.

52 And there were impecunious surgeon-apothecaries, such as Richard Perry, whom Smith described, "he now and then lived a few months, and stored up his credit with a new apprentice-fee – but his business was not productive" (BRO, BBM 4, p. 32). Perry temporarily solved his financial problems by eloping with a fourteen-year-old heiress.

53 On apothecaries more generally, see Juanita Burnby, *A Study of the English Apothecary from 1660–1760, Medical History,* supp. 3, London, 1983.

54 William Holland, *Paupers and Pig Killers. The Diary of William Holland,* ed. Jack Ayres (Harmondsworth: Penguin Books, 1986), p. 27.

55 Ibid., p. 177.

56 Samuel England, Casebooks, Royal College of Physicians, M6, p. 3–4. I am very grateful to Dr. Susan Lawrence for discovering that England was a Somerset practitioner and sharing this reference with me.

57 Irvine Loudon, " 'The Vile Race of Quacks with Which This Country Is Infested,' " in Bynum and Porter, *Medical Fringe and Medical Orthodoxy,* pp. 106–28.

58 Loudon, "The Vile Race."

59 Roy Porter and Dorothy Porter, "The Rise of the English Drugs Industry: The Role of Thomas Corbyn," *Medical History* 33 (1989): 277–95.

60 Roger Langdon, *The Life of Roger Langdon* (London: Elliot Stock, n.d.).

61 Ibid., p. 15.

62 Ibid., p. 19.

63 Ibid., p. 16.
64 Ibid.
65 Sarah Stone, *A Complete Practice of Midwifery* (London: T. Cooper, 1737).
66 Stone's work seems to have been analogous with that of Percival Willughby, who practiced in Derby in the late seventeenth century. Adrian Wilson has analyzed his practice and shows that much of it consisted of emergency cases. Wilson claims that this emphasis was characteristic of *man-* midwifery; I would prefer to make distinctions between what I call primary midwifery (i.e., the first midwife called, or booked, to attend a woman in labor) and consultant midwifery, such as that of Stone and Willughby. (Wilson uses the term "primary" differently.) Although male midwives may have done mostly consultant work, the inverse (that most of the consultant work was done by men) may not be the case. See Adrian Wilson, "William Hunter and the Varieties of Man-Midwifery," in W. F. Bynum and Roy Porter, eds., *William Hunter and the Eighteenth-Century Medical World* (Cambridge University Press, 1985), pp. 343–69.
67 Stone, *Practice of Midwifery,* p. 103.
68 Ibid., p. 63.
69 Ibid., pp. xiii, 155.
70 Ibid., p. xiv. It is interesting to note that, for Stone, dissections were the cardinal difference in male and female midwifery training.
71 See, for example, Jean Donnison, *Midwives and Medical Men* (London: Heinemann, 1977), esp. ch. 2; and Adrian Wilson, "Childbirth in Seventeenth- and Eighteenth-Century England" (Ph.D. diss., University of Sussex, 1982).
72 England, Casebooks, M6, p. 359.
73 *FFBJ,* 9 Jan. 1755, and many subsequent weeks.
74 See, for instance, in Ephemera collection, Wellcome Institute for the History of Medicine; Donnison, *Midwives,* p. 34. On a related theme, see Roy Porter, "A Touch of Danger: The Man-Midwife as Sexual Predator," in G. S. Rousseau and Roy Porter, eds., *Sexual Underworlds of the Enlightenment* (Manchester University Press, 1987), pp. 206–31.
75 John Latimer, *Annals of Bristol in the Eighteenth Century* (Bristol: printed for the author, 1893), p. 336.
76 Wilson, "Childbirth."
77 *FFBJ,* 26 June 1762.
78 BRO, BBM 2, p. 157.
79 Ibid., p. 159.
80 BRO, BBM 1, p. 59.
81 Ward's 1786 cash book, Gloucestershire Record Office, D 1928 A3.
82 BRO, BBM 6, p. 410.
83 Physicians were also the most likely to be included in the directory of 1775 or in Smith's memoirs; these figures are therefore more inclusive than those for either surgeons or apothecaries.
84 BRO, BBM 1, p. 670.

85 Porter, *Health for Sale*, p. 222.
86 On the historical meaning of quackery, see Roy Porter, "The Language of Quackery in England 1660–1800," in Peter Burke and Roy Porter, eds., *The Social History of Language* (Cambridge University Press, 1987), pp. 73–103.
87 BRO, BBM 1, p. 74.
88 BRO, BBM 6, p. 78.
89 *Bristol Journal*, 19 May 1750. Thanks to Dr. Jonathan Barry for this reference.
90 BRO, BBM 2, pp. 234–8. See also, on the more general point, Porter, "Language of Quackery." On the naming of remedies, see Porter, *Health for Sale*, pp. 45, 47, 103.
91 Dyer diary, BCL 20095, 30 Mar. 1756, 5 Sept. 1757.
92 Ibid., 19 May 1751, 9 Oct. 1781.
93 *FFBJ*, 10 March 1770. Plunkett actually practiced in Bath, but advertised frequently in Bristol and came there occasionally.
94 *Bristol Journal*, 20 May 1775.
95 See, for instance, Dyer diary, BCL 20096, 16 Oct., 30 Nov. 1762.
96 Poor Law records, Somerset Record Office, D/P/Stogs/13/2/4, 1798–9.
97 *FFBJ*, 11 May 1782.
98 Deafness: *Gloucester Journal*, 1 Mar. 1736/7, 6 June 1732; *FFBJ*, 8 Feb. 1755. Corns: *Bristol Oracle and Country Advertiser*, 16 June 1744. The relationship between surgery and more general care for the body, verging on that performed by servants, is suggested in this advertisement by the practitioner's offer to cut toenails and "wait on any Gentleman or Ladies, at their own Houses." Dentistry: *FFBJ*, 9 July 1768. Oculist: *FFBJ*, 26 June 1762.
99 Wickland is in Sketchley's Directory of 1775 and Matthew's Directory of 1793, as well as in the christening register of the parish (as a parent), BRO, P/St.P&J/R/1–4.
100 Holland, *Diary*, p. 34.
101 *Gloucester Journal*, 26 Aug. 1793.
102 BRO, BBM 2, pp. 672–6; BRO, BBM 3, pp. 11–12; also *FFBJ*, 2 Jan. 1775; see also BCL 20095 14 Apr. 1784, Blagden inoculating. The "Infirmary" house was in no way officially connected to the Infirmary, but of its three surgeons, only Rodbard did not attain an hospital post.
103 Sarah Champion diary, photocopy in Friends House Library, London, MS. Box D, 20 Mar. 1768.
104 *Bristol Journal*, 9 Dec. 1775.
105 [Dr. Glass], *A Letter from Dr. Glass to Dr. Baker on the Means of Procuring a Distinct and Favourable Kind of Smallpox* (London: W. Johnson, 1767), pp. 8–9.
106 BRO, P/Abs/OP/2 a, b; P/Abs/R/1a. For further details of the health care provided in this parish, see Chapter 5 of this book.
107 BRO, BBM 1, p. 65.
108 Michael Neve, "Orthodoxy and Fringe: Medicine in Late Georgian Bristol," in Bynum and Porter, *Fringe and Orthodoxy*, pp. 40–55.

109 Introduction, Bynum and Porter, *Fringe and Orthodoxy.*
110 Dyer diary, BCL 20095, 24 Feb. 1752.
111 Ibid., 27 July 1756.
112 This is paralleled in contemporary African medical systems, where many different types of healers are available; choices are shaped by a variety of considerations. See, for example, J. E. Janzen, *The Quest for Therapy in Lower Zaire* (Berkeley and Los Angeles: University of California Press, 1978).
113 Lowder letters, BRO 15140, 16 Feb. 1772.
114 Holland, *Diary*, p. 166.
115 Ibid., pp. 166, 152, 167.
116 England, Casebooks, M 5, p. 63.
117 Ibid., p. 134.
118 Beddoes, *Contributions to Medical Knowledge*, p. 388.
119 *'Wilt Thou be Made Whole'* . . . (London: Benjamin Matthews, 1751), p. 30. See also [J. Davies], *A Short Description of the Waters at Glastonbury* (Exeter: Andrew Brice, 1751), p. 21. For more on Glastonbury, a spa for the poor, see Chapter 9.
120 England, Casebooks, M5, p. 47.
121 Ibid., pp. 54–5. Such examples could be cited for almost any early modern English casebook.
122 John Blake, *A Letter to a Surgeon on Inoculation* (London: W. Owen, 1771), p. 18. Blake was a Bristol surgeon, and was replying to Thomas Dimsdale, whose subsequent publication, *Thoughts on General and Partial Inoculators* (London: William Richardson, 1776), also alludes to this practice.
123 Dyer diary, BCL 20095, 17 June 1760.
124 Ibid.
125 Ibid., 19 Mar. 1761.
126 Ibid., BCL 20096, 4 Oct. 1762.
127 Richard Symes, *Fire Analyzed* (Bristol: Thomas Cocking, 1771), p. 7.
128 Ibid., p. 13.
129 Ibid., pp. 63–4.
130 Ibid., pp. 75–6.
131 See, for instance, Marmaduke Berdoe, *An Enquiry into the Influence of the Electric-Fluid, in the Structure and Formation of Animated Beings* (Bath: the author, 1771); John Becket, *An Essay on Electricity* . . . (Bristol: J. B. Becket, 1773).
132 Neil McKendrick, John Brewer, and J. H. Plumb, *The Birth of a Consumer Society: The Commercialization of Eighteenth-Century England* (London: Hutchinson, 1982).
133 Porter, *Health for Sale*, p. 43.
134 Beddoes, *Isaac Jenkins*, p. 14.

CHAPTER 4

1 On the eighteenth-century provincial hospital, John Woodward, *To Do the Sick No Harm* (London: Routledge & Kegan Paul, 1974), is still a

useful starting point. See also Roy Porter, "The Gift Relation: Philanthropy and Provincial Hospitals in Eighteenth-Century England," in Lindsay Granshaw and Roy Porter, eds., *The Hospital in History* (London: Routledge, 1989) Guenter B. Risse, *Hospital Life in Enlightenment Scotland. Care and Teaching at the Royal Infirmary of Edinburgh* (Cambridge University Press, 1986). On the Bristol Infirmary in particular, see G. Munro Smith, *A History of the Bristol Royal Infirmary* (Bristol: Arrowsmith, 1917). See also Michael Neve, "Natural Philosophy, Medicine and the Culture of Science in Provincial England: The Cases of Bristol 1790–1850, and Bath 1750–1820," (Ph.D. diss., University College, London, 1984).

2 On the founding of the Infirmary, see Bristol Record Office, Bristol Biographical Memoirs (hereafter BRO BBM) 1; *An Account of the Hospitals, Alms Houses and Public Schools in Bristol* (Bristol: H. Farley for T. Mills, 1775); Smith, *Bristol Royal Infirmary*.

3 Court of Governors Minutes, Hampshire Record Office (hereafter HRO), 8 Oct. 1737, p. 53.

4 Porter, "Gift Relation."

5 David Owen, *English Philanthropy* (Cambridge, Mass.: Harvard University Press, 1964).

6 Porter, "Gift Relation."

7 *The Adventures of Bampfylde Moore Carew*, in Robert Hays Cunningham, ed., *Amusing Prose Chapbooks* (London: Hamilton Adams, 1889).

8 Gloucestershire Record Office D 1928 A2.

9 Ibid.

10 See Charles Webster, *The Great Instauration* (London: Duckworth, 1975), pp. 288–300.

11 Carew Reynell, *A Sermon Preached Before Contributors to the Bristol Infirmary* (Bristol: S. and F. Farley, 1738), p. 11.

12 Ibid.

13 Court of Governors, HRO, p. 55.

14 Unlike many other infirmaries, in Bristol, the term "governor" can be applied to all who paid the two-guinea annual subscription – all subscribers were entitled to attend the weekly committee that, in effect, ran the hospital.

15 Reynell, *Sermon*, p. 15.

16 Champion family letter-book, BRO 38083 (2) Dec. 1768.

17 Ibid., (3) 29 Sept. 1771.

18 Ibid.

19 Smith, *Bristol Royal Infirmary*, p. 14.

20 John Cary, *A Proposal Offered to the Committee* . . . (London: n.p., [1700]).

21 Paul Slack, *Poverty and Policy in Tudor and Stuart England* (London: Longman Group, 1988), pp. 195–8.

22 Ibid., p. 196.

23 7 & 8 William III c. 32. See also British Library 816.m.54 and 55 for Cary's note on a handbill advertising his scheme.

24 Society for the Promotion of Christian Knowledge Archives, Abstract Letter Book CRI2, letter 2189, 5 Aug. 1709.

25 A. G. Craig, "The Movement for the Reformation of Manners, 1688–1715" (Ph.D. diss., Edinburgh University, 1980).
26 Josiah Woodward, *An Account of the Progress of the Reformation of Manners* . . . (London: J. Downing, 1706), 14th ed., p. 50.
27 Craig, "Reformation of Manners," p. 4.
28 Charles Brent, *Persuasion to a Publick Spirit* (London: John Wyat, 1704), p. 21.
29 E. E. Butcher, *Bristol Corporation of the Poor, 1696–1834* (Bristol: Bristol Record Society Publications, 1932), vol. 3, p. 62.
30 John Cary, *An Account of the Proceedings of the Corporation for the Poor* . . . (London: F. Collins, 1700), p. 11.
31 Ibid., p. 12.
32 Richard T. Vann, *The Social Development of Quakerism 1655–1755* (Cambridge, Mass.: Harvard University Press, 1969), p. 141.
33 Minutes of the Men's Meeting, Society of Friends, BRO 14585 SF/A1/9a, pp. 128–9. When this woman later had an illegitimate child, the minutes noted that she had brought "reproach to our Christian Community."
34 Court of Governors, HRO, p. 55.
35 BRO 35893 1a, 29 Feb. 1739.
36 Court of Governors, HRO, p. 56.
37 [W. A. Greenhill], *The Life of Sir James Stonhouse* (Oxford: John Henry Parker, 1844), p. 22.
38 What follows is pieced together from BRO BBM 3 (diet) and BRO 35893 2b (rules), as well as from miscellaneous details in BRO BBM.
39 Josiah Tucker, *A Sermon Preached in the Parish Church in Bristol* (Bristol: William Crossley, 1746).
40 Ibid., p. 15.
41 BRO BBM, 2, p. 768.
42 John Bellers, *Proposals for Raising a College of Industry* . . . (London: T. Sowle, 1695), p. 13.
43 Matthew Tindall, *The Rights of the Christian Church Asserted* . . . (London: n.p., 1706), p. 134. My thanks to Dr. Tim Hitchcock for this reference.
44 Ibid., p. 117.
45 Reynell, *Sermon*, p. 2.
46 Melvin Endy, *William Penn and Early Quakerism* (Princeton, N.J.: Princeton University Press, 1973), pp. 70–1, 235–6.
47 Ibid., p. 236.
48 Arthur Bedford, *A Sermon Preached to the Societies for the Reformation of Manners* (London: Joseph Downing, 1734), pp. 8–9.
49 Champion family letter book, BRO 38083 (1) 7 Sept. 1764.
50 John Bellers, *An Essay Towards the Improvement of Physick* . . . (London: J. Sowle, 1714), p. 6. On Bellers, see George Clarke, ed., *John Bellers: His Life, Times and Writings* (London: Routledge & Kegan Paul, 1987).
51 Bellers, *Essay*, p. 44.
52 On the uses of charity, see Sandra Cavallo, "Charity, Power, and Patronage in Eighteenth-Century Italian Hospitals: The Case of Turin," in Granshaw and Porter, *Hospital in History*, pp. 93–122.

53 Monica M. Tompkins, "The Two Workhouses of Bristol 1696–1735" (Master's thesis, University of Nottingham, 1962), p. 79.

54 James Johnson, *Transactions of the Corporation of the Poor During 126 Years* (Bristol: P. Rose, 1826), pp. 26–9.

55 Johnson, *Corporation,* p. 138. Johnson, an early nineteenth-century historian of Bristol's Poor Law, claimed that the Guardians from 1696 to 1718 were all High Church. I find this claim most unlikely for the period prior to 1714, because it was subsequently so difficult to run the Corporation without dissenters. Like many others, Johnson managed to obscure the sectarian roots of various approaches to poor relief, because he himself was not without an agenda for reform.

56 Cary, *Proceedings of the Corporation,* p. 3.

57 John Latimer, *Annals of Bristol in the Eighteenth Century* (Bristol: printed for the author, 1893), pp. 85–6.

58 M. G. Jones, *The Charity School Movement* (Cambridge University Press, 1938).

59 Elizabeth Baigent estimates that there were as many as 1,500 Quakers in Bristol at this time; this seems too large, and 1,200 serves as a baseline (Elizabeth Baigent, "Bristol in 1775" (D. Phil. diss., Oxford University, 1985). See also David Pratt, *English Quakers and the First Industrial Revolution* (New York: Garland, 1985), p. 64, who estimates that Quakers were 1,200 to 1,400 in number, or about 1 percent of the city's population. A figure of 5 for household size and the estimated 70 Quaker subscribers in 1750 leads to an estimate of one-third of households subscribing.

60 Kathleen Wilson, "The Rejection of Deference: Urban Provincial Culture in England, 1715–1785" (Ph.D. diss., Yale University, 1985); Peter Borsay, "The English Urban Renaissance: The Development of Provincial Urban Culture, c. 1680–1760," *Social History* 5 (1977): 581–99; idem, *The English Urban Renaissance: Culture and Society in the Provincial Town, 1660–1770* (Oxford: Oxford University Press [Clarendon Press], 1989); Jonathan Barry, "The Cultural Life of Bristol, 1640–1775" (D.Phil. diss., Oxford University, 1985); Paul Langford, *A Polite and Commercial People: England 1727–1783* (Oxford: Oxford University Press [Clarendon Press], 1989); P. J. Corfield, *The Impact of English Towns, 1700–1800* (Oxford University Press, 1982), pp. 143–4. BRO BBM contains much miscellaneous information about urban sociability, drinking, political, debating, musical clubs, and so forth, which indicates the city's highly organized and differentiated social environment.

61 Lewins Mead Poor Book, BRO 6687(3).

62 Cashbook, Penn St. Tabernacle, BRO 35481 PT/F(a).

63 It is impossible to know what Nurse Rattle did for her £5 per annum. From Poor Law records, it seems that nursing was a fairly common occupation for women. There is always the possibility that Nurse Rattle was in fact a wet nurse, but it seems unlikely that the congregation would ever annually retain a wet nurse. More likely, she was just on contract to minister to the poorer members of the group.

64 Barry, "Cultural Life of Bristol."

65 At least two-thirds of the husbands of these recipients were pump-makers, barber-surgeons, confectioners, jewelers, accountants, and the like – probably fairly well-off compared to a laborer or other worker. Of course, for any family, the expenses of a month's lying-in, of special foods for the mother, of household help, midwives' fees, fuel, and baby linens, must have been considerable. BRO 33041 BMC/8/1 contains records of this charity and others.

66 BRO 33041 BMC/6/23.

67 Latimer, *Eighteenth Century*, p. 435.

68 Ibid., p. 183.

69 Stephen MacFarlane, "Social Policy and the Poor in the Later Seventeenth Century," in A. L. Beier and Roger Finlay, eds., *London 1500–1700: The Making of the Metropolis* (London: Longman Group, 1985), pp. 253.

70 Although not frequently noted in discussions of English charity, such partisan divisions have often been discussed in continental charity. See Kathryn Norberg, *Rich and Poor in Grenoble 1600–1814* (Berkeley and Los Angeles: University of California Press, 1985); Cavallo, "Charity, Power, and Patronage."

CHAPTER 5

1 Similar methods of nominal linkage have been used to provide evidence of family structures in both parishes. The Abson Poor Law overseers' accounts for 1764 to 1803 have been linked with parish registers, so that family and occupational data are available for most of the parish's 154 relief recipients (BRO, P/Abs/OP/2a,b; P/Abs/R/1a). In the city, the Infirmary admission book has been sampled for patients from SS. Philip and Jacob and been linked with parish registers, which contain unusually detailed information about occupations and addresses. This group of 1,024 inpatients and outpatients represents 1 out of every 15 patients from the parish for the period from 1771 to 1805 (BRO P/St P&J/R/1–4; 35893 19, 20). For further details, see M. E. Fissell, "The 'Sick and Drooping Poor' in Eighteenth-Century Bristol and its Region," *Social History of Medicine* 2 1989: 35–58.

2 This description of Abson is derived from the following: Samuel Rudder, *A New History of Gloucestershire* (Gloucester: Alan Sutton [reprint], 1977); BRO HA/L/1–4 (records of a suit over tithes); Ralph Bigland, *Historical, Monumental, and Genealogical Collections . . . Gloucestershire* (Frocester: printed for Robert Bigland, 1791–1889); Thomas Rudge, *The History of the County of Gloucestershire* (Gloucester: printed for the author, 1803); Isaac Taylor, *Map of Gloucestershire* (1777), reprinted in *A Gloucestershire and Bristol Atlas* (London: for the Bristol and Gloucestershire Archaeological Society, 1961).

On SS Philip and Jacob, see: John Latimer, *Annals of Bristol in the Eighteenth Century* (Bristol: printed for the author, 1893); Elizabeth Baigent, "Assessed Taxes as Sources for the Study of Urban Wealth,"

Urban History Yearbook (1988): 31–48; James New, "An Account of the Houses and Inhabitants of the Parish of Philip and Jacob in the City of Bristol," MS. 1781, Bristol Central Library (hereafter BCL) 21769; James Johnson, *Transactions of the Corporation of the Poor . . .* (Bristol: P. Rose, 1826), appendices D and E, pp. 170–1.

3 Tim Wales, "Poverty, Poor Relief, and the Life-Cycle: Some Evidence from Seventeenth-Century Norfolk," in Richard M. Smith, ed., *Land, Kinship and Life-Cycle* (Cambridge University Press, 1984), pp. 351–404.

4 Bristol Infirmary, Annual Reports 1740–1806 bound in BRO BBM, vol. 1, vol. 3. These figures have been cross-checked with admissions registers in order to confirm that they do not represent repeat visits rather than admissions.

5 This figure, 5 percent, was calculated in two ways. First, the numbers admitted to hospital, drawn from Annual Reports were compared with the city's population as a whole. Second, a manuscript survey of the population of SS Philip and Jacob parish (New, "An Account") was compared with the numbers of patients from that parish in the admissions registers. Five percent is a figure consonant with early nineteenth-century medical charity; see John V. Pickstone, *Medicine and Industrial Society: A History of Hospital Development in Manchester and Its Region, 1752–1946* (Manchester University Press, 1986), p. 70; Hilary Marland, *Medicine and Society in Wakefield and Huddersfield 1780–1870* (Cambridge University Press, 1987), p. 103. See also I. S. L. Loudon, "The Historical Importance of Outpatients," *British Medical Journal* 1 (1978): 974–7.

6 BRO P/St P&J/4 a, b.

7 On health care and the Old Poor Law generally, see: Dorothy Marshall, *The English Poor in the Eighteenth Century* (London: Routledge & Kegan Paul, 1926), pp. 115–22; Joan Lane, "The Provincial Practitioner and His Services to the Poor 1750–1800," *Bulletin of the Society for the Social History of Medicine* 28 (1981): 10–14; Irvine Loudon, *Medical Care and the General Practitioner, 1750–1850* (Oxford: Oxford University Press [Clarendon Press], 1986), pp. 228–66.

8 This is an estimate based upon a population of 400 to 600, with 154 Poor Law recipients, and the fact that some of those recipients were families, implying more than one actual person on relief.

9 John Skinner, *Journal of a Somerset Rector 1803–34*, ed. Howard Coombs and Peter Coombs, (Oxford University Press, 1984).

10 M. A. Crowther, "Family Responsibility and State Responsibility in Britain Before the Welfare State," *Historical Journal* 25 (1982): 32 especially; and David Thomson, "I am Not My Father's Keeper: Families and the Elderly in Nineteenth-Century England," *Law and History Review* 2 (1984): 265–86, for discussions of the rather more stringent legal definitions of family obligation.

11 Skinner, *Journal*, p. 216.

12 On the Bristol Corporation, see *Some Considerations Offered . . .* (London: 1711); E. E. Butcher, *The Bristol Corporation of the Poor* (Bristol: Bristol Record Society, 1932) vol. 3; John Cary, *An Account of the Proceedings of the Corporation . . .* (London: F. Collins, 1700); Isaac

Cooke, *Address . . . on the Enormous Increase of the Poor Tax in the Said City . . .* (Bristol: 1786); James Johnson, *Transactions of the Corporation of the Poor During 126 Years* (Bristol: P. Rose, 1826); J. C. Prichard, *A History of the Epidemic Fever Which Prevailed in Bristol During the Years 1817, 1818, and 1819* (London: Arch, 1820).

13 BRO 06570, Settlement Examinations, 1748–1820. I have only analyzed those up to 1778, because there are none for the period 1779–1819.

14 The baptismal registers for SS Philip and Jacob include designations of the father's occupation. A random sample of fathers' occupations for 1775 and for 1800 has been compared with those of the Poor Law examinees and the Infirmary patients.

15 E. A. Wrigley and R. Schofield, *The Population History of England, 1541–1871* (London: Edward Arnold, 1981), Table A3.1, p. 529.

16 The population of SS. Philip and Jacob may have been more "mature" than that of the country overall. High infant mortality (ranging from 92 to 259 per 1,000 in the period 1776–1805) and high adult in-migration could have shifted the age structure upward. However, the figures on outpatients suggest that the discrepancy may not be too great. It must also be emphasized that men and women may have used the institution for different purposes. See T. V. Hitchcock, "The English Workhouse: A Study in Institutional Poor Relief in Selected Counties 1696–1750" (D. Phil. diss., Oxford University, 1985), pp. 194–201 for an analysis of gender-differentiated use of workhouses.

17 See David Souden, "Migrants and the Population Structure of Later Seventeenth-Century Provincial Cities and Market Towns," in Peter Clark, ed., *The Transformation of English Provincial Towns* (London: Hutchinson, 1984), pp. 152–4, who shows that even in 1696, Bristol's population was already characterized by a fairly high number of lodgers.

18 James Lackington, *Memoirs of the First Forty-five Years of the Life of J. L . . .* (London: printed for the author, 1792), 2d ed., p. 118.

19 E. A. Wrigley, "The Changing Occupational Structures of Colyton over Two Centuries," *Local Population Studies* 18 (1970): 9–21; Peter Clark, "Migration in England During the Late Seventeenth and Early Eighteenth Century," *Past and Present* 83 (1979): 57–90. See also, Peter Clark and David Souden, eds., *Migration and Society in Early Modern England* (London: Unwin Hyman, 1988).

20 William Holland, *Paupers and Pig Killers, The Diary of William Holland*, ed. Jack Ayres (Harmondsworth: Penguin Books, 1986), p. 58. See the discussion of the effects of nonconformity on completeness of registration of baptisms and burials in Anglican registers in Wrigley and Schofield, *Population History of England*, pp. 89–96, and the local study, M. Slack, "Non-conformist and Anglican Registration in the Halifax Area, 1740–99," *Local Population Studies* 38 (1987): 44–5.

21 See, for an example of this, Richard Symes, *Fire Analyzed* (Bristol: Thomas Cocking, 1771), pp. 67–8.

22 Margaret Pelling, "Illness Among the Poor in an Early Modern Town: The Norwich Census of 1570," *Continuity and Change* 3 (1988): 273–90.

23 Evidence for smallpox comes from the parish register and from the Poor Law accounts. Evidence for all three epidemics comes from a practitioner in a nearby village, who published his findings in a medical journal. J. C. Jenner noted typhus in 1785–6, smallpox in 1785, and ague in 1784–7. In Abson, smallpox came earlier, in 1781–2, and again in 1784–7. It was, needless to add, endemic as well as epidemic. See J. C. Jenner, *London Medical Journal* VII (1786): 163; *London Medical Journal* IX (1788): 47.

24 John V. Pickstone and Stella Butler, "The Politics of Medicine in Manchester 1788–1792," *Medical History* 28 (1984): 227–49.

25 On this diagnostic category, see Irvine Loudon, "Leg Ulcers in the Eighteenth and Early Nineteenth Centuries," *Journal of the Royal College of General Practitioners* 31 (1981): 263.

26 Irvine Loudon " 'The Vile Race of Quacks with Which This Country Is Infested' " in W. F. Bynum and Roy Porter, eds., *Medical Fringe and Medical Orthodoxy 1750–1850* (London: Croom Helm, 1986), pp. 106–28.

27 E. Sigsworth, "Gateways to Death?" in Peter Mathias, ed., *Science and Society 1600–1900* (Cambridge University Press, 1972).

28 BRO, Accounts, St. Peter's, 1796–7.

29 John Woodward, *To Do the Sick No Harm* (London: Routledge & Kegan Paul, 1985); Brian Abel-Smith, *The Hospitals 1800–1948* (Cambridge, Mass.: Harvard University Press, 1964).

CHAPTER 6

1 Oddly enough, the medical staff of the Infirmary was largely Tory by the latter part of the century. Elections to these posts were often characterized by highly political and sectarian battles.

2 The only sources for the names of the governors are annual reports. Because a complete run of these does not exist, I have sampled a selection of years over the century: 1736, 1750, 1762, 1775, 1791, and 1806. People usually signed on and remained subscribers for life, so that any picture of changing interests must remain blurry. The intent is to look at the composition of each year chosen and to compare it as a cohort with the other years sampled.

Occupational data was derived from the earliest Bristol directory (Sketchley's, in 1775), the poll books of 1754 and 1774, Beaven's *Bristol Lists,* Burgess books, and apprentice registers in the Bristol Record Office (hereafter BRO), as well as the BRO name index. There are two problems with this method. First, the reliability of the sources varies irregularly over time. For instance, a great many men were made freemen, and thus registered in burgess books, just prior to the 1774 election. The number of possible sources also increases over time, so that more is known about later cohorts. However, this is balanced by the second problem: the certainty of any given identification.

Because the lists of governors contain only names, I have had to use common-sense guidelines rather than nominal-linkage algorithms. For example, if the subscriber died in the past year, the list usually includes the notation "dec." I have also traced subscribers forward and backward to get a sense of their tenure, which eliminates some possibilities. Ultimately, however, over a third of my sample remains either unknown or undetermined.

Mapping out the sectarian alliances of subscribers is equally problematic. Dissent is probably underrepresented due to methods. A list of Bristol Quakers ca. 1796 and the records of both Quaker and Unitarian burial grounds have been used to indicate dissenters (BRO, SF/R1/5-6, 39461/R/2(a)). Both registers note when outsiders were buried, so I am fairly certain that the people whom I have designated as Quaker or Unitarian were in fact so. But, obviously, a dissenter might well have been buried in an Anglican churchyard for any number of reasons. Ergo, I have probably undercounted dissenters and consequently overcounted "Anglicans" (i.e., leftovers). Although both Methodists and Baptists were strong in Bristol, they curiously were somewhat absent from the Infirmary.

3 Few were women. Even those women who did subscribe were often just taking up their husband's subscription upon widowhood.

4 Roy Porter, "The Gift Relation: Philanthropy and Provincial Hospitals in Eighteenth-Century England," in Lindsay Granshaw and Roy Porter, eds., *The Hospital in History* (London: Routledge, 1989), esp. pp. 158–62.

5 John V. Pickstone, *Medicine and Industrial Society: A History of Hospital Development in Manchester and Its Region, 1752–1946* (Manchester University Press, 1986).

6 Craig Rose, "Politics and the London Royal Hospitals, 1683–92," in Granshaw and Porter, *Hospital in History*, pp. 123–48.

7 Richard Symes, *Fire Analyzed* (Bristol: Thomas Cocking, 1771), pp. 67–8.

8 For information on this sample of patients, see Chapter 5.

9 BRO P/St J/Ch 8(6).

10 John Skinner, *Journal of a Somerset Rector 1803–34*, ed. Howard Coombs and Peter Coombs (Oxford University Press, 1984), p. 230.

11 Ibid., p. 253.

12 Ibid., pp. 35, 293.

13 Thomas Beddoes, *The History of Isaac Jenkins* (Bristol: J. Mills, 1804), p. 12.

14 Of course, by the 1800s when this cautionary tale was written, it may easily be read as a plea for a return to an old-fashioned world of deferential social relationships where everyone knew his or her place.

15 Obviously, I draw upon the work of Edward Thompson here. E. P. Thompson, "Patrician Society, Plebian Culture," *Journal of Social History 7* (1974): pp. 382–405; idem, "Eighteenth-Century English Society: Class Struggle Without Class?" *Social History 3* (1978): p. 133–65; idem, "The Moral Economy of the English Crowd in the Eighteenth Century," *Past and Present 50* (1971): pp. 76–136. For a somewhat different perspective, see Harold Perkin, *The Origins of Modern English Society 1780–1880* (London: Routledge & Kegan Paul, 1969).

16 See BRO, Bristol Biographical Memoirs (hereafter BBM) 4, p. 374.

17 BRO, BBM 14, p. 228; and for midwifery, BRO, BBM 3, p. 18.

18 The only reference I have ever seen to this institution is in BRO, BBM 3, p. 195. No doubt there were other small charities that have escaped historical recognition.

19 Joseph Cottle, *Early Recollections, Chiefly Relating to the Late Samuel Taylor Coleridge* (London: Longman Rees, 1837), vol. 2, p. 41.

20 Thomas Beddoes, *Rules of the Medical Institute for the Benefit of the Sick and Drooping Poor . . .* (Bristol: J. Mills, 1804), p. 24.

21 BRO, BBM 4, report inserted in between pp. 159–60.

22 BRO, BBM 11, p. 154.

23 BRO, BBM 8, p. 373.

24 On this theme, see Lindsay Granshaw, " 'Fame and Fortune by Means of Bricks and Mortar': the Medical Professions and Specialist Hospitals in Britain 1800–1948," in Granshaw and Porter, *Hospital in History*, pp. 199–220.

25 This practice is noted by Smith, BRO, BBM 2, and by an anonymous author, "Hints to Young Practitioners," *Edinburgh Medical and Surgical Journal* 5 (1809): 338.

26 "Hints to Young Practitioners," 339.

27 Elizabeth Baigent, "Bristol in 1775" (D. Phil. diss., Oxford University, 1985).

28 BRO, BBM 2, p. 812. In 1783, the Anchor relieved 113 mothers and another 462 poor people.

29 In some ways, my argument parallels that of Gareth Stedman Jones for London several decades later: Gareth Stedman Jones, *Outcast London* (Oxford University Press, 1971). Although the model of geographical separation, of inspection and moral surveillance I advance for Bristol may seem premature, there are two dimensions intersecting in patterns of charity and welfare over long periods of time. One is the cyclical nature of reform campaigns, often focusing on particular groups and on close personal supervision (think for example of the 1690s), which alternated with periods characterized by a more relaxed attitude. But this cyclical pattern was altered by changes in class relations – what Stedman Jones calls the deformation of the gift – which recast the way in which personal connections could be made between rich and poor, ultimately replacing personal patronage with moral surveillance.

30 BRO 38463 (2).

31 BRO, BBM 8, pp. 127–9. This is their annual Report, 1819.

32 BRO P/St BM/X/1.

33 Ibid.

34 Clifton Dispensary, *First Report*, BRO 16071.

35 BRO P/St BM/X/1 Aug. 1821.

36 Ibid., Nov. 1823, Aug. 1834, Aug. 1820.

37 Among the many discussions relating to this topic, see Leonore Davidoff and Catherine Hall, *Family Fortunes: Men and Women of the English Middle Class, 1780–1850* (London: Hutchinson, 1987); F. K. Prochaska, *Women and Philanthropy in Nineteenth-Century England* (Oxford University Press, 1980).

CHAPTER 7

1 Hampshire Infirmary, Court of Governors Proceedings, Hampshire Record Office, 8 Oct. 1737, p. 52.
2 Bristol Record Office (hereafter BRO), *Rules* 35893 2b.
3 BRO, Bristol Biographical Memoirs (hereafter BBM) 1, pp. 44 et seq.
4 BRO, BBM 3, pp. 174.
5 Ibid., p. 147.
6 BRO, BBM 6, pp. 36.
7 Susan C. Lawrence, "Science and Medicine at the London Hospitals: The Development of Teaching and Research, 1750–1815" (Ph.D. diss., University of Toronto, 1985). Many of the Infirmary's early surgeons had gone, not to London, but to Paris for further education after their apprenticeships. John Castelman, James Ford, and John Page, for example, all trained at the Hôtel-Dieu.
8 BRO, BBM 1, pp. 52–3, an incomplete printed syllabus of the course.
9 BRO, BBM 1, p. 118.
10 BRO, BBM 4(2), p. 527.
11 Ibid., pp. 528–34.
12 Ibid., p. 542.
13 Ibid., p. 262.
14 Erwin Ackerknecht, *Medicine at the Paris Hospital 1794–1848* (Baltimore: Johns Hopkins University Press, 1967); Toby Gelfand, *Professionalizing Modern Medicine: Surgeons and Medical Science and Institutions in the Eighteenth Century* (Westport, Conn.: Greenwood Press, 1980).
15 Russell C. Maulitz, *Morbid Appearances: The Anatomy of Pathology in the Early Nineteenth-Century* (Cambridge University Press, 1987).
16 Lawrence, "London Hospitals."
17 Toby Gelfand, "Hospital Teaching as Private Enterprise," in Roy Porter and W. F. Bynum, eds., *William Hunter and the Eighteenth-Century Medical World* (Cambridge University Press, 1986), p. 135; Lawrence, "London Hospitals"; Othmar Keel, "The Politics of Health and the Institutionalization of Clinical Practice in Europe in the Second Half of the Eighteenth Century," in Bynum and Porter, *William Hunter,* pp. 207–56. See also Bynum's essay "Physicians, Hospitals and Career Structures in Eighteenth Century London," pp. 105–28, in the same volume, for a discussion of physicians' use of the hospital in making their careers. Outside of London, however, I doubt that Bynum's findings would be replicated – in the provinces, many more surgeons held institutional posts than physicians, if only due to the latter's relative scarcity.
18 The following analysis is drawn from a survey of medical occupations in the Apprentice Rolls in the Bristol Record Office.
19 Deed, 1755, BRO 00429. The Surgeons' Hall was evidently a room in the West India Coffee House for a number of years. See also, George Parker, "Early Bristol Medical Institutions," *Bristol and Gloucestershire Archaeological Society* 44 (1922), for a discussion of the Barber-Surgeons Company.

20 An average of 1.16 per year (1700–1724) had fallen to 0.68 per year by the second quarter of the century.
21 See Gelfand, "Hospital Teaching as Private Enterprise," for a similar argument about pupillage versus apprenticeship in London hospitals.
22 BRO, BBM 1, p. 59.
23 BRO, BBM 2, p. 760.
24 BRO Minutes of House Committee Meetings, 15 Nov. 1797, 35983 2b.
25 Ibid., May 1798.
26 BRO, BBM 3, p. 194.
27 BRO Minutes of House Committee Meetings, May 1798, 35983 2b.
28 Ibid.
29 Ibid., 17 Nov. 1802.
30 Ibid., 13 March 1805.
31 Thomas Lee, *An Address to the Subscribers and the Public Supporting the Bristol Infirmary* . . . (Bristol: Emery and Adams, 1805).
32 Thomas Lee, *A Second Address to the Subscribers and the Public Supporting the Bristol Infirmary* (Bristol: Emery and Adams, 1805), p. 4.
33 Ibid., p. 9.
34 *Mirror,* 14 Sept. 1805.
35 Henry Alford, "The Bristol Infirmary in My Student Days," *Bristol Medico-Chirugical Journal* 8 (1890): 167. On body snatching and dissection more generally, see Ruth Richardson, *Death, Dissection and the Destitute* (London: Routledge, 1987).
36 R. Campbell, *The London Tradesman* (London: T. Gardner, 1747), p. 50.
37 Henry Thomson, *Medical Observations and Inquiries* 2 (1762): 351.
38 Alford, "Student Days," p. 190.
39 John Latimer, *Annals of Bristol in the Eighteenth Century* (Bristol: printed for the author, 1893), p. 193.
40 BRO, BBM 1, p. 71.
41 BRO, BBM 5, pp. 353–4.
42 BRO, BBM 4(2), pp. 525–6.
43 BRO, BBM 8, p. 161.
44 BRO, BBM 6, p. 194F; replies from the surgeons are inserted into the memoirs.
45 BRO, BBM 4(2), p. 562.
46 James Bedingfield, *A Compendium of Medical Practice* (Bristol: Highley, 1816), p. 200.
47 Ibid, p. 299.
48 Alford, "Student Days."
49 William Hunter, quoted in C. H. Brock, *William Hunter 1718–1783* (University of Glasgow Press, 1983), p. 13.
50 See Lisa Rosner, "Students and Apprentices: Medical Education at Edinburgh University 1760–1810" (Ph.D. diss., Johns Hopkins University, 1986), for similar career paths of men who attended Edinburgh's medical school.
51 See Chapter 5 for a discussion of the numbers of patients seen in the Infirmary. Obviously, precise figures are impossible to obtain. Suppos-

edly neither Beddoes nor the Dispensary would have seen patients who were eligible for Infirmary admission, but actual practice may have been different. Also, in all eighteenth-century published figures of admission, there is always the chance that they counted visits rather than patients. In these three cases, however, this is unlikely due to the format of records.

52 I am grateful to Dr. W. F. Bynum for suggesting to me that charities might have competed with private practice for patients, although I probably take the argument further than he intended. The idea that charity competed with private practice was, of course, oft-repeated in nineteenth-century discussions of hospitals.

53 "Hints to Young Practitioners," *Edinburgh Medical and Surgical Journal* 5 (1809): 335–9. Many of these suggestions are identical to those of Tobias Smollett in his novel *Ferdinand Count Fathom,* referred to in Roy Porter, "The Language of Quackery in England 1660–1800," in Peter Burke and Roy Porter, eds., *The Social History of Language* (Cambridge University Press, 1987), pp. 73–103. Interestingly, Smollet does not suggest hospitals or charity as means of getting ahead, but rather emphasizes the aspects of public display – a fancy carriage, being called out of public places for "emergencies," and so forth. Smollet was, of course, a doctor, and Fathom visits the Bristol Hotwells in the novel.

54 BRO, BBM 1, pp. 32–3.

55 G. Munro Smith, *A History of the Bristol Royal Infirmary* (Bristol: Arrowsmith, 1917), p. 19.

56 BRO, BBM 1, p. 120.

57 On a slightly later period, see Irvine Loudon's remarks on the importance of doctors' carriages as emblems of social standing. Irvine Loudon, *Medical Care and the General Practitioner 1750–1850* (Oxford: Oxford University Press [Clarendon Press], 1986), pp. 117–25.

CHAPTER 8

1 Alexander Morgan, Casebook, Wellcome Institute for the History of Medicine Library, London, MS. 3631, p. ii.

2 Thomas Beddoes, *On Fever* (Clifton: n.p., n.d.), case #21; James Bedingfield, *A Compendium of Cases from the Bristol Infirmary* (London: Highley, 1816), p. 155.

3 See Stanley Joel Reiser, *Medicine and the Reign of Technology* (Cambridge University Press, 1978), pp. 1–22.

4 Although not entirely in agreement with his interpretation, I obviously draw upon Michel Foucault, *The Birth of the Clinic,* trans. A. Sheridan (New York: Pantheon, 1973), in this discussion. The process he identifies with Paris medicine was not unique to post-Revolutionary France; some of the features of medical knowledge he delineates were characteristic of late eighteenth-century hospitals elsewhere in Europe and were related to their particular social structures.

5 Bedingfield, *Compendium,* p. 6.

6 Nathaniel Bedford, Observations and Cases, Royal College of Surgeons' MS., 42.c.2, p. 1.

7 Bayford, "An Account of Two Aneurysms in the Aorta," *Medical Observations and Inquiries* 3 (1769): 14.

8 Samuel Pye, "The Effect of an Accidental Vomiting," *Medical Observations and Inquiries* 2 (1762): 123. This Samuel Pye was not the Bristolian, although there is a suggestion that they were relatives. Of course, the fact that Pye was a physician also shaped his style of reporting. But a comparison of this case to one reported in the same journal by a Bristol surgeon reveals the same kind of split between private patients' narratives and hospital patients' physical signs. See Abraham Ludlow, "A Case of Obstructed Deglutition," *Medical Observations and Inquiries* 3 (1769): 86. Ludlow is quite explicit, saying that "our patient gave us nearly the following account." This is the same case discussed in Chapter 2, of a man who swallowed a cherry pit, which lodged in his throat.

9 Thomson, "An Account of an Aneurysm," *Medical Observations and Inquiries* 3 (1769): 58.

10 Edward Estlin, Casebook, BRO 35893 (32), p. 457.

11 Bedingfield, *Compendium,* p. 116.

12 Ibid., p. 125.

13 Beddoes, *On Fever.*

14 Bedingfield, *Compendium,* p. 115.

15 Pugh, "A Violent Scorbutic Case," *Medical Observations and Inquiries* 2 (1762): 241.

16 Such signs also spoke to the patient through the medium of the doctor's attention to them.

17 Bedingfield, *Compendium,* p. 89.

18 Ibid., p. 114.

19 Ibid., pp. 146, 94.

20 Hey, "An Account of the Effects of Electricity in the Amaurosis," *Medical Observations and Inquiries* 5 (1776): 2. This article is a good example of the shift from private to hospital medicine; the first case includes parts of the patient's narrative, but the remainder, all hospital cases, rely upon discussions of physical evidence and therapy. In one case, Hey is intrigued by the onset of the disease – but his eliciting of the circumstances of the patient's illness only happens once Hey is interested in the ailment, long after the patient left the Infirmary.

21 See also, for similar examples, Estlin, Casebook, p. 37.

22 Thomas Antrobus, "An Amputation of the Leg," *Medical Observations and Inquiries* 2 (1762): 153. Antrobus was a surgeon at the infirmary in Liverpool.

23 Thomas Laqueur has made almost the opposite point, linking the rise of case histories to humanitarian concerns. But the accretion of detail central to forms of discourse created in the late eighteenth and early nineteenth centuries implied a distance from the actual body of the sufferer so described, in a manner perhaps analogous to pornography. Thomas Laqueur, "Bodies, Details, and the Humanitarian Narrative," in Lynn

Hunt, ed., *The New Cultural History* (Berkeley and Los Angeles: University of California Press, 1989), pp. 176–204.

24 Estlin, Casebook, p. 23.

25 Ibid., p. 21.

26 Ibid., p. 45.

27 Ibid., p. 49.

28 William Cullen, *Synopsis Nosologiae Methodicae* (Edinburgh: Creech, 1769).

29 W. P. Williams and W. A. Jones, "A List of Somerset Dialect," *Somersetshire Archaeological and Natural History Society Proceedings* 18 (1878).

30 Rice Charlton, *Cases of Persons Admitted into the Hospital at Bath under the Care of the Late Dr. Oliver* (Bath: R. Cruttwell, 1774), p. 6.

31 Samuel England, Casebooks, Chirurgery, pp. 69, 87, Royal College of Physicians, M 5, 6. My thanks to Dr. Susan Lawrence for this reference.

32 Bedford, Observations and Cases, p. 22.

33 Estlin, Casebook, p. 63.

34 Marmaduke Berdoe, *An Enquiry into the Influence of the Electrical Fluid in the Structure and Formation of Animated Beings* (Bath: S. Hazard, 1771), p. 149.

35 E. L. Fox, *Surmises Respecting . . . the Cholera* (Bristol: Mills & Son, 1831), p. 4.

36 Ibid.

37 Thomas Beddoes, *Rules of the Preventive Medical Institution* (Bristol: J. Mills, 1804), p. 94. I am very grateful to Mrs. Dorothy Stansfield, Beddoes's recent biographer, for calling this quotation to my attention.

38 The following analysis is drawn from data in the burials register, BROP/St P&J/R/4(b). Eight years were chosen at random from 1782–1825, and all deaths analyzed from them. The burials register listed name, age, cause of death, and whether a pauper or a stranger. It by no means represents all of the deaths within the parish; people could be buried in other churchyards, most notably the Quaker one. However, its inclusion of the cause of death makes it a rare example of lay diagnosis. I have no reason to suspect that the population buried in the churchyard at SS Philip and Jacob was notably at variance with that of the parish overall. The bodies of inmates of St. Peter's (the city workhouse) were often returned to their own parish for burial.

39 The numbers are as follows: Decline, 27 percent of 496 cases were paupers; Debility, all 6 cases were paupers; Natural Decay, 4 out of 5 cases were paupers; Atrophy, all 40 cases were paupers.

40 See *Pharmacopeia in Usum Nosocomii Bristoliensis* (Bristol: Bonner and Middleton, 1777); and Bristol Infirmary, *Manuale Medicaminum Simplicium et Commistorum Formulas Continens in Usum Valetudinarii Bristolensis Accodatum* (Bristol: n.p., 1816).

41 Bristol Record Office Bristol Biographical Memoirs (hereafter BRO BBM) 2, p. 1,012.

42 Bedingfield, *Compendium*, p. 39.

43 Henry Alford, "The Bristol Infirmary in My Student Days 1822–28," *Bristol Medico-Chirurgical Journal* 8 (1890): 189.

44 Ibid., p. 190.
45 Ibid., p. 189.
46 Bedingfield, *Compendium*, p. 10.
47 Ibid., p. 37.
48 Ibid., p. 29.
49 Broughton notes, Bristol University Medical School Library, UA/DM/ 1C1, pp. 125–6.
50 Bedingfield, *Compendium*, p. 10.
51 Ibid., p. 83.
52 Bayford, "Aneurysms," p. 24.
53 Bedingfield, *Compendium*, pp. 147–8.
54 Estlin, Casebook, p. 445.
55 Ibid., p. 411.
56 Ruth Richardson, *Death, Dissection and the Destitute* (London: Routledge, 1987), esp. pp. 3–29.
57 *Felix Farley's Bristol Journal* (hereafter *FFBJ*) 7 July 1770.
58 Martha More, *Mendip Annals*, ed. Arthur Roberts (London: James Nisbet & Co., 1859), p. 65.
59 Dyer diary, Bristol Central Library, 90025.
60 *FFBJ*, 12 June 1762.
61 On the importance and shifting meanings of pauper funerals, see Thomas Laqueur, "Bodies, Death and Pauper Funerals," *Representations* 1 (1983): 109–31. See also Clare Gittings, *Death, Burial, and the Individual in Early Modern England* (London: Croom Helm, 1984), especially ch. 3, which shows the importance of a decent burial even among society's most marginal members.
62 *Farley's Bristol Newspaper*, 16 April 1726.
63 Ibid., 23 April 1726.
64 *Bristol Oracle*, 2 July 1743.
65 BRO, BBM 8, p. 49.
66 In BRO, BBM 8, in between pp. 39 and 40 and pp. 53 and 54, there are newspaper clippings, a broadside, and a poster offering a reward, from which I draw the following account.
67 Ibid., pp. 43–53, for details of this incident.
68 Ibid., p. 46.
69 Both of these cases come from clippings in BRO, BBM 8, p. 60.
70 Here I obviously draw upon the ideas of Douglas Hay, "Property, Authority and the Criminal Law," Douglas Hay, et al., eds., *Albion's Fatal Tree*: Crime and Society in Eighteenth-Century England (Harmondsworth: Penguin Books, 1977). Hay argues that the discretionary power of the court in extending mercy served to reinforce the hegemonic powers of the ruling classes who controlled the courts. Although this contention has been criticized, the overall point that I wish to emphasize – that surgeons, in performing the dissection of felons' bodies, allied themselves with the ruling classes – still holds. See also, Joanna Innes and John Styles, "The Crime Wave: Recent Writings on Crime and Criminal Justice in Eighteenth Century England," *Journal of British Studies* 25 (1986): 380–435.

71 The actual legal status of the dead body, as Richardson has documented, was curious – it was not legally property and hence could not be stolen. Nevertheless, as bodies became commercial items, bought, sold, and stolen, they acquired a commodity value.

72 W. H. Harsant, "Medical Bristol in the Eighteenth Century," *Bristol Medico-Chirurgical Journal* 17 (1899): 4.

73 G. Munro Smith, *A History of the Bristol Royal Infirmary* (Bristol: Arrowsmith, 1917), pp. 268 et seq.

74 The interrelationships of forensic medicine, anatomical dissection, and the collection of curiosities are complex in Bristol in this period. I have used the word "dissect" because it seems the most descriptive of what surgeons were doing. Very few autopsies, it seems, were performed in Bristol, even by contemporary standards. In the sketchy coroners' records that survive, there are no examples of autopsies performed to determine cause of death; usually, bodies were fished out of the river, and death was declared to be due to drowning. The second confusion, between what was regarded as "legitimate" dissection and mere curiosity-seeking, was emphasized in the long newspaper battle over illicit dissection at the Mint. Thomas Rigge, a physician, called in authorities from Guy's and St. Thomas's hospitals in London to prove the rights of medical men to ascertain cause of death. His opponents claimed that there was a difference between "examining" and "mutilating for the sake of a curiosity in a bottle." This was an obvious snipe at Richard Smith, Sr., Rigge's co-conspirator in breaking into the deadhouse, since he ran an anatomical museum. Smith, Jr.'s treatment of Horwood's body suggests that, in the case of the Smiths, father and son, Rigge's anonymous opponent had a legitimate point.

75 Estlin, Casebook, p. 358.

76 Smith's notes on the case, including a phrenological examination of Horwood, are in BRO 35893.

77 Bedingfield, *Compendium*, p. 13.

78 Joseph Wilde, *The Hospital: A Poem in Three Books* (Norwich: Stevenson, Matchelt, and Stevenson, 1810).

CHAPTER 9

1 On popular culture and the disappearance of the supernatural, Keith Thomas, *Religion and the Decline of Magic* (New York: Scribner, 1971), remains the key work. See also Michael MacDonald, "Religion, Social Change, and Psychological Healing in England 1600–1800," in W. J. Sheils, ed., *The Church and Healing, Studies in Church History* 19 (1982): 101–26. Others who place the disappearance of the supernatural somewhat later in time than does Thomas include: Jonathan Barry, "Piety and the Patient, Medicine and Religion in Eighteenth-Century Bristol," in Roy Porter, ed., *Patients and Practitioners* (Cambridge University Press, 1985), pp. 145–76; Charles Phythian-Adams, "Rural Culture," in G. E. Mingay, ed., *The Victorian Countryside* (London: Routledge & Kegan Paul, 1981), pp. 616–25; James Obelkevich, *Religion and*

Rural Society: South Lindsey, 1825–1875 (Oxford: Oxford University Press [Clarendon Press], 1976). For a French parallel, see Judith Devlin, *The Superstitious Mind: French Peasants and the Supernatural in the Nineteenth Century* (New Haven, Conn.: Yale University Press, 1987).

2 Obviously, for historians of religion, many of the generalizations that follow may be too broad, but it is important to recognize that sectarian divisions we take for granted had little meaning for the eighteenth century. Seekers after religious enlightenment often became associated with a series of groups. For example, William Dyer, the Bristol clerk, attended John Wesley's services, participated in a Behmenist circle in the city, and was often involved with Quaker activities – he pursued his own path toward awakening and saw commonalities rather than differences among his fellow seekers. On religion in this period, see A. D. Gilbert, *Religion and Society in Industrial England* (London: Longman Group, 1978); Michael Watts, *The Dissenters* (Oxford: Oxford University Press [Clarendon Press], 1978); Gordon Rupp, *Religion in England 1688–1791* (Oxford: Oxford University Press [Clarendon Press], 1986).

3 Clarke Garrett, *Spirit Possession and Popular Religion from the Camisards to the Shakers* (Baltimore: Johns Hopkins University Press, 1987), see esp. pp. 3–6, 44, 78–9. A similar point has been made by Hillel Schwartz, *The French Prophets* (Berkeley and Los Angeles: University of California Press, 1980). See especially Schwartz's discussion of the popular mockery puppet-theater renditions of the French Prophets' meetings.

4 Charles R. Cherry, "Enthusiasm and Madness: Anti-Quakerism in the Seventeenth Century," *Quaker History* 73 (1975): 1–24.

5 Schwartz, *French Prophets*, p. 49.

6 John Lacy, *The Prophetical Warnings of John Lacy, Esq.; Pronounced under the Operation of the Spirit* (London: 1707), vol. 2, p. 98, quoted in Schwartz, *French Prophets*, p. 255.

7 On enthusiasm and medicine more generally, see Michael Heyd, "The Reaction to Enthusiasm in the Seventeenth Century: Towards an Integrative Approach," *Journal of Modern History* 53 (1981): 258–80; Johanna Geyer-Kordesch, "Passions and the Ghost in the Machine: Or What Not to Ask About Science in Seventeenth- and Eighteenth-Century Germany," in Roger French and Andrew Wear, *The Medical Revolution of the Seventeenth Century* (Cambridge University Press, 1989), pp. 145–63; David Harley, "Mental Illness, Magical Medicine and the Devil in Northern England, 1650–1700," in the same volume, pp. 114–44; George Rosen, " 'Enthusiasm' a Dark Lanthorn of the Spirit," *Bull. Hist. Med.* 42 (1968): 393–421; George Williamson, "The Restoration Revolt Against Enthusiasm," *Studies in Philology* 30 (1933): 571–603; Truman Guy Steffan, "The Social Argument Against Enthusiasm," *Studies in English* 21 (1941): 39–63.

8 Schwartz, *French Prophets;* Clarke Garrett, *Respectable Folly: Millenarians and the French Revolution in France and England* (Baltimore: Johns Hopkins University Press, 1975); Garrett, *Spirit Possession;* James K. Hopkins, *A Woman to Deliver Her People. Joanna Southcott and English*

Millenarianism in an Era of Revolution (Austin: University of Texas Press, 1982); E. P. Thompson, *The Making of the English Working Class* (New York: Vintage Books, 1966); J. F. C. Harrison, *The Second Coming: Popular Millenarianism 1780–1850* (London: Routledge & Kegan Paul, 1979); Richard H. Popkin, ed., *Millenarianism and Messianism in English Literature and Thought, 1650–1800* (Leiden: Brill, 1988); T. V. Hitchcock, "Radical Millenarianism in Early Eighteenth-Century England," unpublished manuscript.

9 On Whiston, see James E. Force, *William Whiston, Honest Newtonian* (Cambridge University Press, 1985).

10 See Garrett, *Spirit Possession;* and Schwartz, *French Prophets.*

11 John Wesley, *The Journal of the Reverend John Wesley,* ed. Nehemiah Curnock (London: Charles H. Kelly, 1909–1916), vol. 2, p. 226.

12 John Free, *Rules for the Discovery of False Prophets: or the Dangerous Impositions of the People called Methodists . . .* (Oxford: n.p., 1758).

13 Ibid., p. 2.

14 Ibid., p. 9.

15 William Dodwell, *The Nature, Mischiefs and Remedy of Superstition Illustrated* (Oxford: n.p., 1754), p. 53.

16 Ibid., pp. 18–19.

17 Michael MacDonald, "The Secularization of Suicide in England 1660–1800," *Past and Present* 111 (1986): 86.

18 David Hume, *An Enquiry Concerning the Human Understanding,* section XI, "Of a Particular Providence and a Future State," and section X, "Of Miracles," ed., L. A. Selby-Bigge, rev. P. H. Nidditch (Oxford University Press, 1975). On the miracles controversy, see James Allen Herrick, "Miracles and Reasonableness in the Eighteenth Century" (Ph. D. diss., University of Wisconsin, 1986). See also Donald T. Siebert, "Johnson and Hume on Miracles," *Journal of the History of Ideas* 36 (1975): 343–7 and the rejoinder by James E. Force, "Hume and Johnson on Prophecy: The Context of Hume's essay 'Of Miracles,' " *Journal of the History of Ideas* 43 (1982): 463–75.

19 James E. Force, "Hume and the Relation of Science to Religion Among Certain Members of the Royal Society," *Journal of the History of Ideas* 45 (1984): 517–36.

20 *Daily Advertiser,* 26 March 1753.

21 Garrett, *Spirit Possession,* p. 83. John Raimo has traced Bristol's penchant for dissent back to the early fifteenth century, when the city harbored Lollards. More significant for the current discussion is Raimo's illustration of the continuities among the behaviors of Bristol Quakers in the 1650s, French Prophets in the early decades of the eighteenth century, and Wesleyan Methodists, all of whom used the body as a powerful symbol of divine will. John Raimo, "Spiritual Harvest: The Anglo-American Revival in Boston, Massachusetts, and Bristol, England, 1739–1742" (Ph. D. diss., University of Wisconsin, 1974); see also Barry, "Piety and the Patient."

22 On quietism, Watts, *The Dissenters,* pp. 461–2; Melvin Endy, *William Penn and Early Quakerism* (Princeton, N.J.: Princeton University Press,

1981), pp. 216–17, 236–8; F. B. Tolles, "Quietism vs. Enthusiasm: The Philadelphia Quakers and the Great Awakening," *Pennsylvania Magazine of History and Biography* 69 (1945): 26–49; May Drummond, *Internal Revelation the Source of Saving Knowledge,* ed. J. Nelson (London: Reading, 1736).

23 Wesley, *Journal,* vol. 2, p. 183.

24 Ibid., p. 298.

25 Ibid., p. 210.

26 John Wesley, *Primitive Physick* (Bristol: n.p. [1747]), p. iv.

27 *Gentleman's Magazine* 21 (1751): 295.

28 Ibid., p. 415.

29 Ibid.

30 Thomas Carte, *History of England* (London: 1747); *The Spirit of the Whigs and Jacobites Compared* (London: 1746); both cited in J. C. D. Clark, *English Society 1688–1832* (Cambridge University Press, 1985), pp. 160–3. Tucker's exposure of Lovell's death was also reprinted in that arbiter of polite culture, the *Gentleman's Magazine* 18 (1748). See also John Latimer, *Annals of Bristol in the Eighteenth Century* (Bristol: printed for the author, 1893), pp. 117–18; Barry, "Piety and the Patient"; *Bristol Oracle,* 23 Jan. 1748; *Bristol Weekly Intelligencer,* 31 Aug. 1751; I owe these last two references to the kindness of Dr. Jonathan Barry.

31 On Tucker, see George Shelton, *Dean Tucker and Eighteenth-Century Economic and Political Thought* (London: Macmillan Press, 1981). Tucker provides a link between the last vestiges of 1690s–style reforms of manners, mid-century definitions of "politeness" and the later evangelical attack on forms of popular culture – like Sir James Stonhouse, another such Bristolian, he was a friend of Hannah More. Of course, some people thought that Methodists were Jacobites in disguise. See Rupp, *Religion in England,* p. 373; John Walsh, "Methodism and the Mob in the Eighteenth Century," in Derek Baker, ed., *Studies in Church History* 9 (1972).

32 Samuel Werenfels, *A Dissertation on Superstition in Natural Things* (London: printed and sold by J. Robinson, 1748), p. 70. Werenfels belongs to an earlier generation – he was professor in the faculty of theology at Basle from 1696 and died in 1740. He was connected to an earlier reformation-of-manners movement, having links to the SPCK. See Eamon Duffy, "*Correspondence Fraternelle;* The SPCK, the SPG and the churches of Switzerland in the War of the Spanish Succession," in Derek Baker, ed., *Reform and Reformation: England and the Continent, c1500–c1750 Studies in Church History* 16 (1979). On Mapp, see Roger Cooter, "Bones of Contention? Orthodox Medicine and the Mystery of the Bone-Setter's Craft," in W. F. Bynum and Roy Porter, eds., *Medical Fringe and Medical Orthodoxy, 1750–1850* (London: Croom Helm, 1987), pp. 158–73.

33 *Gentleman's Magazine* 21 (1751): 504.

34 This position takes issue with an essay of Roy Porter's that argues medicine was not subject to the reforms of popular culture that such expressions as holidays, calendar customs, and games and recreations

were. He shows the extent of "lay" knowledge and interest in medicine through the lens of the *Gentleman's Magazine*. He is partly correct, but what he overlooks is that, although the *Gentleman's Magazine* may have mirrored lay interest on one level, it participated in the repression of plebian medicine on another. By serving as an arbiter of polite culture, it created and maintained boundaries of "credulity" and "sense" that disparaged the everyday health care of major portions of the population. Roy Porter, "Lay Medical Knowledge in the Eighteenth Century: The Evidence of the *Gentleman's Magazine*," *Medical History* 29 (1985): 138–68.

35 *Bristol Weekly Intelligencer*, 23 June 1750.

36 William Cadogan, *An Essay on Nursing and the Management of Children* . . . (London: J. Roberts, 1747), p. 3.

37 Ibid., p. 4.

38 Harrison, *Second Coming*. See especially ch. 3.

39 M. J. Naylor, *The Inanity and Mischief of Vulgar Superstitions, in Four Sermons* (Cambridge: Flower, 1795), pp. iv–v.

40 Ibid., p. v.

41 Ibid., p. 94.

42 *Methodism and Popery Dissected and Compared . . . Remarks on the Nature and Affinity Between Enthusiasm and Superstition* (London: Fielding and Walker, 1779).

43 For another example, see William Reid's denunciation of millenarians and political radicals, in which he claims that the evils of methodistical preachers are unparalleled "since the business of out-door preaching was *lain* down by Oliver's preachers" (William Reid, *The Rise and Dissolution of the Infidel Societies in this Metropolis* . . . [London: J. Hatchard, 1800], p. 41).

44 MacDonald, "Suicide," p. 94.

45 Simon Schaffer, "Natural Philosophy and Public Spectacle in the Eighteenth Century," *History of Science* 21 (1983): 31.

46 Thus, for example, the replacement of historical interpretation based upon ages and eras with one based upon progress and advance (see Schaffer, "Natural Philosophy," pp. 31) could allow writers like Naylor and others to draw lessons from the recent past.

47 Natural philosophers, however, did have links with healing through electricity. See, for example, Phillippe de Loutherberg's electrical clinic, mentioned in Schaffer, "Natural Philosophy," pp. 30–1. It was no accident that electricity, the mediator between matter and spirit, the seen and unseen worlds, was often at the center of healing associated with radical religion and natural philosophy. See Barry, "Piety and the Patient," on Richard Symes's career as an electrical healer in Bristol. Wesley, of course, was deeply involved with electrical healing.

48 On Brothers, see Harrison, *Second Coming*, pp. 57–85; Garrett, *Respectable Folly;* Thompson, *Making of the English Working Class*, pp. 116–19, and more generally, pp. 350–400. Primary sources include Brothers's own writings, *A Revealed Knowledge of the Prophecies and the*

Times (London: n.p., 1794), and those of his disciples, as well as notices in *The Times,* particularly 4 March 1795.

49 *The Times,* 4 March 1795.

50 William Bryan, *A Testimony of the Spirit of Truth Concerning Richard Brothers . . .* (London: n.p., 1795), p. 17.

51 Ibid., p. 30.

52 Ibid.

53 Ibid., pp. 36–8. See also, E. E. Butcher, *The Bristol Corporation of the Poor* (Bristol: Bristol Record Society Publications, 1932), vol. 3, p. 125, for a reference to this institution.

54 Bryan, *Testimony,* p. 36.

55 See J. F. C. Harrison, "Early Victorian Radicals and the Medical Fringe," in Bynum and Porter, *Fringe and Orthodoxy,* pp. 198–215.

56 Quoted in Ford K. Brown, *Fathers of the Victorians: The Age of Wilberforce* (Cambridge University Press, 1961), p. 76.

57 Brown, *Fathers of the Victorians;* see also M. G. Jones, *Hannah More* (Cambridge University Press, 1952).

58 M. J. D. Roberts, "The Society for the Suppression of Vice and Its Early Critics, 1802–1812," *The Historical Journal* 26 (1983): 159–76.

59 *Morning Post,* 12 June 1772.

60 Mr. Gurney, *The Trial of Joseph Powell at the Sessions-House, Clerkenwell* (London: C. & F. Rivington, 1808).

61 Ibid., pp. 9–10.

62 Ibid., p. 16.

63 William Blake was horrified by Blair's actions – see his letter of 14 Oct. 1807, reprinted in J. Bronowski, ed., *William Blake, A Selection of Poems and Letters* (Harmondsworth: Penguin Books, 1958), p. 242. My thanks to Dr. J. V. Pickstone for this reference.

64 *Times,* 31 Oct. 1808, p. 4 col. 3.

65 Hannah More, *Tawny Rachel, or the Fortune Teller* (London: J. Marshall, published for the Cheap Repository Tracts, n.d.), p. 3. See, more generally, Victor Neuberg, *Popular Literature. A History and Guide* (Harmondsworth: Penguin Books, 1977); R. K. Webb, *The British Working-Class Reader, 1790–1848: Literacy and Social Tension* (London: n.p., 1955).

66 More, *Tawny Rachel,* p. 4.

67 Ibid., p. 15.

68 Hannah More, *Black Giles the Poacher* (London: J. Marshall, for the Cheap Repository Tracts, n.d.), p. 11.

69 Susan Pedersen, "Hannah More Meets Simple Simon: Tracts, Chapbooks, and Popular Culture in Late Eighteenth-Century England," *Journal of British Studies* 25 (1986): 84–113. See also, Deborah M. Valenze, "Prophecy and Popular Literature in Eighteenth-Century Literature," *Journal of Ecclesiastical History* 29 (1978): 75–92.

70 On Mrs. Williams, see the collection of advertisements in the British Library, 1881.b.6., pp. 178–80.

71 See the collections of advertisements in the British Library, 1881.b.6; C.103.k.11, as well as miscellaneous advertisements listed in the ESTC.

72 Deborah M. Valenze, *Prophetic Sons and Daughters: Female Preaching and Popular Religion in Industrial England* (Princeton, N.J.: Princeton University Press, 1985).
73 Harrison, *Second Coming*, pp. 45–6, 122–4.
74 Ibid., p. 123.
75 William Hey, "An Account of the Effects of Electricity in the Amaurosis," *Medical Observations and Inquiries* 5 (1776): esp. 21–3.
76 The following account is taken from Joseph Easterbrook, *An Appeal to the Public Respecting George Lukins* . . . (Bristol: n.p., n.d.); Samuel Norman, *Authentic Anecdotes of George Lukins* . . . (Bristol: G. Routh, 1788); *A Narrative of the Extraordinary Case of George Lukins* . . . (Bristol: Bulgin and Rosser, 1788); I have been unable to locate copies of Samuel Norman, *Great Apostle Unmasked*, or of the chapbook version of Lukins's life. For historical approaches to this incident, see Henry D. Rack, "Doctors, Demons and Early Methodist Healing," in Sheils, *The Church and Healing*, especially pp. 147–9.
77 Norman, *Authentic Anecdotes*.
78 Ibid., p. 14.
79 Ibid., pp. 14–15.
80 Ibid., p. 17.
81 Ibid.
82 Ibid., p. 19.
83 Ibid., pp. 26–7.
84 See Hopkins, *A Woman to Deliver her People;* Thompson, *Making of the English Working Class;* Harrison, *Second Coming*.
85 Richard Reece, *A Correct Statement of the Circumstances That Attended the Last Illness and Death of Mrs. Southcott* . . . (London: Sherwood, Neely and Jones, 1815). See also, P. Mathias, *The Case of Joanna Southcott* . . . (printed for the author, n.d.); Elias Carpenter, *A Complete Refutation of the Statements and Remarks published by Dr. Reece* . . . (London: n.p., 1815); Six Female Physicians, *The Extraordinary Case of a Picadilly Patient: Or, Dr. Reece Physick'd. by Six Female Physicians* (London: for the authoresses, 1815).
86 Reece, *Correct Statement*, p. vii.
87 *The Times*, 30 Aug. 1814.
88 Mathias, *Joanna Southcott*, p. 4.
89 Reece, *Correct Statement*, pp. 8, 96–7.
90 *An Address to the Public From the Society for the Suppression of Vice* . . . (London: printed for the Society, 1803), p. 91.

CHAPTER 10

1 Christopher Lawrence, "Incommunicable Knowledge: Science, Technology and the Clinical Art in Britain 1850–1914," *Journal of Contemporary History* 20 (1985): 503–20, can be read as evidence that certain features of the early modern patient/practitioner relationship persisted in elite British medicine into the twentieth century.

Bibliography

PRIMARY SOURCES

MANUSCRIPT SOURCES

Bodleian Library, Oxford

John Johnson Collection.

Bristol Central Library

William Dyer diary. 1762.

James New, An Account of the Houses and Inhabitants of the Parish of Philip and Jacob in the City of Bristol, MS. 1781.

Bristol Record Office

Abson and Wick parish records.

John Bennett, MS. autobiography.

Bristol Royal Infirmary records.

Champion family letter-book.

Edward Estlin, casebook.

Lewins Mead Poor Book.

Penn St. Tabernacle, cashbook.

Settlement Examinations, 1748–1820.

Society of Friends, Minutes of the Men's Meeting.

Friends House Library, London

Sarah Champion diary (photocopy).

Gloucestershire County Record Office

Danvers Ward's cashbook, 1786.

Remedy book, p218 MI1.

Hampshire County Record Office

Records of Winchester Infirmary.

Society for the Promotion of Christian Knowledge

Abstract Letter Books.

Somerset County Record Office

John Cannon diary.

University of Bristol Medical School

Arthur Broughton, MS. lecture notes.

"Coughs and Colds" MS.

Royal College of Physicians

Samuel England, casebooks.

Royal College of Surgeons

Nathaniel Bedford, observations and cases.

Wellcome Institute for the History of Medicine Library

Alexander Morgan, casebook.

Ephemera Collection.

Remedies (MS. 3576).

PRINTED SOURCES

An Account of the Hospitals, Alms Houses and Public Schools in Bristol. Bristol: H. Farley for T. Mills, 1775.

Addington, John. "Cases of Gonorrhea Treated with Muriate of Quicksilver," In *Contributions to Physical and Medical Knowledge, Principally from the West Country.* Edited by Thomas Beddoes. Bristol: Biggs and Cottle, 1799.

An Address to the Public From the Society for the Suppression of Vice. . . . London: Printed for the Society, 1803.

The Adventures of Bampfylde Moore Carew. In *Amusing Prose Chapbooks,* edited by Robert Hays Cunningham. London: Hamilton Adams, 1889.

Alford, Henry. "The Bristol Infirmary in My Student Days 1822–28," *Bristol Medico-Chirurgical Journal* 8 (1890): 165–91.

Antrobus, Thomas. "An Amputation of the Leg," *Medical Observations and Inquiries* 2 (1762): 152–5.

"Aristotle," *Complete Works.* London: L. Hanes, 1772.

Mr. Bayford. "An Account of Two Aneurysms in the Aorta," *Medical Observations and Inquiries* 3 (1769): 14–27.

Becket, John. *An Essay on Electricity. . . .* Bristol: J. B. Becket, 1773.

Beddoes, Thomas. *The History of Isaac Jenkins.* Bristol: J. Mills, 1804.

Hygiea, or Essays Moral and Medical . . . . Bristol: J. Mills, 1802.

Observations on the Nature and Cure of Calculus, Sea Scurvy, Consumption, Catarrh and Fever. . . . London: J. Murray, 1793.

On Fever. Clifton: n.p., n.d.

Rules of the Medical Institute for the Benefit of the Sick and Drooping Poor. . . . Bristol: J. Mills, 1804.

[Bedford, Arthur.] *Letter to the Bishop of Gloucester from a Bristol Clergyman.* London: H. Hills, 1704.

Bedford, Arthur. *A Sermon Preached to the Societies for the Reformation of Manners.* London: Joseph Downing, 1734.

Bedingfield, James. *A Compendium of Medical Practice.* Bristol: Highley, 1816.

Bellers, John. *An Essay Towards the Improvement of Physick. . . .* London: J. Sowle, 1714.

Proposals for Raising a College of Industry. . . . London: T. Sowle, 1695.

Berdoe, Marmaduke. *An Enquiry into the Influence of the Electric-Fluid, in the Structure and Formation of Animated Beings.* Bath: The author, 1771.

Bigland, Ralph. *Historical, Monumental, and Genealogical Collections . . . Gloucestershire.* Frocester: Printed for Robert Bigland, 1791–1889.

Blake, John. *A Letter to a Surgeon on Inoculation.* London: W. Owen, 1771.

Blake, William. *William Blake, A Selection of Poems and Letters.* Edited by J. Bronowski. Harmondsworth: Penguin Books, 1958.

Blondel, James. *The Power of the Mother's Imagination over the Fetus Examin'd. . . .* London: John Brotherton, 1729.

Brent, Charles. *Persuasion to a Publick Spirit.* London: John Wyat, 1704.

Bristol Infirmary, *Manuale Medicaminum Simplicium et Commistorum Formulas Continens in Usum Valetudinarii Bristolensis Accodatum.* Bristol: n.p., 1816.

Pharmacopeia in Usum Nosocomii Bristolensis. Bristol: Bonner and Middleton, 1777.

Brothers, Richard. *A Revealed Knowledge of the Prophecies and the Times.* London: n.p., 1794.

Bryan, William. *A Testimony of the Spirit of Truth Concerning Richard Brothers. . . .* London: n.p., 1795.

Bourne, Henry. *Observations on Popular Antiquities . . . John Brand.* London: William Baynes, 1810.

Butcher, E. E. *Bristol Corporation of the Poor, 1696–1834.* Bristol: Bristol Record Society Publications, vol. 3, 1932.

Cadogan, William. *An Essay on Nursing and the Management of Children. . . .* London: J. Roberts, 1747.

Campbell, R. *The London Tradesman.* London: T. Gardner, 1747.

Cary, John. *An Account of the Proceedings of the Corporation for the Poor. . . .* London: F. Collins, 1700.

A Proposal Offered to the Committee. . . . London: n.p., [1700].

Charlton, Rice. *Cases of Persons Admitted into the Hospital at Bath under the care of the late Dr. Oliver.* Bath: R. Cruttwell, 1774.

Clifton Dispensary. *First Report.* 1813.

Cooke, Isaac. *Address . . . on the Enormous Increase of the Poor Tax in the Said City. . . .* Bristol: 1786.

Cottle, Joseph. *Early Recollections, Chiefly Relating to the Late Samuel Taylor Coleridge.* London: Longman Rees, 1837.

Cullen, William. *Synopsis Nosologiae Methodicae.* Edinburgh: Creech, 1769.

Culpeper, Nicholas. *Culpeper's Last Legacy,* London: Nathaniel Brooke, 1671.

The English Physician Enlarged. London: A. & J. Churchill, 1698.

[Davies, J.] *A Short Description of the Waters at Glastonbury.* Exeter: Andrew Brice, 1751.

Davis, William. *A New Almanack Made in Wiltshire.* London: n.p., 1692.

Dimsdale, Thomas. *Thoughts on General and Partial Inoculators.* London: William Richardson, 1776.

Dodwell, William. *The Nature, Mischiefs and Remedy of Superstition Illustrated.* Oxford: n.p., 1754.

Drummond, May. *Internal Revelation the Source of Saving Knowledge.* London: Printed for U. Reading, 1736.

Easterbrook, Joseph. *An Appeal to the Public Respecting George Lukins. . . .* Bristol: n.p., [1788].

Falconer, William. *An Account of the Efficacy of the Aqua Mephitica Alkalina.* London: T. Cadell, 1792.

The Five Strange Wonders of the World, or A New Merry Book of All Fives. Tewkesbury: Printed and sold by S. Harwood, n.d.

Fox, E. L. *Surmises Respecting . . . the Cholera.* Bristol: Mills & Son, 1831.

Free, John. *Rules for the Discovery of False Prophets: Or the Dangerous Impositions of the People Called Methodists. . . .* London: Printed for the author by E. Owen, 1758.

[Dr. Glass.] *A Letter from Dr. Glass to Dr. Baker on the Means of Procuring a Distinct and Favourable Kind of Smallpox.* London: W. Johnson, 1767.

Mr. Gurney. *The Trial of Joseph Powell at the Sessions-House, Clerkenwell.* London: C. & F. Rivington, 1808.

Hey, William. "An Account of the Effects of Electricity in the Amaurosis." *Medical Observations and Inquiries* 5 (1776): 1–31.

"Hints to Young Practitioners." *Edinburgh Medical and Surgical Journal* 5 (1809): 338.

Holland, William. *Paupers and Pig Killers. The Diary of William Holland.* Edited by Jack Ayres. Harmondsworth: Penguin Books, 1986.

Hume, David. *An Enquiry Concerning the Human Understanding.* Edited by L. A. Selby-Bigge, rev., P. H. Nidditch. Oxford: 1975.

Jenner, J. C. *London Medical Journal* 7 (1786): 163.

London Medical Journal 9 (1788): 47.

Johnson, James. *Transactions of the Corporation of the Poor during 126 Years.* Bristol: P. Rose, 1826.

Lackington, James. *Memoirs of the First Forty-five Years of the Life of J. L. . . . ,* 2d ed. London: Printed for the author, 1792.

Langdon, Roger. *The Life of Roger Langdon.* London: Elliot Stock, n.d.

Lee, Thomas. *An Address to the Subscribers and the Public Supporting the Bristol Infirmary. . . .* Bristol: Emery and Adams, 1805.

A Second Address to the Subscribers and the Public Supporting the Bristol Infirmary. Bristol: Emery and Adams, 1805.

Ludlow, Abraham. "A Case of Obstructed Deglutition." *Medical Observations and Inquiries* 3 (1769): 85–101.

Mathias, P. *The Case of Joanna Southcott. . . .* Printed for the author, n.d.

Maubray, John. *The Female Physician Containing All the Diseases Incident to That Sex, in Virgins, Wives, and Widows. . . .* London: J. Holland, 1724.

Methodism and Popery Dissected and Compared . . . Remarks on the Nature and Affinity Between Enthusiasm and Superstition. London: Fielding and Walker, 1779.

The Miracle of Miracles. Reprinted in *Chapbooks of the Eighteenth Century*, edited by John Ashton. Welwyn Garden City: Seven Dials Press, 1969.

More, Hannah. *Black Giles the Poacher*. London: J. Marshall, for the Cheap Repository Tracts, n.d.

Tawny Rachel, or the Fortune Teller. London: J. Marshall, for the Cheap Repository Tracts, n.d.

More, Martha. *Mendip Annals*, edited by Arthur Roberts. London: James Nisbet, 1859.

A Narrative of the Extraordinary Case of George Lukins. . . . Bristol: Bulgin and Rosser, 1788.

Naylor, M. J. *The Inanity and Mischief of Vulgar Superstitions, in Four Sermons*. Cambridge: Flower, 1795.

Norman, Samuel. *Authentic Anecdotes of George Lukins*. . . . Bristol: G. Routh, 1788.

Prichard, J. C. *A History of the Epidemic Fever Which Prevailed in Bristol during the Years 1817, 1818, and 1819*. London: Arch, 1820.

Mr. Pugh. "A Violent Scorbutic Case." *Medical Observations and Inquiries* 2 (1762): 241–244.

Pye, Samuel. "The Effect of An Accidental Vomiting." *Medical Observations and Inquiries* 2 (1762): 121–129.

Reece, Richard. *A Correct Statement of the Circumstances That Attended the Last Illness and Death of Mrs. Southcott*. . . . London: Sherwood, Neely and Jones, 1815.

Reid, William. *The Rise and Dissolution of the Infidel Societies in This Metropolis*. . . . London: J. Hatchard, 1800.

Reynell, Carew. *A Sermon Preached Before Contributors to the Bristol Infirmary*. Bristol: S. and F. Farley, 1738.

Rudder, Samuel. *A New History of Gloucestershire*. Gloucester: Alan Sutton reprint, 1977.

Rudge, Thomas. *The History of the County of Gloucestershire*. Gloucester: Printed for the author, 1803.

Salmon, William. *Synopsis Medicinae, or a Compendium of Astrological, Galenical and Chymical Physick*. . . . London: William Godbird for Richard Jones, 1671.

Sholl, Samuel. *A Short Historical Account of the Silk Manufacture in England*. . . . London: Stower, 1811.

Skinner, John. *Journal of a Somerset Rector 1803–34*, edited by Howard Coombs and Peter Coombs. Oxford University Press, 1984.

Smith, Charles Manby. *The Working Man's Way in the World*. . . . London: William and Frederick Gash, n.d.

Smythson, Hugh. *The Compleat Family Physician*. London: Harrison, 1781.

Some Considerations Offered. . . . London: n.p., 1711.

Stone, Sarah. *A Complete Practice of Midwifery*. London: T. Cooper, 1737.

Strange and Wonderful News. . . . n.p., n.d.

A Strange and Wonderful (Yet True) Relation of . . . Abraham Moon a Pretended Quaker. London: R. Lee, n.d.

Symes, Richard. *Fire Analyzed*. Bristol: Thomas Cocking, 1771.

Thomson, Henry. "Observations on a Dislocated Shoulder." *Medical Observations and Inquiries* 2 (1762): 340–59.

Mr. Thompson. "An Account of an Aneurysm." *Medical Observations and Inquiries* 3 (1769): 57–63.

Tindall, Matthew. *The Rights of the Christian Church Asserted. . . .* London: n.p., 1706.

Tucker, Josiah. *A Sermon Preached in the Parish Church in Bristol.* Bristol: William Crossley, 1746.

A Warning to Married Women. London: Printed for A. M. W. D. and T. Thackray, n.d.

Werenfels, Samuel. *A Dissertation on Superstition in Natural Things.* London: Printed and sold by J. Robinson, 1748.

Wesley, John. *The Journal of the Rev. John Wesley,* edited by Nehemiah Curnock. London: Charles H. Kelly, 1909–1916.

Primitive Physick. London: Printed and sold by Thomas Trye, 1747.

Wilde, Joseph. *The Hospital: A Poem in Three Books.* Norwich: Stevenson, Matchelt, and Stevenson, 1810.

Willis, Thomas. *The London Practice of Physick, or the Whole Practical Part of Physick contained in the Works of Dr. Willis.* London: Thomas Basset and William Crooke, 1685.

Willis's Oxford Case Book (1650–52), edited by Kenneth Dewhurst. Oxford: Sanford Publications, 1981.

"Wilt Thou be made Whole" . . . . London: Benjamin Matthews, 1751.

Wiseman, Richard. *Severall Chirurgical Treatises.* London: E. Flesher and J. Macock, for R. Royston, 1676.

Woodward, Josiah. *An Account of the Progress of the Reformation of Manners . . . ,* 14th edn. [sic]. London: J. Downing, 1706.

Young, Arthur. *A Six Weeks' Tour through the Southern Counties of England and Wales.* London: W. Nicoll, 1768.

SECONDARY SOURCES

Abel-Smith, Brian. *The Hospitals 1800–1948.* Cambridge, Mass.: Harvard University Press, 1964.

Ackerknecht, Erwin. *Medicine at the Paris Hospital 1794–1848.* Baltimore: Johns Hopkins University Press, 1967.

Ademuwagun, Z. A., et al., eds. *African Therapeutic Systems.* Waltham, Mass.: Crossroads Press, 1979.

Alexander, John K. *Render Them Submissive: Responses to Poverty in Philadelphia, 1760–1800.* Amherst: University of Massachusetts Press, 1980.

Baigent, Elizabeth. "Bristol in 1775." D. Phil. diss., Oxford University, 1985.

"Assessed Taxes as Sources for the Study of Urban Wealth." *Urban History Yearbook* (1988): 31–48.

Barry, Jonathan. "The Cultural Life of Bristol, 1640–1775." D.Phil. diss., Oxford University, 1985.

"Piety and the Patient: Medicine and Religion in Eighteenth-Century Bristol." In *Patients and Practitioners,* edited by Roy Porter, pp. 145–76. Cambridge University Press, 1985.

Beier, A. L. and Roger Finlay, eds.. *London 1500–1700: The Making of the Metropolis*. London: Longman Group, 1985.
Beier, Lucinda. *Sufferers and Healers: The Experience of Illness in Seventeenth-Century England*. London: Routledge & Kegan Paul, 1987.
Borsay, Peter. " 'All the Town's a Stage': Urban Ritual and Ceremony 1660–1800." In *The Transformation of English Provincial Towns 1600–1800*, edited by Peter Clark, pp. 228–58. London: Hutchinson, 1984.
The English Urban Renaissance: Culture and Society in the Provincial Town, 1660–1770. Oxford: Oxford University Press (Clarendon Press), 1989.
"The English Urban Renaissance: The Development of Provincial Urban Culture, c. 1680–1760." *Social History* 5 (1977): 581–99.
Boucé, Paul-Gabriel. "Imagination, Pregnant Women, and Monsters in Eighteenth-Century England and France." In *Sexual Underworlds of the Enlightenment*, edited by G. S. Rousseau and Roy Porter, pp. 86–100. Manchester: Manchester University Press, 1987.
Brock, C. H. *William Hunter 1718–1783*. Glasgow: University of Glasgow Press, 1983.
Brody, Harold. *Stories of Sickness*. New Haven, Conn.: Yale University Press, 1987.
Brown, Ford K. *Fathers of the Victorians: The Age of Wilberforce*. Cambridge University Press, 1961.
Burke, Peter. *Popular Culture in Early Modern Europe*. London: Temple Smith, 1978.
Burnby, Juanita. *A Study of the English Apothecary from 1660–1760, Medical History*, supp. 3. London, 1983.
Bushaway, Bob. *By Rite: Custom, Ceremony, and Community in England, 1700–1880*. London: Junction Books, 1982.
Bynum, W. F. "Physicians, Hospitals and Career Structures in Eighteenth Century London." In *William Hunter and the Eighteenth-Century Medical World*, edited by W. F. Bynum and Roy Porter, pp. 105–128. Cambridge University Press, 1985.
"Treating the Wages of Sin: Venereal Disease and Specialism in Eighteenth Century Britain." In *Medical Fringe and Medical Orthodoxy 1750–1850*, edited by W. F. Bynum and Roy Porter, pp. 5–28. London: Croom Helm, 1987.
Bynum, W. F., and Roy Porter, eds. *Medical Fringe and Medical Orthodoxy 1750–1850*. London: Croom Helm, 1987.
William Hunter and the Eighteenth-Century Medical World. Cambridge University Press, 1985.
Cavallo, Sandra. "Charity, Power, and Patronage in Eighteenth-Century Italian Hospitals: The Case of Turin." In *The Hospital in History*, edited by Lindsay Granshaw and Roy Porter, pp. 93–122. London: Routledge, 1989.
"Patterns of Poor Relief and Patterns of Poverty in Eighteenth-Century Italy: The Evidence of the Turin Ospedale di Carità." *Continuity and Change* 5 (1990): 1–33.
Chavunduka, G. L. *Traditional Healers and the Shona Patient*. Gwelo: Mambo Press, 1978.
Clark, J. C. D. *English Society 1688–1832*. Cambridge University Press, 1985.
Clark, Peter. "Migration in England During the Late Seventeenth and Early Eighteenth Century." *Past and Present* 83 (1979): 57–90.

Clark, Peter, ed. *The Transformation of English Provincial Towns 1600–1800*. London: Hutchinson, 1984.

Clark, Peter, and David Souden, eds. *Migration and Society in Early Modern England*. London: Unwin Hyman, 1988.

Clarke, George, ed. *John Bellers: His Life, Times and Writings*. London: Routledge & Kegan Paul, 1987.

Cooter, Roger. "Bones of Contention? Orthodox Medicine and the Mystery of the Bone-Setter's Craft." In *Medical Fringe and Medical Orthodoxy*, edited by W. F. Bynum and Roy Porter, pp. 158–73. London: Croom Helm, 1987.

Corfield, P. J. *The Impact of English Towns, 1700–1800*. Oxford University Press, 1982.

Craig, A. G. "The Movement for the Reformation of Manners, 1688–1715." Ph. D. diss., Edinburgh University, 1980.

Crowther, M. A. "Family Responsibility and State Responsibility in Britain Before the Welfare State." *Historical Journal* 25 (1982).

Curry, Patrick. *Prophecy and Power, Astrology in Early Modern England*. London: Polity Press, 1989.

Daston, Lorraine, and Katherine Park. "Unnatural Conceptions: The Study of Monsters in Sixteenth and Seventeenth Century France and England." *Past and Present* 92 (1981): 20–54.

Davidoff, Leonore, and Catherine Hall. *Family Fortunes: Men and Women of the English Middle Class, 1780–1850*. London: Hutchinson, 1987.

Devlin, Judith. *The Superstitious Mind: French Peasants and the Supernatural in the Nineteenth Century*. New Haven, Conn.: Yale University Press, 1987.

Donnison, Jean. *Midwives and Medical Men*. London: Heineman, 1977.

Duden, Barbara. *Geschichte unter der Haut: Ein Einsacher Artz und seine Patientinnen um 1730*. Stuttgart: Klett and Cotta, 1987.

Earle, Peter. *The Making of the English Middle Class*. London: Methuen, 1989.

Endy, Melvin. *William Penn and Early Quakerism*. Princeton, N.J.: Princeton University Press, 1981.

Feierman, Steven. "Struggles for Control: The Social Roots of Health and Healing in Modern Africa." *African Studies Review* 28 (1985): 73–147.

Fissell, Mary E. "The 'Sick and Drooping Poor' in Eighteenth-Century Bristol and its Region." *Social History of Medicine* 2 (1989): 35–58.

Force, James E. "Hume and Johnson on Prophecy: The Context of Hume's Essay 'of Miracles.' " *Journal of the History of Ideas* 43 (1982): 463–75.

"Hume and the Relation of Science to Religion Among Certain Members of the Royal Society." *Journal of the History of Ideas* 45 (1984): 517–36.

William Whiston: Honest Newtonian. Cambridge University Press, 1985.

Foucault, Michel. *The Birth of the Clinic*. Translated by Alan Sheridan. New York: Pantheon, 1973.

Discipline and Punish: The Birth of the Prison. Translated by Alan Sheridan. London: Allen Lane, 1977.

French, Roger, and Andrew Wear, eds. *The Medical Revolution of the Seventeenth Century*. Cambridge University Press, 1989.

Garrett, Clarke. *Respectable Folly: Millenarians and the French Revolution in France and England*. Baltimore: Johns Hopkins University Press, 1975.

Spirit Possession and Popular Religion from the Camisards to the Shakers. Baltimore: Johns Hopkins University Press, 1987.

Gelfand, Toby. " 'Invite the Philosopher, as Well as the Charitable': Hospital Teaching as Private Enterprise in Hunterian London." In *William Hunter and the Eighteenth-Century Medical World,* edited by W. F. Bynum and Roy Porter, pp. 129–52. Cambridge University Press, 1985.

Professionalizing Modern Medicine: Surgeons and Medical Science and Institutions in the Eighteenth Century. Westport, Conn.: Greenwood Press, 1980.

Geyer-Kordesch, Johanna. "Passions and the Ghost in the Machine: Or What Not To Ask About Science in Seventeenth- and Eighteenth-Century Germany." In *The Medical Revolution of the Seventeenth Century,* edited by Roger French and Andrew Wear, pp. 145–63. Cambridge University Press, 1989.

Gilbert, A. D. *Religion and Society in Industrial England*. London: Longman Group, 1978.

Gittings, Clare. *Death, Burial, and the Individual in Early Modern England*. London: Croom Helm, 1984.

Gould-Martin, Katherine. "Hot Cold Clean Poison and Dirt: Chinese Folk Medical Categories." *Social Science & Medicine* 12 (1978): 39–46.

Granshaw, Lindsay. " 'Fame and Fortune by Means of Bricks and Mortar': the Medical Professions and Specialist Hospitals in Britain 1800–1948." In *The Hospital in History,* edited by Lindsay Granshaw and Roy Porter, pp. 199–220. London: Routledge, 1989.

Granshaw, Lindsay, and Roy Porter, eds. *The Hospital in History*. London: Routledge, 1989.

[Greenhill, W. A.] *The Life of Sir James Stonhouse*. Oxford: John Henry Parker, 1844.

Harley, David. "Mental Illness, Magical Medicine and the Devil in Northern England, 1650–1700." In *The Medical Revolution of the Seventeenth Century,* edited by Roger French and Andrew Wear, pp. 114–44. Cambridge University Press, 1989.

Harrison, J. F. C. "Early Victorian Radicals and the Medical Fringe." In *Medical Fringe and Medical Orthodoxy,* edited by W. F. Bynum and Roy Porter, pp. 198–215. London: Croom Helm, 1987.

The Second Coming: Popular Millenarianism 1780–1850. London: Routledge & Kegan Paul, 1979.

Hay, Douglas. "Property, Authority and the Criminal Law." In *Albion's Fatal Tree Crime and Society in Eighteenth-Century England,* edited by Douglas Hay, Peter Linebaugh, John G. Rule, E. P. Thompson, and Cal Winslow, pp. 17–64. Harmondsworth: Penguin Books, 1977.

Helman, Cecil. " 'Feed a Cold, Starve a Fever' – Folk Models of Infection in an English Suburban Community, and Their Relation to Medical Treatments." *Culture, Medicine and Psychiatry* 2 (1978): 107–37.

Herrick, James Allen. "Miracles and Reasonableness in the Eighteenth Century." Ph. D. diss., University of Wisconsin, 1986.

Herzlich, Claudine, and Janine Pierret. *Illness and Self in Society*. Translated by Elborg Forster. Baltimore: Johns Hopkins University Press, 1987.

Heyd, Michael. "The Reaction to Enthusiasm in the Seventeenth Century: Towards an Integrative Approach." *Journal of Modern History* 53 (1981): 258–80.

Hitchcock, T. V. "The English Workhouse: A Study in Institutional Poor Relief in Selected Counties 1696–1750." D. Phil. diss., Oxford University, 1985.

"Radical Millenarianism in Early Eighteenth-Century England." Unpublished manuscript.

Holmes, Geoffrey. *Augustan England: Professions, State and Society 1680–1730*. London: Routledge & Kegan Paul, 1982.

Hopkins, James K. *A Woman to Deliver Her People. Joanna Southcott and English Millenarianism in an Era of Revolution*. Austin: University of Texas Press, 1982.

Horwitz, Henry. " 'The Mess of the Middle Class' Revisited: The Case of the 'Big Bourgeoisie' of Augustan London." *Continuity and Change* 2 (1987): 263–96.

Hufton, Olwen. *The Poor of Eighteenth Century France 1750–1789*. Oxford: Oxford University Press (Clarendon Press), 1974.

Innes, Joanna, and John Styles. "The Crime Wave: Recent Writings on Crime and Criminal Justice in Eighteenth Century England." *Journal of British Studies* 25 (1986): 380–435.

Janzen, J. E. *The Quest for Therapy in Lower Zaire*. Berkeley and Los Angeles: University of California Press, 1978.

Jewson, N. D. "The Disappearance of the Sick-Man from Medical Cosmology, 1770–1870." *Sociology* 10 (1976): 225–44.

"Medical Knowledge and the Patronage System in Eighteenth Century England." *Sociology* 8 (1974): 369–85.

Jones, Colin. *Charity and Bienfaisance: The Treatment of the Poor in the Montpellier Region, 1740–1815*. Cambridge University Press, 1982.

Jones, M. G. *The Charity School Movement*. Cambridge University Press, 1938.

Hannah More. Cambridge University Press, 1952.

Keel, Othmar. "The Politics of Health and the Institutionalization of Clinical Practice in Europe in the Second Half of the Eighteenth Century." In *William Hunter and the Eighteenth-Century Medical World,* edited by W. F. Bynum and Roy Porter, pp. 207–56. Cambridge University Press, 1985.

Kleinman, A. *Illness Narratives: Suffering, Healing, and the Human Condition*. New York: Basic Books, 1988.

Lane, Joan. "The Medical Practitioners of Provincial England in 1783." *Medical History* 28 (1984): 353–71.

"The Provincial Practitioner and His Services to the Poor 1750–1800." *Bulletin of the Society for the Social History of Medicine* 28 (1981): 10–14.

Langford, Paul. *A Polite and Commercial People: England 1727–1783*. Oxford: Oxford University Press (Clarendon Press), 1989.

Laqueur, Thomas. "Bodies, Death and Pauper Funerals." *Representations* 1 (1983): 109–31.

"Bodies, Details, and the Humanitarian Narrative." In *The New Cultural History,* edited by Lynn Hunt, pp. 176–204. Berkeley and Los Angeles: University of California Press, 1989.

Latimer, John. *Annals of Bristol in the Eighteenth Century*. Bristol: Printed for the author, 1893.

Lawrence, Christopher. "Incommunicable Knowledge: Science, Technology and the Clinical Art in Britain 1850–1914." *Journal of Contemporary History* 20 (1985): 503–20.

"Ornate Physicians and Learned Artisans: Edinburgh Medical Men, 1726–1776." In *William Hunter and the Eighteenth-Century Medical World,* edited by W. F. Bynum and Roy Porter, pp. 153–76. Cambridge University Press, 1985.

Lawrence, Susan C. "Science and Medicine at the London Hospitals: The Development of Teaching and Research, 1750–1815." Ph. D. diss., University of Toronto, 1985.

Loudon, Irvine. "Leg Ulcers in the Eighteenth and Early Nineteenth Centuries." *Journal of the Royal College of General Practitioners* 31 (1981): 263.

Medical Care and the General Practitioner, 1750–1850. Oxford University Press, 1986.

"The Historical Importance of Out-patients." *British Medical Journal* 1 (1978): 979–90.

" 'The Vile Race of Quacks with Which This Country Is Infested.' " In *Medical Fringe and Medical Orthodoxy 1750–1850,* edited by W. F. Bynum and Roy Porter, pp. 106–28. London: Croom Helm, 1987.

MacDonald, Michael. *Mystical Bedlam: Madness, Anxiety, and Healing in Seventeenth-Century England.* Cambridge University Press, 1981.

"Religion, Social Change, and Psychological Healing in England 1600–1800." In *The Church and Healing, Studies in Church History* 19 (1982): 101–26.

"The Secularization of Suicide in England 1660–1800." *Past and Present* 111 (1986): 50–100.

McGrath, Patrick, ed. *Bristol in the Eighteenth Century.* Newton Abbot: David Charles, 1972.

MacFarlane, Stephen. "Social Policy and the Poor in the Later Seventeenth Century." In *London 1500–1700. The Making of the Metropolis,* edited by A. L. Beier and Roger Finlay, pp. 252–77. London: Longman Group, 1985.

McKendrick, Neil, John Brewer, and J. H. Plumb. *The Birth of a Consumer Society: The Commercialization of Eighteenth-Century England.* London: Hutchinson, 1982.

Malcolmson, Robert W. *Popular Recreations in English Society 1700–1850.* Cambridge University Press, 1973.

Marland, Hilary. *Medicine and Society in Wakefield and Huddersfield 1780–1870.* Cambridge University Press, 1987.

Marshall, Dorothy. *The English Poor in the Eighteenth Century.* London: Routledge & Kegan Paul, 1926.

Maulitz, Russell C. *Morbid Appearances: The Anatomy of Pathology in the Early Nineteenth Century.* Cambridge University Press, 1987.

Nash, Gary B. "Poverty and Poor Relief in Pre-Revolutionary Philadelphia." *William and Mary Quarterly* 33 (1976): 3–30.

"Urban Wealth and Poverty in Pre-Revolutionary America." *Journal of Interdisciplinary History* 6 (1976): 545–84.

Neuberg, Victor. *Popular Literature. A History and Guide.* Harmondsworth: Penguin Books, 1977.

Neve, Michael. "Natural Philosophy, Medicine and the Culture of Science in Provincial England: The Cases of Bristol 1790–1850, and Bath 1750–1820." Ph.D. diss., University College London, 1984.

"Orthodoxy and Fringe: Medicine in Late Georgian Bristol." In *Medical Fringe and Medical Orthodoxy 1750–1850*, edited by W. F. Bynum and Roy Porter, pp. 40–55. London: Croom Helm, 1987.

Norberg, Kathryn. *Rich and Poor in Grenoble 1600–1814*. Berkeley and Los Angeles: University of California Press, 1985.

Obelkevich, James. *Religion and Rural Society: South Lindsey, 1825–1875*. Oxford: Oxford University Press (Clarendon Press), 1976.

Owen, David. *English Philanthropy*. Cambridge, Mass.: Harvard University Press, 1964.

Parker, George. "Early Bristol Medical Institutions." *BGAS* 44 (1922).

Pedersen, Susan. "Hannah More Meets Simple Simon: Tracts, Chapbooks, and Popular Culture in Late Eighteenth-Century England." *Journal of British Studies* 25 (1986): 84–113.

Pelling, Margaret. "Appearance and Reality: Barber-Surgeons, the Body, and Disease." In *London 1500–1700: The Making of the Metropolis*, edited by A. L. Beier and Roger Finlay, pp. 82–112. London: Longman Group, 1985.

"Illness Among the Poor in an Early Modern Town: The Norwich Census of 1570." *Continuity and Change* 3 (1988): 273–90.

"Occupational Diversity: Barber-Surgeons and the Trades of Norwich, 1550–1640." *Bulletin of the History of Medicine* 56 (1982): 484–511.

Pelling, Margaret, and Charles Webster. "Medical Practitioners." In *Health, Medicine and Mortality in the Sixteenth Century*, edited by Charles Webster, pp. 165–236. Cambridge University Press, 1979.

Perkin, Harold. *The Origins of Modern English Society 1780–1880*. London: Routledge & Kegan Paul, 1969.

Phythian-Adams, Charles. "Rural Culture." In *The Victorian Countryside*, edited by G. E. Mingay, pp. 616–25. London: Routledge, 1981.

Pickstone, John V. *Medicine and Industrial Society: A History of Hospital Development in Manchester and Its Region, 1752–1946*. Manchester: Manchester University Press, 1986.

Pickstone, John V., and Stella Butler. "The Politics of Medicine in Manchester 1788–1792." *Medical History* 28 (1984): 227–49.

Pole, Stephen. "Crime, Society and Law Enforcement in Hanoverian Somerset." Ph. D. diss., Cambridge University, 1983.

Popkin, Richard H., ed. *Millenarianism and Messianism in English Literature and Thought, 1650–1800*. Leiden: Brill, 1988.

Porter, Dorothy, and Roy Porter. *Patient's Progress: The Doctor and Doctoring in Eighteenth-Century England*. Oxford: Polity Press, in association with Basil Blackwell, 1989.

Porter, Roy. "The Gift Relation: Philanthropy and Provincial Hospitals in Eighteenth-Century England." In *The Hospital in History*, edited by Lindsay Granshaw and Roy Porter, pp. 149–78. London: Routledge, 1989.

Health For Sale: Quackery in England, 1650–1850. Manchester: Manchester University Press, 1989.

"The Language of Quackery in England 1660–1800." In *The Social History of Language,* edited by Peter Burke and Roy Porter, pp. 73–103. Cambridge University Press, 1987.

"Lay Medical Knowledge in the Eighteenth Century: The Evidence of the *Gentleman's Magazine.*" *Medical History* 29 (1985): 138–68.

" 'The Secrets of Generation Display'd': *Aristotle's Master-piece* in Eighteenth-Century England." In *'Tis Nature's Fault: Unauthorized Sexuality During the Enlightenment,* edited by Robert Purks Maccubbin, pp. 1–21. Cambridge University Press, 1987.

"A Touch of Danger: The Man-Midwife as Sexual Predator." In *Sexual Underworlds of the Enlightenment,* edited by G. S. Rousseau and Roy Porter, pp. 206–31. Manchester University Press, 1987.

Porter, Roy, ed. *Patients and Practitioners: Lay Perceptions of Medicine in Pre-Industrial Society.* Cambridge University Press, 1985.

Porter, Roy, and Dorothy Porter. "The Rise of the English Drugs Industry: The Role of Thomas Corbyn." *Medical History* 33 (1989): 277–95.

In Sickness and in Health: The British Experience, 1650–1850. London: Fourth Estate, 1988.

Pratt, David. *English Quakers and the First Industrial Revolution.* New York: Garland, 1985.

Rack, Henry D. "Doctors, Demons and Early Methodist Healing." In *The Church and Healing, Studies in Church History,* edited by W. J. Shiels, 19: 137–52.

Raimo, John. "Spiritual Harvest: The Anglo-American Revival in Boston, Massachusetts, and Bristol, England, 1739–1742." Ph. D. diss., University of Wisconsin, 1974.

Reiser, Stanley Joel. *Medicine and the Reign of Technology.* Cambridge University Press, 1978.

Richardson, Ruth. *Death, Dissection and the Destitute.* London: Routledge & Kegan Paul, 1987.

Risse, Guenter B. *Hospital Life in Enlightenment Scotland. Care and Teaching at the Royal Infirmary of Edinburgh.* Cambridge University Press, 1986.

Roberts, M. J. D. "The Society for the Suppression of Vice and Its Early Critics, 1802–1812." *The Historical Journal* 26 (1983): 159–76.

Rogers, Nicholas. "Money, Land and Lineage: The Big Bourgeoisie of Hanoverian London." *Social History* 4 (1979): 437–54.

Roodenburg, Herman W. "The Maternal Imagination. The Fears of Pregnant Women in Seventeenth-Century Holland." *Journal of Social History* 21 (1988): 701–16.

Rose, Craig. "Politics and the London Royal Hospitals, 1683–92." In *The Hospital in History,* edited by Lindsay Granshaw and Roy Porter, pp. 123–48. London: Routledge, 1989.

Rosenberg, Charles E. *The Care of Strangers: The Rise of America's Hospital System.* New York: Basic, 1988.

"Disease in History: Frames and Framers." *Milbank Quarterly* 67, supp. 1 (1989): 1–15.

"Medical Text and Social Context: William Buchan's *Domestic Medicine.*" *Bulletin of the History of Medicine* 57 (1983): 22–42.

"The Therapeutic Revolution." *Perspectives in Biology and Medicine* 20 (1977): 485–506

Rosen, George. " 'Enthusiasm': A Dark Lanthorn of the Spirit." *Bulletin of the History of Medicine* 42 (1968): 393–421.

Rosner, Lisa. "Students and Apprentices: Medical Education at Edinburgh University 1760–1810." Ph. D. diss., Johns Hopkins University, 1986.

Rupp, Gordon. *Religion in England 1688–1791*. Oxford: Oxford University Press (Clarendon Press), 1986.

Schaffer, Simon. "Natural Philosophy and Public Spectacle in the Eighteenth Century." *History of Science* 21 (1983): 1–43.

Schwartz, Hillel. *The French Prophets: The History of a Millenarian Group in Eighteenth-Century England*. Berkeley and Los Angeles: University of California Press, 1980.

Sheils, W. J. ed. *The Church and Healing, Studies in Church History* 19 (1982).

Shelton, George. *Dean Tucker and Eighteenth-Century Economic and Political Thought*. London: Macmillan, 1981.

Siebert, Donald T. "Johnson and Hume on Miracles." *Journal of the History of Ideas* 36 (1975): 343–7.

Sigsworth, E. "Gateways to Death?" In *Science and Society 1600–1900*, edited by Peter Mathias, Cambridge University Press, 1972.

Slack, M. "Non-Conformist and Anglican Registration in the Halifax Area, 1740–99." *Local Population Studies* 38 (1987): 44–5.

Slack, Paul. "Mirrors of Health and Treasures of Poor Men: The Uses of the Vernacular Medical Literature of Tudor England." In *Health, Medicine, and Mortality in the Sixteenth Century*, edited by Charles Webster, pp. 237–73. Cambridge University Press, 1979.

Poverty and Policy in Tudor and Stuart England. London: Longman Group, 1988.

"Poverty and Politics in Salisbury 1597–1600." In *Crisis and Order in English Towns*, edited by Peter Clark and Paul Slack. London: Routledge & Kegan Paul, 1972.

Smith, Ginnie. "Prescribing the Rules of Health: Self-Help and Advice in the Late Eighteenth Century." In *Patients and Practitioners*, edited by Roy Porter, pp. 249–82. Cambridge University Press, 1985.

Smith, G. Munro. *A History of the Bristol Royal Infirmary*. Bristol: Arrowsmith, 1917.

Smith, Richard M., ed. *Land, Kinship and Life-Cycle*. Cambridge University Press, 1984.

"The Structured Dependence of the Elderly as a Recent Development: Some Skeptical Historical Thoughts." *Ageing and Society* 4 (1984): 413–15.

Snell, K. D. M. *Annals of the Labouring Poor, Social Change and Agrarian England 1660–1900*. Cambridge University Press, 1985.

Souden, David. "Migrants and the Population Structure of Later Seventeenth-Century Provincial Cities and Market Towns." In *The Transformation of English Provincial Towns*, edited by Peter Clark, pp. 133–68. London: Hutchinson, 1984.

Spufford, Margaret. "First Steps in Literacy; The Reading and Writing Experiences of the Humblest Seventeenth-Century Spiritual Autobiographers." *Social History* 4 (1979): 407–35.

Steffan, Truman Guy. "The Social Argument Against Enthusiasm." *Studies in English* 21 (1941): 39–63.

Thomas, Keith. *Religion and the Decline of Magic*. New York: Scribner, 1971.

Thompson, E. P. "Eighteenth-Century English Society: Class Struggle Without Class?" *Social History* 3 (1978): 133–65.

"Patrician Society, Plebian Culture." *Journal of Social History* 7 (1974): 382–405.

The Making of the English Working Class. New York: Vintage Books, 1966.

Thomson, David. "I Am Not My Father's Keeper: Families and the Elderly in Nineteenth-Century England." *Law and History Review* 2 (1984): 265–86.

Tolles, F. B. "Quietism vs. Enthusiasm: The Philadelphia Quakers and the Great Awakening." *Pennsylvania Magazine of History and Biography* 69 (1945): 26–49.

Tompkins, Monica M. "The Two Workhouses of Bristol 1696–1735." Master's thesis, University of Nottingham, 1962.

Valenze, Deborah M. "Prophecy and Popular Literature in Eighteenth-Century Literature." *Journal of Ecclesiastical History* 29 (1978): 75–92.

Prophetic Sons and Daughters: Female Preaching and Popular Religion in Industrial England. Princeton, N.J.: Princeton University Press, 1985.

Vann, Richard T. *The Social Development of Quakerism 1655–1755*. Cambridge, Mass.: Harvard University Press, 1969.

Vincent, David. *Bread, Knowledge and Freedom, A Study of Nineteenth-Century Working Class Autobiography*. London: Methuen, 1981.

Wales, Tim. "Poverty, Poor Relief, and the Life-Cycle: Some Evidence from Seventeenth-Century Norfolk." In *Land, Kinship and Life-Cycle,* edited by Richard M. Smith, pp. 351–404. Cambridge University Press, 1984.

Walsh, John. "Methodism and the Mob in the Eighteenth Century." In *Studies in Church History,* edited by Derek Baker, 9 (1972).

Watts, Michael. *The Dissenters*. Oxford: Oxford University Press (Clarendon Press), 1978.

Wear, Andrew. "Puritan Perceptions of Illness in Seventeenth Century England." In *Patients and Practitioners,* edited by Roy Porter, pp. 55–99. Cambridge University Press, 1985.

Webb, R. K. *The British Working-Class Reader, 1790–1848: Literacy and Social Tension*. London: 1955.

Webster, Charles. *The Great Instauration*. London: Duckworth, 1975.

Webster, Charles, ed. *Health, Medicine and Mortality in the Sixteenth Century*. Cambridge University Press, 1979.

Williamson, George. "The Restoration Revolt Against Enthusiasm." *Studies in Philology* 30 (1933): 571–603.

Williams, Gareth. "The Genesis of Chronic Illness: Narrative Reconstruction." *Sociology of Health and Illness* 6 (1984): 175–200.

Williams, W. P., and W. A. Jones. "A List of Somerset Dialect." *Somerset Archaeological and Natural History Society Proceedings* 18 (1878).

Wilson, Adrian. "Childbirth in Seventeenth- and Eighteenth-Century England." Ph.D. diss., University of Sussex, 1982.

"William Hunter and the Varieties of Man-Midwifery." In *William Hunter and the Eighteenth-Century Medical World,* edited by W. F. Bynum and Roy Porter, pp. 343–69. Cambridge University Press, 1985.

Wilson, Kathleen. "The Rejection of Deference: Urban Provincial Culture in England, 1715–1785." Ph. D. diss., Yale University, 1985.

Woodward, John. *To Do the Sick No Harm.* London: Routledge & Kegan Paul, 1974.

Wrigley, E. A. "The Changing Occupational Structures of Colyton over Two Centuries." *Local Population Studies* 18 (1970): 9–21.

Wrigley, E. A., and R. Schofield. *The Population History of England, 1541–1871.* London: Edward Arnold, 1981.

Yoder, P. Stanley, ed. *African Health and Healing Systems: Proceedings of a Symposium.* Los Angeles: Crossroads Press, 1982.

Index

Printed in the United States
By Bookmasters

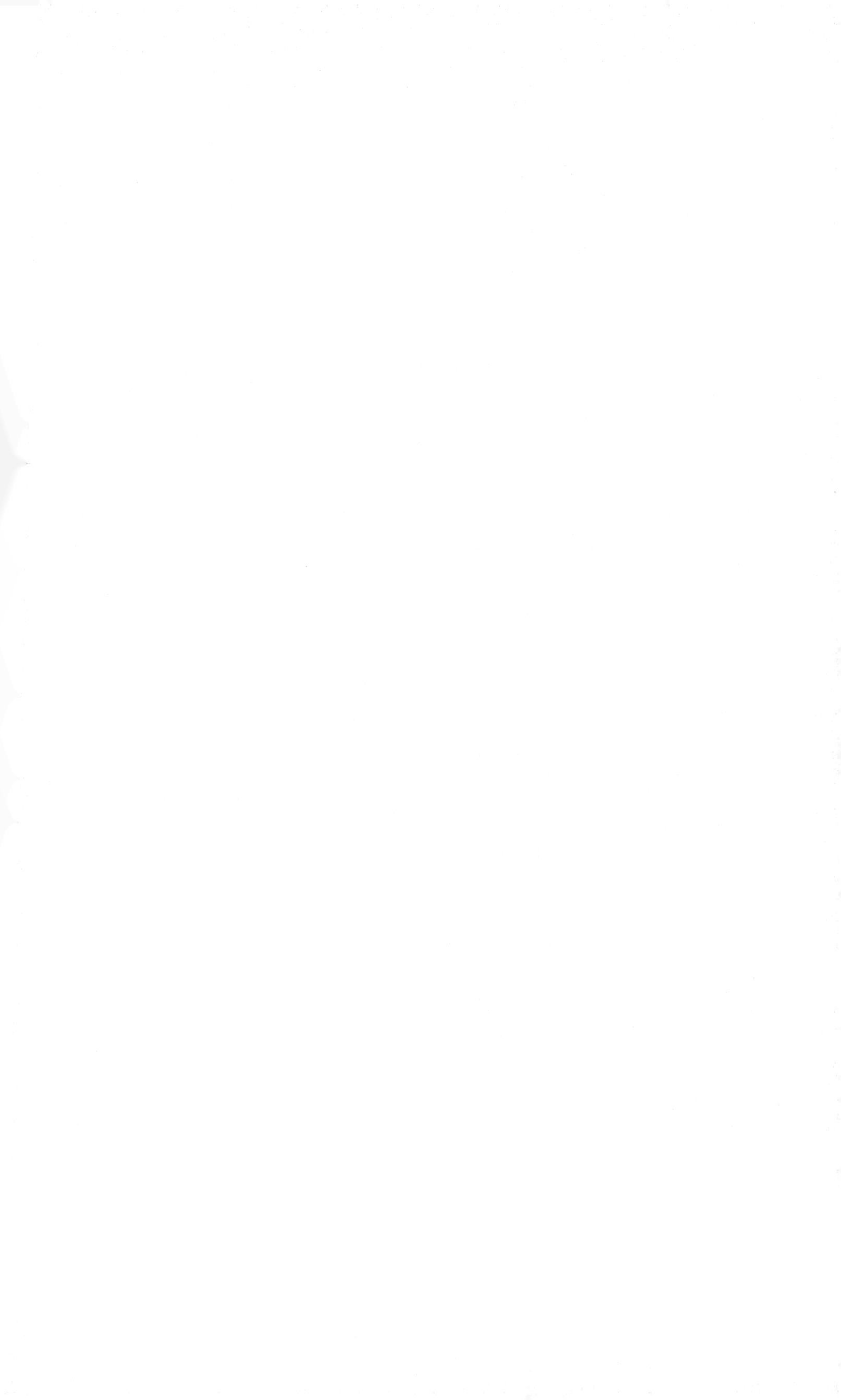